Edition 9

PSYCHIATRIC NURSING

Marguerite Lucy Manfreda, R.N., M.A.

Associate Professor of Nursing, Black Hawk College, Moline, Illinois. Formerly Director, School of Nursing, Swedish-American Hospital, Rockford, Illinois; Assistant Director of Nursing in Charge of Education, Essex County Overbrook Hospital, Cedar Grove, New Jersey; Director of Psychiatric Nursing Affiliation Program, Elgin State Hospital, Elgin, Illinois; Director of Nursing Education, Institute of Living, Hartford, Connecticut; Night Superintendent, Institute of Living, Hartford, Connecticut; Nursing Arts Instructor, Hartford Hospital, Hartford, Connecticut; Staff Nurse, Yale Institute of Human Relations, New Haven, Connecticut; Staff Nurse and Nursing Assistant to Researcher, New York State Psychiatric Institute and Hospital, New York.

F. A. DAVIS COMPANY, PHILADELPHIA

PSYCHIATRIC NURSING

Dedicated to

MISS FLORENCE E. NEWELL, R.N., M.A.

Teacher, Administrator, Consultant, Friend

Formerly Consultant to the Illinois Department of Mental Health

Preface

Changes made in the ninth edition of *Psychiatric Nursing,* including new and revised chapters, reflect contemporary developments and the more obvious movement toward community psychiatry that began about ten years ago.

The front section of the book contains information related to psychiatric facilities, services, and preventive approaches that has been compiled and reprinted with the permission of the National Association for Mental Health.

There are five newly prepared chapters in this edition. Chapter 5, "Orientation to Modern Developments and Psychiatric Nursing," is an account of legislative actions and reports that have influenced changes in the patient population of mental hospitals, long term care facilities, and the education of nurses.

"The Changing Role of the Nurse," Chapter 6, demonstrates the concept that professional nursing is more than a performance of perfunctory activities. The expanded nursing role practiced in a contemporary mental health center is outlined. It serves as a demonstration of how the nursing role has changed and what is expected in the ability performance of professional nurses.

Chapter 8, "Nursing in Community Mental Health Centers," is a discussion of the philosophy underlying the establishment of mental health centers and their role and relationship with other community agencies in providing the five essential psychiatric services that qualify their existence and operation.

The public health role of the psychiatric nurse is focused upon in Chapter 9, "The Extending Community Nursing Role." Psychiatric nursing is discussed as a service that extends into the home as well as many other types of health care facilities. This is in accord with the national trend to make health care readily accessible to people at the community level.

The content of Chapter 28, "Family Therapy," is devoted to the concepts underlying family therapy as part of the treatment program, its historical development, and the technics of conducting family therapy sessions. Some examples of sessions in action are presented.

Chapter 42, "Mental Retardation: Nursing Care," has been rewritten to include more recent information concerning the etiology of specific types of mental retardation. It includes the observations of some professionals regarding a general laxity in using research information to humanize the care of the mentally retarded. The nursing role and nursing approaches are discussed.

Revised chapters include Chapter 24, "Recording Observations and Behavior," where new content on the nursing care plan is presented, and a sample nursing care plan is included. Information on psychedelic drugs has been added to Chapter 31, "Drug Addiction Causing Dependence Behavior: Nursing Care." In accordance with changes made in the American Psychiatric Association classification, *involutional melancholia* is now discussed in Chapter 34, "Moods of Elation and Depression in Affective Behavior: Nursing Care," instead of as a separate disorder.

New illustrations posed for by personnel from cooperating hospitals and many new references appear in the ninth edition. The author is hopeful that this revision will be useful and helpful to readers of *Psychiatric Nursing.*

Marguerite Lucy Manfreda, R.N., M.A.

Acknowledgments

During the ninth edition of *Psychiatric Nursing,* the author received helpful cooperation and assistance from several colleagues and friends. Grateful acknowledgment is made to the following members of Swedish-American Hospital School of Nursing, Rockford, Illinois, faculty, and other staff members. Mrs. Jeanette Wade, R.N., Psychiatric Nursing Instructor, prepared the sample nursing care plan that appears in Chapter 24, "Recording Observations and Behavior." Mrs. Wade, Miss Marilyn Miller, R.N., Assistant Director School of Nursing, and Mrs. Diane Sworm, R.N., Psychiatric Department Head Nurse, reviewed some of the new chapters. Helpful assistance was also given by Mrs. Shirley Powell, R.N., Miss Josephine DiRaimondo, librarian, and Mrs. Dorothy Rudin, secretary. Mr. George Oster, M.S.W., Psychiatric Social Worker, wrote the chapter on "Family Therapy." Mr. Donald Andresen, Audiovisual Director, prepared photographs.

Mrs. Lucilla Warren, R.N., Psychiatric Nursing Service Administrator, and Mrs. Marie Babrick, R.N., Director School of Psychiatric Technician Nursing, Arkansas State Hospital, Little Rock, Arkansas, reviewed some of the new chapters and assisted with the planning of photographs. Mrs. Manolia Schult, R.N., State of Illinois, Department of Public Health, also reviewed some of the new chapters. Miss Marilyn Keener, R.N., Chairman, Department of Nursing, Black Hawk College, Moline, Illinois, gave helpful assistance with the final preparation of the ninth edition. Names of persons who reviewed specific chapters appear at the end of each chapter read by them.

The author wishes to thank all members of the administrative staffs of the hospitals that permitted photographs to be shown in the text, as well as the personnel in those hospitals who posed for the photographs. Names of these hospitals appear with the legend beneath each photograph.

The cooperation given by publishers of various periodicals and books named in the credit footnotes is greatly appreciated.

Marguerite Lucy Manfreda, R.N., M.A.

Contents

Anxiety. Coping with Anxiety. Security Operations. Anxiety is a Nursing Problem. Using Anxiety for Learning in Nursing.

Repression. Suppression. Rationalization. Denial. Compensation. Overcompensation. Substitution. Displacement. Introjection. Sublimation. Projection. Identification. Conversion. Condensation. Isolation. Symbolism. Undoing. Regression. Phantasy.

Symptoms That May Be Part of a Pattern.

Patterns of Withdrawal. Pattern Variations and Interpretations. Approach to Withdrawn Patients. Patterns of Aggression. Pattern Variations and Interpretations. Approach to Aggressive Behavior.

Some Basic Emotional Needs.

Hygiene. Nutrition. Treatment of Physical Complaints.

Nursing and Its Heritage. The Nurse's Spiritual Philosophy. Expressing Religious Sentiments. Spiritual Aid to Patients and Families. Religion. Religious Services. Conversion. Prayer. Articles and Emblems of Faith. Religious Literature. Fasting. Holy Communion. Baptism. Anointing of the Sick. Calling the Clergy. The Incurable Patient. The Dying Patient. Spiritual Aid in the Community.

Learning and Implementation of Concepts. There Is an Interrelation Between Mind and Body. Every Individual Has Intrinsic Worth and Dignity. Every Living Organism Possesses a Dynamic Life-Giving Force. Human Beings Have Common Physical and Emotional Needs. Communication Is the Basis of Social Exchange. Perceptions of Reality Are Individualistic. Self-Awareness Influences One's Understanding of Other Persons. Self-Concepts Are Influenced by Social Interchanges. Ideation, Feelings, Moods, and Actions Constitute Behavior. All Behavior Is Meaningful. Behavior Is Never Static. Emotional Equilibrium (Homeostasis) May Alter with Internal and External Changes and Demands. Stress and Strain May Be Produced by Both Internal and External Changes and Demands. Coping with Stress and Strain Is an Individualistic Ability. Illness Can Be a Learning Experience.

Interests and Aptitudes Represent Growth Potentialities. Human Growth and Personality Development Represent the Result of a Complex Process. Knowledge of Personality Development Structure Provides a Framework for Studying Behavior. Individual Concepts of Specific Illnesses May Be of Cultural, Social, or Familial Origin. Changes Which Alter or Threaten the Capacity Functioning of the Human Body Evoke Physical and Emotional Reactions. Attitudes Influence Behavior. Attitudes Can Be Changed. Rehabilitation Is a Vital Part of Therapy. Rehabilitation Is Influenced by Self-Participation. Rehabilitation Is Influenced by Family Participation. Social Institutions Arise To Meet Society's Needs. Community Education Influences Society's Reactions. Society Is Improved Through Joint Efforts. Treatment and Care of the Mentally Ill Are Now Considered Moral, Social, and Community Responsibilities.

Insulin Therapy. Combined Therapy. Nursing Care During Somatic Therapies.

rotic and Psychotic Behavior. Incidence. Clinical Types. Prevention. Detection of Early Symptoms. Nursing Care. Helping Parents. Criteria for Institutionalization. Community Assistance. Teaching Parents to Protect and Assist the Child. Employment.

Facts About Mental Illness*

20,000,000 Persons Affected By Mental and Emotional Illness

It is estimated that as least one person in every ten (a total of 20,000,000 in the United States) will at some time in his life have some form of mental or emotional illness (from mild to severe) that could benefit from professional help. At least as many people are hospitalized with mental illness as with all other diseases combined, including cancer and heart disease.

Doctors recognize emotional problems to be an important factor in many physical illnesses, even heart disease. Over 50% of all medical and surgical cases have such a complication. In a large number of cases seen by general practitioners, the major problem is an emotional one.

Persons Under Psychiatric Care in Hospitals

During 1967, an estimated 1,600,000 persons were under care in public and private mental hospitals, psychiatric services of general hospitals, and Veterans Administration psychiatric facilities. (This includes patients in hospitals at the beginning of the year, plus those admitted during the year.)

On any one day of the year, about 490,000 persons are *resident* in public and private mental hospitals. Currently, slightly over 1,000,000 persons are admitted during the year to public and private mental hospitals and psychiatric services of general hospitals.

Quick and Proper Treatment Helps Assure Recovery

At least 7 out of 10 patients admitted to a mental hospital can leave

* Reprinted with permission of the National Association for Mental Health.

partially or totally recovered with prompt and proper treatment. One large health insurance company reports that the average length of hospitalization for holders of its insurance is only 13 days, and about 80% leave the hospital within the first year. In 1947 a person with schizophrenia, the most prevalent mental crippler, faced a 50-50 chance of being hospitalized for more than a year. Today, provided he enters an adequately staffed institution, his chance for release within the year is increased to four out of five.

Mental Illness Affects Children

Mental illness occurs at all ages, including childhood. It is conservatively estimated that 1,400,000 children in the U.S. are in need of psychiatric care. Of these, only about one-third receive such care.

The latest annual figures (1967) show that 12,610 children under 18 years of age were admitted to public mental hospitals for the first hospitalization for serious mental disorder. On any given day in that year, there were 12,056 children with serious mental disorders in our public mental hospitals.

In private mental hospitals, first admissions of children under 18 totaled 3,876.

Conservatively estimated, an additional 465,000 children were served in psychiatric clinics in 1967 for less severe mental disorders.

Outpatient Psychiatric Clinics

In 1967, there were 2,259 public and private out-patient psychiatric clinics in the United States. Many of these are part-time, and most of them have long waiting lists. An estimated 1,345,000 children and adults are served in these clinics. About 900 of these clinics are in the northeastern states, principally in urban areas.

Informed mental health professionals estimate that a full-time clinic is needed for every 50,000 people. This would mean about 4,000 or about twice as many as now exist.

Community Mental Health Centers

The community mental health center is a new type of facility for treatment and prevention of mental illness where people with emotional problems can get comprehensive and continuing treatment in their own communities.

Community mental health centers are planned and run by people in the community, with initial help from the Federal government. As of July 1969, Federal grants totaling $292.2 million have been awarded for construction and staffing of 376 centers. However, the entire cost of funding these centers, when state, local, private, and other sources are included, approached $890 million as of July 1969. (It is projected that by 1970, 500 community mental health centers will have been funded; by 1980, 2000.)

When all 376 community mental health centers are in operation (185 were estimated to be in operation as of July 1969), they will provide service to 26 percent of the nation's population (or more than 52 million persons). Each community mental health center serves a designated area ranging in size from 75,000 to 200,000 persons. These centers are located in all states, the District of Columbia, and Puerto Rico.

To be eligible for Federal support, these centers must provide five *essential* services—inpatient care, outpatient care, partial hospitalization, emergency service, and consultation and education. Many of these centers provide additional services—diagnosis, precare and aftercare, rehabilitation, training, research and evaluation, and special services for specific patient groups.

Number of Hospital Facilities

In 1967 there were 527 mental hospitals in the United States. They include 264 state hospitals, 43 county hospitals, 40 Veterans Administration neuropsychiatric hospitals, and 180 private psychiatric hospitals.

Approximately 617 community general hospitals, or about one out of every ten, have separate units for treating psychiatric patients. Another 681 general hospitals admit psychiatric patients to their regular medical facilities.

Quality of Care For the Mentally Ill

Only custodial care is received by the great majority of patients in state mental hospitals. A very small percentage receive intensive psychiatric treatment, even though research has demonstrated that some patients who have been in the hospital as long as 5, 10, or 20 years recover when they receive intensive treatment. The reason for this situation is that few state hospitals get the necessary funds to provide adequate staff and equipment for intensive treatment. A key index of this inadequacy is the amount which the hospital spends per day for the maintenance of each patient. (Maintenance covers the salary of all personnel, treatment supplies, plus equipment, food, clothing, and overhead.) Latest figures show that the average daily expenditure for maintenance in public mental hospitals is $8.84 per patient. One state spends as little as $3.99. By contrast for the same period, authoritative sources estimate short-term general hospitals spend more than $44 per patient per day, private psychiatric hospitals $33 and VA psychiatric services more than $16 per patient per day.

Psychiatrists Serving the Mentally Ill

A 1965 national survey of psychiatrists showed that the median number of hours of service, paid and unpaid, provided by psychiatrists is 50 hours per week. Nearly 75 percent spent some time in direct service to patients. Smaller percentages spent some time in consultation, teaching, administration, and research. Less than 50 percent are self-employed in their principal employment. Just over 60 percent indicated general or adult psychiatry as their primary subfield, 8 percent indicated psychoanalysis, and 8 percent child psychiatry.

The latest available figures from the American Psychiatric Association show that there are about 22,000 psychiatrists and 3,810 psychiatric residents. However, they are not distributed proportionately to the population; for example, there are five states which have one-third of the country's population but one-half of the country's psychiatrists.*

Cost of Mental Illness

According to a recent study published in The American Journal of Psychiatry, mental illness cost the U.S. about 20 billion dollars. Half of this cost was borne by individuals other than the mentally ill. Cost of direct treatment was almost 3 billion—about 75% of this is expended by governmental agencies, and the rest is accounted for by private insurance carriers, private industry and private philanthropy.

Business authorities conservatively estimate that the annual loss to industry directly related to emotional disorders is staggering, amounting to 10 billion dollars each year.

* New York, 20 percent; California, 14 percent; Pennsylvania, 6 percent; and Massachusetts and Illinois, 5 percent each.

Can Mental Illness Be Prevented?*

Great advances have been made in the treatment of mental illness. Many more facilities for treatment have been built. Old facilities are constantly being improved. But what about prevention? Can mental illness be prevented? Our knowledge is limited. We know very little about the causes of mental illness, and until we know much more, we cannot identify any sure way to prevent mental illness. However, we do know certain facts:

1. We know there is a clear relationship between mental illness and inadequate prenatal, obstetrical, and early infant care.

Therefore, we can prevent some forms of mental illness by protecting the brains of infants. We can do this by making adequate medical care available to all expectant mothers and new babies.

2. We know there is a distinct relationship between mental illness and the presence of a number of stressful situations or circumstances ("multiple unendurable stresses").

While each of us has a degree of intolerance to stress, the presence of a number of sources of significant emotional pain results in a greater likelihood of emotional breakdown.
Available evidence demonstrates, for example, that the combination of hunger, crowding, discrimination, and hopelessness in our city ghettos takes its toll in the far higher prevalence of mental illness.
Therefore, we can prevent mental illness by working to change environmental factors which create unendurable stress.

*Reprinted with permission from the National Association for Mental Health

3. We know there is an obvious relationship between "labeling" and the prevalence of mental illness.

Although it may not seem to be a great scientific deduction, it is clear that much of what is thought of as "mental illness", or is called "mental illness", simply does not belong within the definition.

Therefore, we can, in a sense, "prevent mental illness" by simply improving our understanding of individual behavior, and avoiding attaching illness labels to behavior which is simply different.

For example, if we could broaden our tolerance of eccentric behavior, we would automatically slash the rolls of the "mentally ill". If we would recognize that the forgetfulness or vagueness of many elderly people is caused by hardening of the arteries, and not by some sort of mental breakdown, we would gain a similar result. And this wouldn't just be a "nice thing to do", because it would help to remove artificially created obstacles to a happy life, and would help to prevent the terrible tragedy of unnecessary long-term hospitalization.

4. We also know there is evidence which suggests that certain mental health education activities will help to prevent mental illness.

While there is no solid proof that any single form of mental health education will guarantee results, we do know that in selected situations mental health education helps, especially when it is applied toward solving some of the problems caused by the relationships described above.

For example, education for mental health can increase an individual's ability to cope with some of life's experiences and developmental crises, such as adolescence, marriage, prenatal stress, childbirth, aging and death. Selected consultation and education services can help physicians, other mental health workers and teachers identify possible problems early enough to allow for appropriate intervention and to avoid mental illness labeling.

Therefore, we can prevent mental illness by having education programs of proven value available to those who would benefit from them, and by continuing research aimed at identifying new and effective mental health education programs.

Other Things We Can Do

The four approaches described in this leaflet can help to prevent mental illness before it really starts. There are other things we can do to prevent mild problems from becoming serious illnesses, and to prevent mental illness from striking the same individual again.

For example, early identification of emotional or mental disorders through proper diagnosis followed by quick and adequate treatment can remove or control an emotional problem before it develops any further.

In addition, well-trained personnel and good rehabilitation facilities in every community can help the individual who has been ill return to his rightful place in society, reduce the consequences of his illness, and help him to avoid becoming ill again.

And there is one more thing YOU can do to help prevent mental illness. You can *join and support your Mental Health Association.*

Glossary

ABERRATION. A deviation from the normal.

AFFECT. A subjective feeling state. A more consistent, more persistent feeling tone.

ALIENIST. A legal term for a qualified psychiatrist considered competent to testify upon the subject of insanity.

AMBIVALENCE. Coexisting, but contrasting, feeling tones (e. g., love and hate).

AMNESIA. A partial or complete loss of memory.

APATHY. Absence of interest or emotion in a situation which would ordinarily arouse a response.

APPERCEPTION. Use of any of the special senses (sight, hearing, smell, taste, touch) to recognize objects or things in the environment, and to interpret their place or use therein.

ASTHENIC. Referring to a body physique which is slender, flat, long-chested, and with poor musculature development.

ATHLETIC. Referring to a body physique which is broad in the shoulders, and deep-chested. In addition, the abdomen is flat, the neck thick, and the muscles well developed.

AUTISM. Subjective thinking with much introspection, resulting in phantasy, delusions and hallucinations.

CHOREA. A disease characterized by irregular involuntary movements of the arms, legs or whole body.

CLONIC SPASM. Jerking movements of parts of the body, seen following the tonic (stiffening) phase of a convulsion.

CONFLICT. Two opposing incompatible drives or action systems requiring the individual to make a choice between the possible responses.

CONVERSION. The expression of an emotional conflict as a physical symptom, thus relieving the patient of anxiety and unpleasant feelings.

CYCLOTHYMIA. Mildly fluctuating mood shifts resembling manic-depressive states.

DELUSION. A false belief which cannot be changed by the introduction of evidence, or appeal to the person's reason or intellect owing to its affective motivation.

DEPERSONALIZATION. Loss of feeling of personal identity with one's self. The patient may say that he feels like an empty shell, a ghost, as if floating in space, unlike himself any more, etc.

DETERIORATION. Progressive impairment of one's intellect, memory and emotions.

DIPSOMANIA. A periodic overwhelming desire for alcoholic drinks.

DISORIENTATION. The inability to identify the date, time, place, etc; being unaware of one's true surroundings.

EGO. The conscious self which deals with reality.

EGOCENTRIC. Self-centered.

EMOTION. A combination of feeling plus the physiologic expression (*ex.*, goose pimples, nausea).

EMPATHY. Appreciating another's feelings, without experiencing the same emotional reaction.

ENVIRONMENT. All of the external conditions and influences which effect the life, development and behavior of the person.

EXHIBITIONISM. A display of the body or its parts for the purpose of attracting sexual interest.

EXTROVERT. An individual who focuses his interest and directs his energies outward from the self.

FEELING. A pure state of feeling, such as love and hate.

FETISHISM. Adoring or loving something which serves as a substitute for the original love object, such as a lock of hair, a handkerchief, glove, etc.

FUNCTIONAL MENTAL ILLNESS. A psychiatric disorder in which an organic change cannot be observed as a cause or consistent accompaniment.

FUROR. Frenzied feeling state.

HALLUCINATION. A false sensory perception associated with the special senses. The patient will insist that he hears voices, sees persons or objects in the environment, etc., when actually there is no external stimulus to account for them.

HEDONIST. A person who seeks pleasure as his goal.

HETEROSEXUAL. Sexual attraction toward a person of the opposite sex.

HOMOSEXUAL. Sexual attraction toward a person of the same sex.

HYPERACTIVE. Excessive physical and mental activity.

ID. Refers to the unconscious part of the personality, containing the primitive drives and desires.

IDENTIFICATION. A mental mechanism by which an individual unconsciously attempts to pattern himself after another person (*ex.*, a hero or celebrity admired).

ILLUSION. A misinterpretation through one of the special senses, of someone or something in the environment (*e.g.*, patient insists a gray sock on the floor is a mouse).

INCEST. Sexual relations between two people closely linked by blood ties, as sister and brother.

INSOMNIA. Inability to fall asleep.

INTELLIGENCE QUOTIENT. The relationship between mental and chronological age, often called the I.Q.

INTROVERT. An individual whose thoughts and energies are turned inward upon the self.

INVOLUTIONAL. Referring to the period of life known as the menopause.

KLEPTOMANIA. An uncontrollable impulse to steal petty and often useless articles.

LIBIDO. A psychoanalytic term referring to the psychic drive or energy usually associated with the sexual instinct but which may also be asexual.

LUCID INTERVAL. A remission of symptoms in mental illness when the patient's reasoning and judgment appear to be normal for a brief period.

MALINGERER. A person who deliberately pretends an illness or disability.

MASOCHISM. Gaining sexual pleasure from being physically subdued and hurt.

MENTAL MECHANISMS. Psychological

methods of thinking or acting which serve to solve conflicts and meet the needs of the personality.

MULTIPLE PERSONALITY. A major dissociative reaction in which the person adopts two or more different personalities which are separate and compartmentalized. There is a total amnesia for the one or ones not in awareness.

MUTISM. Lack of verbal response which may be due to voluntary or involuntary causes.

NARCISSISM. Unconscious self love which is normal during early childhood but pathological when observed to the same extent in adulthood.

NEGATIVISM. In psychiatry, resistance, active or passive opposition to stimuli such as viewpoints, suggestions, requests, etc.

NEUROLOGIST. A doctor who specializes in the study and treatment of diseases of the nervous system.

NEUROSIS. A functional mental illness in which organic causes cannot be demonstrated. Used interchangeably with the term, psychoneurosis.

NYMPHOMANIA. An insatiable desire in women for heterosexual relations.

OBSESSION. Constant and inescapable preoccupation with an idea or emotion.

ORGANIC MENTAL ILLNESS. A psychiatric disorder caused by or accompanied by physical change in body tissues.

ORIENTED. The ability to identify the time, place, person, etc; being aware of one's true surroundings.

PALSY. Weakness or paralysis of a muscle or group of muscles.

PEDOPHILIA. Sexual love for children.

PERVERSION. A maladjustment in which the sexual object or method of deriving sexual satisfaction deviates from the accepted social pattern.

PHOBIA. An abnormal, marked fear of some nondangerous object or situation.

PREOCCUPIED. Being deeply engaged in thought with an obvious absence of interest in what is happening in the immediate environment.

PSYCHE. The mind.

PSYCHIATRY. The study of the causes and treatment of mental illness.

PSYCHOANALYSIS. An approach developed by Doctor Sigmund Freud in which the attempt is made to relate unresolved conflicts and abnormal behavior to repression causes in the unconscious mind.

PSYCHOBIOLOGIC. An approach encouraged by Doctor Adolph Meyer which stresses the relationship between the patient's conscious drives and his environment. Actually, it is a psychosociality rather than the study of the life of the psyche.

PSYCHODYNAMICS. Mental forces which influence development and motivate behavior.

PSYCHOSIS. Mental illness during which the patient may lose contact with reality and demonstrate bizarre behavior.

PYKNIC TYPE. Referring to a rotund body physique with thick shoulders, short neck, broad head, and a tendency to accumulate fat.

PYROMANIA. A morbid, uncontrollable impulse to set fires.

REACTION FORMATION. The development of a character trait to an extreme degree to conceal the presence of an opposite character trait. A synonym for the mental mechanism overcompensation.

REGRESSION. The inability to function on a socially mature level of behavior, thus going backward to an earlier level of behavior (e.g., being completely dependent to the point of being bathed, dressed and fed by another as when an infant).

REJECTION. Refusal to accept. When used in psychiatry, it usually refers to a feeling state of not being accepted.

REMISSION. The temporary period of relief from the symptoms of an illness.

RETARDATION. Slowing down in actions, thoughts, or both, such as slowness in eating, dressing, walking, responding verbally, etc.

SADISM. Deriving sexual satisfaction by inflicting pain upon others.

SCHIZOID. Resembling the illness of schizophrenia. Used as an adjective: schizoid personality, schizoid symptoms, etc.

SECLUSIVE. Drawing away from the association of other persons and remaining by one's self.

SIBLINGS. Brothers and sisters in a family.

SOMA. The body.

SOMATIC. An adjective referring to the body (*e.g.,* somatic complaints).

SOMNAMBULISM. Sleep-walking.

STEREOTYPY. Aimless, repetition of verbal, intellectual, emotional or motor activities.

SUBCONSCIOUS. That part of the mind which can be recalled and brought to awareness at will. (Syn. Preconscious.)

SUPEREGO. The critical, censoring portion of one's personality (the conscience) which tends to check the socially unacceptable, primitive urges of the id.

TONIC SPASM. The sustained contraction of the affected muscles, such as is observed during the "stiffening" phase of a convulsion.

TOXIC PSYCHOSIS. A mental illness caused primarily by an infection, accumulated drugs, alcohol or other poisonous agents.

TRANSIENT. Fleeting; that which comes and goes.

TRANSVESTISM. Wearing the clothing of the opposite sex.

UNCONSCIOUS. The reservoir of the mind containing the memories, experiences and emotions which cannot be recalled into immediate awareness.

REFERENCES

Committee on Public Information: A Psychiatric Glossary. American Psychiatric Association, Washington, D. C., 1957.

Hinsie, L., and Campbell, R.: Psychiatric Dictionary. New York, Oxford University Press, 1960.

Pearson, Manuel M.: Strecker's Fundamentals of Psychiatry. J. B. Lippincott Co., Philadelphia, 1963, p. 99.

UNIT 1

Information About Mental Illness

CHAPTER 1

Concepts of
Mental Health and Mental Illness

MISCONCEPTIONS REGARDING DEFINITIONS

The terms "mental health" and "mental illness" are used so widely in contemporary society that there appears to be a generalized belief that mental health and mental illness are states of human existence having precise definitions. However, investigations of the literature and thinking related to current concepts of mental health and mental illness do not support such a conclusion. There is a lack of agreement among eminent authorities concerning exactly what aspects of human behavior constitute a state of mental health or mental illness.

Haggerty says that many people think first of mental illness when they hear the term "mental health." This response obviously represents a tendency to consider the mention of mental health as an indication that there is an absence of mental illness. Obviously there is harbored the misconception that mental health and mental illness are relative states, the presence of one condition indicating an absence of the other. No single characteristic of an individual's behavior by itself is evidence of positive mental health. Neither may the lack of any one characteristic be considered to represent evidence of mental illness.[1]

An intensive study of the literature related to current concepts of positive mental health was conducted by the Joint Commission on Mental Illness and Health. Doctor Marie Jahoda, director of the study, postulated that much of the disagreement related to the question of what does constitute mental health is due to failure to establish whether one is speaking about mental health as an enduring attribute of an individual or as a momentary attribute of personal functioning. The report states:

In speaking of a person's mental health, it is advisable to distinguish between attributes and actions. The individual may be classified as more or less healthy in a long term view of his behavior or, in other words, according to his enduring attributes. Or, his actions may be regarded as more or less healthy—that is, appropriate—from the viewpoint of single immediate, short-term situation.

Another interesting observation is that there are in the literature references to "healthy" or "sick" societies as well as diagnostic classifications of a whole society. In respect to this misconception, we read:

Mental health is an individual and personal matter. It involves a living human organism or, more precisely, the condition of an individual human mind. A social environment or culture may be conducive either to sickness or health, but the quality produced is characteristic only of a person; therefore, it is improper to speak of a "sick society" or a "sick community." [2]

CONCEPTS OF POSITIVE MENTAL HEALTH

The report to the Joint Commission on Mental Illness and Health reveals that many scientific investigators value certain individual aspects of human behavior as indicators of positive mental health. Upon investigation of these various selective behaviors it has been discovered that they can be grouped into six major conceptual approaches toward a definition of mental health. The diversity of interpretations surrounding each approach in the literature adds dimension to individual concepts. Together, the six conceptual approaches are impressive enough to suggest that they might be utilized as a guide to the evaluation of an individual's mental status. The explanatory summary of the concepts presented herein merely represents an attempt by the author to convey some understanding of their relative aspects to the reader. It should not be construed as being all inclusive or equal to reading the official report, with its findings and conclusions, to which the reader is referred.[2]

ATTITUDES TOWARD THE INDIVIDUAL SELF

This concept involves aspects related to a person's self-awareness, acceptance, confidence, level of self-esteem; sense of personal identification in relation to role, groups, weaknesses, strengths, sex, vocation, other individuals, etc.

GROWTH, DEVELOPMENT, SELF-ACTUALIZATION

Considered important is what a person does with his abilities and potentialities over a period of time. Future goals and movement towards them are viewed. Investment in living involving one's outside interests, relationships, concern with an occupation, ideas, and other persons adds dimension to this concept.

INTEGRATIVE CAPACITY

The relatedness of all processes and attributes in an individual which influence unified or synchronized personal functioning is the core of this concept. Other aspects concern the ability of the individual to tolerate anxiety and frustration during resistance to stress. Psychoanalysts view this concept as meaning a balance of psychic forces (id, ego, superego).

AUTONOMOUS BEHAVIOR

This concept is related to the individual's ability to personally regulate his decision-making and actions so that these functions are relatively independent of physical and social influences. Another aspect of this concept is the ability to refuse to conform when to do so is a social expectation that conflicts with one's value system.

PERCEPTION OF REALITY

How the individual views and reacts toward the world around him is the focus of this concept. The ability to perceive reality while being free of needs which could distort individual perceptions is an aspect of this concept.

MASTERY OF ONE'S ENVIRONMENT

This concept involves the ability to adapt, adjust, and behave appropriately in situations and in accordance with culturally approved standards so that satisfactions are achieved in love, work, play, and interpersonal relations. The ability to solve problems with expressions of appropriate feeling tones and direct attack is another aspect of this concept.

FACTORS INFLUENCING EVALUATIONS OF BEHAVIOR

When we reflect upon the breadth and depth of the conceptual approaches offered, it is apparent that no one concept by itself defines adequately mental health. Systematic research is needed to clarify further the interpretations made and to observe whether or not interrelations exist between the concepts which would make their consolidation into a lesser number of mental health indicators possible. The extent of the usefulness of concepts is limited owing to factors which are known to influence evaluations of behavior.

Social values may influence concepts of mental health and mental illness. Values may be focused upon certain aspects of personality functioning. For instance, an individual may manifest good interpersonal relations with co-workers as well as interest, satisfaction and achievement in his work with evidence of movement toward continued accomplishment. His vocational achievement may be valued highly; however, he may be inadequate when judged in relation to his family relationships and outside interests. Such observations lend credence to the postulate that no one person possesses consistently all of the characteristics of positive mental health all of the time.[1]

Individual social groups have different standards for judging whether behavior is healthy or unhealthy. These standards vary with the time, place, culture, and expectations of the social group. Behavior viewed as deviant in one social group may be tolerated in another or actually rewarded in certain social groups. For instance, stealing may be considered a moral and legal offense in a social group. In another group, individuals may be taught to steal and be recognized and rewarded for their skill. In a social group oriented toward psychiatric evaluation, stealing may be regarded as the action of a mentally ill person.

Frames of reference used by individuals, as well as by members of one's primary group, to evaluate behavior are not always comparable.[3] The individual may compare his feelings and behavior with how he thinks others feel and behave, or with how he has felt and behaved in the past. Family members, employers, community residents and physicians who interact with the person focus upon the behavior observed during interaction and its relationship to significant aspects of living. An employer may focus on the employee's ability to concentrate and perform efficiently and productively on the job and to relate well to others. Relatives may be attentive to attitudes, viewpoints expressed and situational behavior observed in the family environment. Community residents may judge an individual's behavior in relation to the standards, expectations and requirements for behavior which prevail in the local society. Through his own volition or the pressure of significant others, the person may be placed under medical observation. Psychiatrists tend to evaluate behavior according to the particular school of thought which each one follows. The focus of evaluation may be on long-term or situational behavior or the identification of healthy as well as unhealthy aspects of personality functioning. The focus of evaluation may influence either a diagnosis of mental illness, reaction to a crisis situation, or a specific defect in personality functioning. Treatment approaches revolve around the diagnosis based on behavior evaluations.

DIAGNOSTIC PROBLEMS

The technics and psychological tests used to assess and diagnose behavior yield data from which inferences regarding behavior and its motivation are made. There may be differences in the interpretations made of data. This is in contrast to the many laboratory tests used to diagnose other types of illness which yield specific data related to physiological functioning of the human organism.

When psychiatrists agree that a person is mentally ill they use as the basis for inference the observation of highly complex behavior patterns whose physiological correlates are usually unknown. When a person has lost contact with reality, hallucinates, or is completely unwilling to perform functions for survival, general agreement is quickly reached. Agreement is not as readily reached when the patient manifests less obvious symptoms, such as loss of confidence feelings, anxiety, insecurity, or fears. Many persons considered to be mentally ill do not manifest consistently extreme behavior symptoms.

It is interesting to view with contemplation the usability of the concepts as well as the results of their study. The observation that behavior may be viewed from the long-term or situational viewpoint lends support to the recommendation of modern psychiatrists that intensive treatment centers are needed to treat episodes of deviant situational behavior. Members of the interdisciplinarian health team may find the multiple concepts of positive mental health offered helpful in making behavior evaluations while being aware of the factors which influence and limit their usability. Epidemiologists do not believe that definitions of mental health and mental illness are prerequisites for research into the communicable aspects of mental disorders. They urge psychiatrists to formulate some agreed-upon classification of mental disorders to serve as the basis for research into the etiology and prevention of mental disorders.[4]

Conceiving of mental health as the opposite of mental illness may be the easiest approach to a definition, but its diversity of interpretations poses problems for additional research.

SUGGESTED REFERENCES

Backscheider, J.: The influence of socio-cultural factors on the mentally ill patient. Perspect. Psychiat. Care 3: 12, 1965.

Glasser, W.: Mental Health or Mental Illness. Harper & Brothers, New York, 1960, pp. 1, 187.

Heckel, R., and Jordan, R.: Psychology—The Nurse and the Patient. C. V. Mosby Co., St. Louis, 1967, p. 291.

Jahoda, M.: Current Concepts of Positive Mental Health. Monograph Series #1, Joint Commission on Mental Illness and Health. Basic Books, Inc., New York, 1958.

King, S.: Beliefs and attitudes about mental illness. Chap. 5 in Perceptions of Illness and Medical Care. Russell Sage Foundation, New York, 1962, p. 134.

Kolb, L.: Noyes' Modern Clinical Psychiatry, ed. 7. W. B. Saunders Co., Philadelphia, 1968, p. 80.

Macgregor, F.: Social Sciences and their relation to problems of health and illness. Chap. 2 in Social Science in Nursing. Russell Sage Foundation, New York, 1960, p. 35.

Mechanic, D.: Some factors in identifying and defining mental illness. Ment. Hyg. 46:66 (Jan.), 1962.

Plunkett, R., and Gordon, J.: Epidemiology and Mental Illness. Monograph #6, Joint Commission on Mental Illness and Health. Basic Books, Inc., New York, 1960.

FOOTNOTES

1. Haggerty, T.: (Report of radio address.) Quarterly Journal of the World Federation for Mental Health 13: 144 (Aug.), 1961.
2. Jahoda, M.: Current Concepts of Positive Mental Health. Monograph Series #1, Joint Commission on Mental Illness and Health. Basic Books, Inc., New York, 1958, pp. x–xi.
3. Mechanic, D.: Some factors in identifying and defining mental illness. Ment. Hyg. 46: 66 (Jan.), 1962.
4. Plunkett, R., and Gordon, J.: Epidemiology and Mental Illness. Monograph #6, Joint Commission on Mental Illness and Health. Basic Books, Inc., New York, 1960.

For reviewing this chapter, grateful acknowledgment is made to Miss Elizabeth Maloney, R.N., and Miss Emma Manfreda, R.N.

CHAPTER 2

Causes of Mental Disorders

The facts and phenomena concerning mental disorders appear to be multiple and complex, thus preventing us from identifying any one specific etiologic factor as the sole cause of mental illness.

In certain conditions, such as cerebral arteriosclerosis, general paresis, and the traumatic psychoses, investigators have offered partially satisfactory explanations of the basic causes of these disorders. In other psychiatric conditions, notably schizophrenia, manic depressive psychoses, paranoia, and the like, a definite, causative factor continues to elude scientific research.

Because man is composed of an inseparable soma and psyche, the causes of mental illness appear to involve man's complete physical and mental health.

For purposes of discussion, we may divide the known etiologic aspects into three categories: predisposing, precipitating, and psychic causes.

PREDISPOSING CAUSES

Predisposing causes are those conditions which make the individual susceptible to the effect of the later, precipitating cause, and thus more likely to develop a psychosis. It is generally believed that no human being can escape completely all predisposition to mental disorder. In most instances, however, the predisposition is not strong enough to extinguish the individual resistance of the person.

INHERITANCE

The inheritance factor has always been a controversial one. Some psychiatrists place much emphasis upon its importance. Others condemn the amount of attention directed toward inheritance as an etiologic possibility. In a few psychiatric conditions, direct inheritance has been well demonstrated. Huntington's chorea is known to be the result of direct inheritance. Questions have arisen among doctors, however, concerning a definite inheritance factor in epilepsy and other conditions. Genetic evidence has been demonstrated in individual family histories, particularly in the manic depressive psychoses group. Many of these patients' histories bear a record of this same illness in the family picture. Some psychiatrists, however, discount this observation by pointing out that there is hardly a family in existence which does not have, somewhere within its past or present history, evidence of psychiatric affliction.

AGE

There are three periods in life when persons appear to be constitutionally vulnerable to mental disorder: adolescence, the menopause, and the senile periods. We are much aware that during these periods the body undergoes very definite physiological changes. Combined with the stress and strain of everyday living and its inevitable problems, change may prove vastly overwhelming for some persons. Thus, we discover in mental hospitals and facilities a large number of patients who are afflicted with early schizophrenia and the involutional and senile psychoses.

SEX

Generally speaking, sex in itself does not predispose one to, or protect one against, mental disorder. Statistical graphs indicate an increase in the incidence of mental illness in women during the child-bearing and menopause periods; this may well be attributed to the changes and stress of these times instead of sex specifically. With the increase in the life span, women are living longer than men, and we find many of them afflicted with the senile disorders.

ENVIRONMENTAL AND SOCIAL FACTORS

Serious predisposing factors may develop in the environment and social setting of an individual. The mores and customs of one's culture may become problematical, particularly if a person migrates to a different environment and becomes involved in the assimilation process.

The economic and social conditions of the period may be frightening, threatening, and predisposing toward later mental illness. Financial depression with its accompanying deprivations, war with its fears and family member separations, and new inventions such as the atom and hydrogen bombs with their accompanying threats of annihilation may deter the individual from satisfying the normal human instincts of marriage and a home and children.

Health, sanitation conditions in the home, and community contacts may all figure prominently in the development of predisposition toward mental illness.

Very important environmental social factors are the feelings which exist in relationships between family members. A child who feels emotionally insecure and unwanted is potentially the victim of psychiatric disorder in later life. The child who is over-protected and unable to emancipate himself from parental control may become predisposed to later mental disorder.

OCCUPATION

Occupations may predispose one to mental disorders, both directly and indirectly. Contact with certain chemicals being produced by industry may directly affect the central nervous system of an individual and result in the expression of mental symptoms. Lead and carbon bisulfide are examples of such chemicals. Some authorities point to the incidence of drug addiction observed in doctors and nurses as being influenced probably by the access these persons have to drugs. Alcoholics are often associated with groups which find it necessary to entertain and indulge in social drinking.

PREVIOUS ATTACK

One attack of mental illness may predispose a person to the second and additional attacks. In certain medical diseases we know that one attack of a specific illness protects the person against further attacks. This is particularly true of such childhood diseases as measles and chickenpox. Perhaps the only immunities known of in psychiatry are in a few psychoneurotic patients who have been skillfully treated. In the psychoses, particularly manic depressive psychoses, we know that one attack is usually the commencement of a series of recurrences.

PRECIPITATING CAUSES

The precipitating etiologic factor is best described as the exciting cause of a psychiatric disorder. Oftentimes, the precipitating occurrence is just prior to the development of the disorder, although it is only casually related, the predisposing causes having rendered the individual susceptible.

Some persons, in discussing precipitating causes, describe them as highly emotional and critical situations. The sudden unexpected death of a loved one, personal failure, divorce, financial losses have all been cited as examples of precipitating causes.

PHYSICAL PRECIPITATING CAUSES

Infection, Fever, Exhaustion

Some infectious illnesses are accompanied by a rise in body temperature and toxic reactions. Psychiatric symptoms may develop, depending upon the individual's predisposition to these bodily changes. Some persons have been known to become delirious while experiencing a relatively low temperature of 100 degrees Fahrenheit, while others have remained in good contact with reality when the temperature elevation was well above 100 degrees Fahrenheit. Delirious reactions of extreme restlessness, fear, misidentification, and uncooperativeness may be quite marked and represent problematical behavior symptoms when contrasted with the physical changes observed.

Physical exhaustion with accompanying psychiatric symptoms may be observed as complications of long, debilitating, infectious diseases in some persons. Exhaustion may also develop from severe emotional stress and strain. During World War II, men in the armed forces were treated by psychiatrists for emotional disorders known as combat and flight fatigue.

Intoxicants

Narcotics, alcohol, bromides, barbiturates and benzedrine, when taken in large amounts over a long period of time, may accumulate in the body and cause the individual to manifest psychiatric symptoms. Most investigators believe, however, that persons who take these drugs are already endowed with a predisposing sociopathic or neurotic personality structure.

Organic Conditions

Brain tumors, paralysis agitans, multiple sclerosis, vascular hemorrhage, Pick's disease, Alzheimer's disease, and other conditions known to be accompanied by definite organic changes in cells and tissues are often associated precipitating psychiatric symptoms.

Trauma

Acute delirium may follow brain injury. Sometimes a few or several months following the date of injury, pronounced changes in an individual's personality and behavior are noted.

PSYCHIC PRECIPITATING CAUSES

The psychic precipitating causes of mental disorder are considered by many investigators to be the more dynamic, motivating and damaging causes of mental illness. While it is possible to identify the physical etiologic factors through laboratory examinations and specific tests, the psychic or emotional precipitating factors are not as easily identified or understood. It is impossible to weigh exactly the emotions of love, hate, depression, fear and the many other emotional manifestations we observe in the mentally ill.

Conflicts between one's conscious and unconscious drives may be expressed in an individual's behavior reaction to such everyday incidents as disappointment, rejection, deprivation, marital difficulties, failure in one's ambitions, inferiorities, and economic reverses. All of these, and many other life incidents, produce uncomfortable feelings of tension and anxiety which, when continued for long periods, are believed to break down the person's constitutional resistance. Disorganization of one's personality may result. Since it has been observed that patterns of behavior and reaction to conflict are acquired in early childhood, many investigators believe that behavior patterns observed in the mentally ill have their roots in childhood experiences.

SUGGESTED REFERENCES

Kolb, L.: Noyes' Modern Clinical Psychiatry, ed. 7. W. B. Saunders Co., Philadelphia, 1968, p. 116.
O'Hara, P., and Reith, H.: Understanding mental illness. Chapter 12 in Psychology and the Nurse. W. B. Saunders Co., Philadelphia, 1966, p. 212.
Pearson, M.: Strecker's Fundamentals of Psychiatry. J. B. Lippincott Co., Philadelphia, 1963, p. 13.

CHAPTER 3

Legal Aspects of Hospitalization

During the past decade there has developed a noticeable trend toward making admission of the mentally ill to hospitals a procedure to be conceived of as an opportunity for patients to receive early medical treatment and care. The individual states have made statutory provisions for various types of hospital admission and discharge procedures for the mentally ill. Generally speaking, admission to a hospital may be voluntary or involuntary. A written application for admission as well as an examination of the patient is required. The statutes stipulate who may make the application as well as who may examine the patient to determine his mental status, need for hospitalization, and treatment. The length of time that a patient may be confined in a hospital under voluntary and involuntary applications and the rights and privileges of the patients admitted are also stated in the law. Nurses should refer to the statutes of the particular states in which they practice to learn the specific provisions enacted for the hospitalization and discharge of the mentally ill.

NURSE'S RESPONSIBILITY

The nurse caring for a mentally ill patient is expected to know and anticipate the various types of hazards which may develop as a result of the individual patient's mental status. The nurse can be held liable if, in the opinion of the court, the nurse was negligent in providing protection and care constituting prevention against the development of any situation injurious to the patient. Suicidal attempts as well as accidental injuries, occurring in the hospital or, in the case of a patient's unauthorized absence, outside the hospital bounds, would be considered from this viewpoint.

TYPES OF ADMISSION

VOLUNTARY ADMISSION

This is considered the most desirable way to obtain treatment in a mental hospital. Any resident citizen of lawful age may go to a private or state hospital and make written application for admission. In some states a parent or legal guardian may request voluntary admission for a person if the individual is too ill to carry out the details of the procedure but is willing to have the application made and to be admitted. The hospital cannot accept persons making voluntary application unless it is certain that the individual understands and is willing to abide by the requirements for hospitalization as well as for subsequent discharge.

Voluntary admission is widely favored because it is believed that a person who recognizes that he is mentally ill and seeks hospitalization is likely to participate actively in his treatment. Its availability encourages patients and their families to obtain treatment during an early stage of illness when the promise of recovery is greatest. It is also believed that voluntary admission reduces the unfavorable emotional reactions which patients sometimes show towards involuntary hospitalization.

Patients admitted to a mental hospital on a voluntary application do not, as a rule, lose their civil rights (see p. 18). Usually there is no interference with the patients' rights to vote, sign personal papers, and perform duties essential in the management of their property and estates. The laws of a few states provide for the appointment of a temporary guardian by the court.

Written notice to the hospital superintendent is the usual requirement made of the voluntarily admitted patient who wishes to be discharged from the hospital. In some states the hospital must release the patient upon receipt of his written notification. In others the patient may be required to remain for a specified time, ranging from 48 hours to 30 days, dependent upon the individual state's statutory provisions. This requirement enables the hospital authorities to notify the patient's relatives if, in their opinion, the patient should remain in the hospital for further treatment. The family may be helpful in encouraging the patient to withdraw his written notification for discharge. If the patient refuses to withdraw his notice, the hospital is obligated to release him from the institution unless authorized persons initiate involuntary hospitalization action, thereby changing the original voluntary status of the patient.

INVOLUNTARY ADMISSION

While the term "involuntary hospitalization" suggests actual compulsion, it should be recognized that this element of action is not always present. A patient may be so ill that he may be unresponsive or too indecisive to act in his own interest to meet his mental health needs. Someone must take the action necessary for the person to be admitted and to receive treatment in the hospital. On other occasions the individual may lack the insight necessary to recognize his need for hospitalization and treatment, or the person may become acutely ill to the extent of being irrational and unable to protect himself or society from his uncontrollable impulses. These are the major reasons why involuntary hospitalization for the mentally ill is sometimes essential.

Most states have more than one type of involuntary procedure permitting the removal of a person judged to be mentally ill from his normal surroundings to a hospital authorized to detain the patient. In some instances a court order is required to effect the patient's removal to the hospital, but in others a court order is not necessary.

Application

The statutes designate who may make application to hospitalize allegedly mentally ill persons. In some jurisdictions the statutes authorize any person to make the application. In other states only citizens may initiate such action. The right to file an application may be limited in the statutes to any one or more of the following groups: spouses, relatives, friends, guardians, public officials, physicians, and superintendents of general hospitals.[1]

Examination

An examination of the patient's mental status is required. The statutes specify the time limit within which the examination must be made as well as the qualifications of physicians and other persons who examine the patient. The determination of whether the patient's mental condition warrants involuntary hospitalization for a specified or unspecified period of time is usually made by a court, an administrative tribunal, or a specified number of physicians acting within the statutory provisions of the particular state in which the patient resides.

TEMPORARY INVOLUNTARY ADMISSION

Temporary involuntary admission is a more recent development intended for observational, diagnostic, and short-term therapy purposes. Emergency conditions do not prevail when this type of involuntary hospitalization is effected. Dependent upon the individual state's statutory provisions, the allegedly mentally ill person may be hospitalized for a determinate (specified) period of time. In some states the specified maximum period of time is 60 days. In no state does the specified maximum period of time exceed a six month period. At the end of the observational period the patient must be released or an application must be filed by the proper authority for indeterminate (unspecified) involuntary hospitalization. The advantage of temporary involuntary admission is that some persons may recover sufficiently within the specified time period to be discharged, or if further treatment is necessary, patients so admitted may become willing to make voluntary application.

Some of the states require that all applications to temporarily involuntarily hospitalize an individual be approved by a court order. Other states require that a court order be obtained only if the person protests involuntary hospitalization. Temporary involuntary hospitalization for a specified number of days, usually 60 days, is required in other states before a petition may be filed to obtain a court order to hospitalize any patient for an indeterminate period of time.[1]

EMERGENCY ADMISSION

Almost all of the states have statutory provisions for the emergency hospitalization of persons considered unable to protect themselves and society from their uncontrollable impulses. In those states not having emergency detention statutory provisions, mentally ill persons are often taken into custody by the police and kept in jail. Medical authorities are opposed strongly to this practice as well as to the transportation of patients to hospitals in police conveyances. Emergency detention has only limited, short-range goals. It is provided to suppress and prevent conduct likely to be injurious to the patient, society, and property.

In states having statutory provisions for emergency detention of the mentally ill, some formal application is required in order to initiate the action. Persons permitted to file the application are authorized by the statutes. Authorization is granted in some states to any reputable citizen. In others it is limited to attending physicians, town selectmen, and law enforcement and health officers. A few states require judicial approval of emergency detention, with approval being vested in local magistrates, county clerks, or board of health or board of county commissioners. In other jurisdictions, judicial certification is dispensed with and medical certification by one or two physicians, dependent upon the statutes, is required instead. The power to certify is usually not limited to psychiatrists, but is granted to all general practitioners. Most states do not permit the certifying physician to be one who is a close relative of the patient or who is on the payroll of the treatment institution. The period of time for which the person may be kept in a mental hospital as well as the time during which the subsequent medical examination is to be completed is specified in the statutes and varies from state to state.

FORMAL (COURT) COMMITMENT

This procedure provides for indeterminate hospitalization of the patient after a formal judicial hearing.

CIVIL RIGHTS

The term "civil rights" designates such privileges as the right to buy, sell and maintain property, to possess a driver's license, to vote, to hold office, to practice a profession, and to engage in a business. Freedom is considered to be the prime civil right of an individual. Formal commitment of an individual to a mental hospital obviously suspends this right. Therefore, commitment procedures must be followed exactly as stipulated in the statutes. Failure to do so would support an individual's claim that he was illegally deprived of his freedom.

HABEAS CORPUS PROCEEDINGS

Habeas corpus proceedings represent a valuable human right; they date back to the English Common Law which we have inherited. The courts assume jurisdiction over the person whose behavior becomes so abnormal that he is considered to be incompetent to administer his own affairs. The Constitution of the United States provides for habeas corpus proceedings. Any person, deprived of his liberty, is entitled to be brought before a court of law where those individuals who would restrain the person must defend their action. Any patient may force court action when illegal detention is alleged. The objective of a writ of habeas corpus is to effect the release of the person from the institution. The writ is directed to the executive having charge of the hospital. It requires that the body of the person alleged to be held unlawfully in restraint of his liberty in that institution be brought before the court where inquiry is to be made into the issue. On the date of the hearing to determine the sanity and alleged unlawful restraint of the individual, all persons having an interest in the matter are entitled to be heard. The court may impanel a jury to determine the issue before the law. If the patient is judged to be sane he may be discharged from the hospital. A writ of habeas corpus may be issued on behalf of any patient committed as insane who later alleges that he has regained his sanity and is being illegally detained.

PRIVILEGES OF PATIENTS

The study conducted by the American Bar Foundation revealed that the majority of states did not have statutory provisions related to the patient's visitation and correspondence rights.[1] In the absence of statutory provisions the hospitals assume responsibility for the details of these privileges because the patients are considered to be wards of the state. The institution determines who may visit individual patients, the hours of visitation, and whether or not letters shall be censored. Visitors and incoming mail are sometimes restricted when the physician believes that they may be emotionally distressing to patients. Sometimes individual patients request that certain persons not be permitted to visit. Outgoing mail may be censored on occasions to prevent patients from sending letters which might produce an embarrassing situation for the patient and family. Some of the statutes designate the office of certain individuals to whom patients may send uncensored mail, such as the state governor, attorney general, and mental hygiene commissioner. Under these provisions mail addressed to these persons must always be posted. Hospitals usually have United States Post Office mailboxes located on the institution grounds for the convenience of patients who have access to them and mail their own correspondence.

HOSPITAL CHARTS

Hospital charts are usually obtainable by the court by issuing a subpoena to the physician under whose supervision the record was made. The responsible physician is required to identify the record in court. Entries made in the record may be accepted as evidence upon the testimony of the supervising physician. Medical personnel who performed tests and examinations under the orders and supervision of the physician may testify concerning their own entries. In many but not all states, confidential information discussed between the physician and patient during the course of treatment is regarded as privileged communication and is not admissible as evidence in a court of law.[2]

CONSENT FOR TREATMENT

Consent for treatment is not mandatory in all states. However, written consent of the voluntary patient or of the person legally responsible for the involuntary hospitalized patient should be obtained before certain physical treatments may be performed. Every person, as a human being, is presumed to have a "natural" right—to be protected from assault, insult, and slander. Treatment, such as electrotherapy or psychosurgery, might be construed as an assualt if performed without proper written consent upon a person judged to be mentally competent. Nurses assisting physicians with such treatments should inquire to ascertain if the consent has been obtained. Such action can be a helpful reminder to the responsible physician.

MAKING CONTRACTS

Contracts made during lucid intervals are valid and binding. "From the legal point of view a lucid interval is not a perfect restoration to reason, but a restoration so far as to be able, beyond doubt, to comprehend and do the act with such perception, memory and judgment as to make it a legal act."[3] If the court determines that the patient was mentally incompetent at the time of making a contract, the contract is assumed to be invalid. The court retains the right to cancel a deed or contract made by any individual who is shown to have been mentally incompetent and unable to protect his own interests or to resist importunity in the making of a contract. Hospitals usually make an administrative officer responsible for the witnessing of written agreements and contracts made by patients. Nurses requested to witness agreements and contracts should always refer the requesting parties to the hospital superintendent.

MAKING WILLS

An individual's mental ability to make a will is known as testamentary capacity. A person making a will must know (1) that he is making a will, (2) the nature and extent of his property, and (3) the natural objects of his bounty; that is, the patient must know what he is doing, of what he is disposing, and to whom he is bestowing his property. A will made during a lucid interval by a psychiatric patient is valid. A will may not be considered invalid simply because the patient was confined to a mental hospital or was psychotic. Persons contesting the will of a deceased person who was mentally ill prior to death must prove that this individual's illness impaired one of the three essential elements of his testamentary capacity. Psychiatrists may be called upon to testify concerning a patient's testamentary capacity at the time a will was made; in some instances, however, the psychiatrist may not have known the testator. Evidence of testamentary capacity may be sought from nursing notes in the hospital record or from questions directed to witnesses. For instance, a note that the patient called the nurse "Cousin Jenny" might be interpreted as a misidentification of an object of the patient's natural bounty.

Nurses caring for patients in the home may be asked to witness the patient's will. They should be aware of the criteria established to determine one's testamentary capacity and to make observations of the situation associated with the three essential elements of testamentary capacity. Oral testimony is often influential in determining a court's judgment. To testify effectively a witness must (1) observe events intelligently, (2) remember them clearly, (3) be free of emotions which may motivate the witness to suppress or distort the truth, and (4) be articulate in verbalizing descriptions of the events observed.

MARRIAGE

A marriage is considered valid if the persons entering into the relationship possess sufficient mental capacity to consent to the marriage. The usual test of an individual's mental capacity to enter into a marriage relationship seeks to determine whether or not the person understands the nature of the marriage relation as well as the duties and obligations involved. The mental capacity of the person at the time of marriage determines the validity of the marriage, and not the mental condition before or after the marriage.

Some states prohibit the marriage of epileptic, mentally ill and mentally deficient persons. There are jurisdictions which require that a medical certificate testifying to the absence of the statutes' prohibited conditions be produced before a marriage license can be issued.

DIVORCE

Mental disability as a ground for divorce has always been a controversial subject. The number of states permitting the spouse of a mentally ill patient to sue for divorce on grounds of postnuptial mental illness has increased slowly. At the present time more than half of the states have such statutory provisions. There is substantial similarity between the statutes of these jurisdictions regarding divorce under such circumstances. The similarities exist in the statutes' regulations that the mental disability shall have existed for a specified number of years (usually three to five years), that the condition shall be incurable, and that its incurability must be established by medical testimony. Some states require that the incurability of the illness be established by more than one medical expert.

Although very few states do allow mentally ill spouses to sue for divorce it is generally believed that the advisability of permitting this action should be considered cautiously. This is because it is recognized that mentally ill persons often view situations in an entirely different light when ill than they would should they recover. If they recover they may not wish to have a divorce. The majority of courts do not recognize the right of a patient's guardian to institute divorce proceedings on behalf of the patient. The judicial opinion in these actions has been that the power conferred by the statutes upon the guardian to sue in the patient's behalf does not apply to divorce proceedings. An additional opinion held is that a divorce action is such a personal matter that it cannot be maintained by an individual who is not a party to the marriage. Another reason cited is that a petition in a divorce proceeding must be verified personally and that mentally ill persons are incapable of doing this.[1]

GUARDIANSHIP, PROPERTY CONTROL

According to the various statutes, the terms "guardian," "conservator," "committee," and "curator" all designate guardianship. Relatives, friends, or a corporation (such as a trust company or a trust company officer) may be appointed to act under the supervision and control of the court to manage the estate of the patient who is mentally incompetent.

In some states a guardian is automatically named by the court during the one legal commitment procedure, even though the condition of mental incompetency has not been established previously. In other states two separate proceedings are required (1) to determine the patient's incompetency and (2) to appoint a guardian. There are states in which commitment automatically adjudicates the patient to be mentally incompetent. In these instances the appointment of a guardian becomes an administrative instead of a judicial procedure. Many of the states provide for the commitment of a patient who is mentally ill and in need of treatment. The condition of mental incompetency must be established before a guardian may be appointed. A separate and additional procedure is required to name a guardian.

Relatives are usually the persons who initiate proceedings for appointment of a guardian. However, anyone having an interest in preserving the estate of the individual considered unable to manage his own affairs may petition the court for the appointment of a guardian. For instance, if a psychotic individual is squandering money, a creditor may ask the court to appoint a guardian. The state may petition for the naming of a guardian if a patient having assets is mentally incapable of signing the checks required to reimburse the state hospital. Following appointment, the guardian is billed for the patient's care.

Many states grant the mental hospital varying degrees of control over the patient's property or money, not to exceed a specified amount or value, whether or not the patient has a guardian. This authority provides an extra guarantee for the hospital that it will receive payments due for the patient's hospitalization. Although hospitals are not subject to the same accounting requirements applicable to guardians, this authority does provide considerable safeguards against dissipation of the patient's property.

DISCHARGE FROM THE HOSPITAL

Because medical science has made considerable progress in the treatment and rehabilitation of the mentally ill, discharge procedures have become an important part of hospital administration. Patients may be released subject to certain conditions (conditional discharge) or be granted an unconditional discharge (absolute discharge).

CONDITIONAL DISCHARGE

A patient who has improved may be granted a conditional discharge. The usual condition required is that the patient receive out-patient treatment from a local clinic or psychiatrist or return periodically to the hospital for follow-up care.

The philosophy underlying conditional discharge is that it is a means of helping the patient to bridge the gap between hospital care and sustaining one's self in the community. A considerable number of patients have been able to become self-supporting upon conditional discharge. Patients who do not make satisfactory adjustments during the trial period may have to return later to the hospital as resident patients. Because the patient is still under the legal supervision of the hospital, it is not necessary to initiate a new admission procedure. This is considered an advantage.

Most of the states provide for conditional release. The period of release is usually one year, although it may range from 30 days to an indefinite period of time. At the end of the conditional period, the hospital reviews the progress and adjustment made by the patient. Depending upon the conclusion reached, the conditional period may be extended or the patient may receive an absolute discharge from the facility.

ABSOLUTE DISCHARGE

Absolute discharge terminates the legal relationship between the hospital and patient. Patients so discharged may not return to the hospital unless a new admission procedure is initiated.

In all states the patient's discharge from the hospital is considered an administrative function and is made the responsibility of the mental institution's chief administrative officer or the central state agency having control of the mental hospitals. In most states the central agency is known as the Department of Mental Health. States vesting this authority in the hospital administrator may or may not require the administrator to notify the central department of all discharge actions contemplated. On the institutional level the usual procedure to determine a patient's eligibility for conditional as well as absolute discharge consists in having the patient's attending physician examine the patient before a recommendation to discharge the patient is made to the chief administrator. The chief administrator or his assistant interviews the patient in a conference attended by other responsible staff members. A written decision citing the observations made and the reasons for approving or disapproving the patient's discharge is made.

Some states do provide for the absolute discharge of patients who have not improved and those whose improvement appears unlikely. Under these circumstances it is considered advisable to grant an absolute discharge to only those patients not considered potentially hazardous to themselves or society. For instance, senile patients who have not improved or who appear unlikely to improve have been so discharged. Arrangements are made with relatives or a guardian prior to discharge for the satisfactory care of the patient. The individual statutes specify who must be notified when an absolute discharge is to be granted to a patient designated as "unimproved." The hospital administrator may be required to notify the responsible state agency, a relative, guardian, or the sheriff serving the county in which the patient is to reside.

JUDICIAL DISCHARGE

More than half of the states have enacted legislation which permits a patient, his guardian, or his relatives to appeal to the court for the patient's discharge from a mental hospital when the hospital does not approve of the discharge. Some of the states require that the application to the court be accompanied by a medical certificate attesting to the patient's competency. The statutes in other states stipulate that the court must order a medical examination of the patient. In some jurisdictions a notice of the application must be given to the patient's family, guardian, or superintendent of the supervising institution, dependent upon the specifications contained in the statutes. Existing legislation does not require that all interested parties be given a full opportunity to appear and present their views. Some of the states providing for judicial discharge entitle the court to require security, oftentimes a bond, as a guarantee of the patient's future conduct.

Research studies have been commenced to ascertain the factors which influence the differences of opinions held by the hospital and court when judicial discharge is granted.[4]

All states recognize the patient's right to seek discharge from a mental hospital through habeas corpus proceedings if the patient believes he is being improperly detained (see p. 18).

SUGGESTED REFERENCES

Davidson, H.: Forensic Psychiatry. The Ronald Press Company, New York, 1965.
Dolan, M.: Violent patients! you and the law. R. N. 68: 42 (Aug.), 1968.
Freedman, A., and Kaplan, H.: Comprehensive Textbook of Psychiatry. The Williams & Wilkins Co., Baltimore, 1967, p. 1588.
Goldstein, A., and Katz, J.: Psychiatrist-patient privilege: The gap proposal and the Connecticut statute. Am. J. Psychiat. 118: 733 (Feb.), 1962.
Hershey, L.: Medical records and the nurse. Am. J. Nurs. 63: 110 (Feb.), 1963.
Kolb, L.: Noyes' Modern Clinical Psychiatry, ed. 7. W. B. Saunders Co., Philadelphia, 1968, p. 606.
Lindman, F., and McIntyre, D.: The Mentally Disabled and the Law. The University of Chicago Press, Chicago, 1961.
Mezer, R., and Rheingold, P.: Mental capacity and incompetence: a psycho-legal problem. Am. J. Psychiat. 118: 827 (March), 1962.
Rappeport, G. and Gruenwald, F.: Evaluation and follow-up of state hospital patients who had sanity hearings. Am. J. Psychiat. 118: 1078 (June), 1962.
Regan, W.: The legal side of confidential information. RN 28: 73 (June), 1965.
Stachyra, M.: Mental health and the law—nurses, psychotherapy and the law. Ment. Health Digest (April), 1970.

FOOTNOTES

1. Lindman, F., and McIntyre, D.: The Mentally Disabled and the Law. The University of Chicago Press, Chicago, 1961, pp. 23, 37, 155, 200-201, 203-204.
2. Goldstein, A., and Katz, J.: Psychiatrist-patient privilege: the gap proposal and the Connecticut statute. Am. J. Psychiat. 118: 733 (Feb.), 1962.
3. Hinsie, L., and Campbell, R.: Psychiatric Dictionary. Oxford University Press, New York, 1960, p. 432.
4. Rappeport, G., and Gruenwald, F.: Evaluation and follow-up of state hospital patients who had sanity hearings. Am. J. Psychiat. 118: 1078 (June), 1962.

For reviewing this chapter, grateful acknowledgement is made to Doctor Henry Davidson, Doctor William Longley, Doctor Daniel Manelli, and Mrs. Esther Mackenzie, R.N.

Introduction to Psychiatry and Psychiatric Nursing

CHAPTER 4

Psychiatry and Its Heritage

It is said that the attitude of a people toward mental disorders is a fairly accurate indication of the stage of civilization attained by the group. The history of psychiatry bears evidence that social attitudes and viewpoints have always influenced treatment and care of the mentally ill.

Medicine and religion have been associated as far back as authentic records exist. For many centuries they were inseparable, and religious beliefs often accounted for the interpretation placed upon the appearance of mental illness.

PRIMITIVE PEOPLE

Primitive people believed that the mentally ill were possessed of demons who invaded the human body as a form of punishment for sins which the afflicted person had committed. This theory was enlarged to such an extent that there was a demon assigned to each of 36 parts of the body. Treatment based upon such a conviction led to the use of methods which were designed to drive the evil spirits out of the body.

Anthropologists have discovered skulls which present evidence that trephine operations were performed in primitive times. The conclusion has been reached that such procedures may have been utilized to relieve headache or mental disorder. More brutal measures, such as starving and beating patients, were also used. The intentions underlying these practices were said to represent attempts to make the body unattractive and uninhabitable to demons. History also reveals that many so-called "possessed" individuals were abandoned, as misfits or worthless, to the forests where they were devoured by animals and that others were burned at the stake.

29

This latter practice appeared to be prompted by the belief that the mentally ill were allied with the devil and capable of casting spells.[1]

ANCIENT PEOPLE (2600–600 B.C.)

The ancients also believed in the demonological theory which gave rise to a group of healers who were a curious mixture of priest, physician, psychologist, and magician. These persons had the confidence of the people and expressed the ability to interpret the desires and trends of the unseen forces. Their methods consisted of mystic rites, incantations, exorcisms, and other mysterious actions in the temples. Beating, starving, fumigating and attacking the external body, simultaneously with vocal chanting and the tendering of burnt offerings to supernatural powers, were common practices. These healers were established as competent in their art in many countries, including China, India, Scotland and England.

With the passing of the centuries, more physical remedies, such as herbs, vegetables, and ointments, accompanied incantations. Precious stones, thought to be imbued by supernatural agencies with magical power, were also prescribed. Through an agelong process of selection and elimination, however, the most efficacious remedies naturally survived.

Existing records contain some interesting information relative to the conditions of health and disease of ancient people. There were attempts to systematize demonology. Melancholia and hysteria were obviously known. Hoang-Ti of China observed alterations in the pulse of the mentally ill. Knowledge of the nervous system was very elementary; in fact, the bone marrow and brain were thought to be composed of the same substances.

In the famous Egyptian Ebers Papyrus written in the year 1550 B.C., mental disorders were mentioned as being dependent upon evil spirits. Descriptions of senile deterioration, alcoholism, melancholia and hysteria, although not specifically called by these names, are obvious in these writings.

The Vedas or "Works of Wisdom" of the early Hindus, particularly the Ayur-Veda (1400 B.C.), contain the first classification of mental disorders. This outline was based upon the supposed varieties of demoniacal possession, of which there were believed to be seven kinds.

The Sushruta-Samhita, another of the Vedas, contained instructions and qualifications for the nurse. According to them, the nurse should be cool-headed, pleasant, kind-spoken, strong and attentive to the needs of the sick, and indefatigable in following the physician's instructions.

The descriptions of patients are most interesting. One is spoken of as alcoholic, spiteful, hot-tempered, proud and claiming to be a god. Another who sang, danced and bedecked himself with trinkets is described. A third patient is depicted as being filthy, naked and without his memory.

The early Hebrew accounts reveal that Saul, King of Israel, suffered recurrent attacks of melancholia and mania which terminated in his suicide. There is also mention of David's illness and the lycanthropic illness (believing oneself to be a wolf or some other animal and acting like one) of Nebuchadnezzar of Babylonia.

Ancient Greek dramatists referred to insanity as "the ancient wrath." Mental disorders were regarded as divine or demoniacal visitations. A psychotic person was either revered as a holy object or avoided as a devil, depending upon the peaceful or blasphemous expressions of his mental content. The demonological theory held sway but was not ascribed to a particular cause. Various types of demons, such as ghosts of dead human beings and animals, and human enemies were thought to possess the power to cast spells or carry out the wishes of the gods.

The classics of the poets, particularly those of Homer, and the writings of the historian Herodotus contain many references to mental illness which were attributed to a number of legendary persons. Hera, the wife of Zeus and queen of heaven, was believed to possess the power to cause insanity and demonstrated this power on some of the drama characters. Hallucinations were regarded as phantoms or specters communicating with the person instead of false sensory impressions.

We have records which indicate that in the temple of Aesculapius in Greece some remedial features were used for the treatment of mental disease which are employed today. One of the ancient writings found in this temple is as follows: "As often as they had phrenetic patients or such as were unhinged they did make use of nothing so much for the cure of them and restoration of their health as symphony, sweet harmony, and concert voices." The treatment was suggestion, kindness, occupation, music and recreation. Hypnotism and temple sleep were much in vogue.

Epilepsy was familiar to the ancients and was diagnosed in Cambyses, the King of Persia.

Juvenal, the Roman satirist, spoke of senile dementia as being worse than the loss of a limb. He lamented that this condition affected the memory so that the person was unable to remember names and faces of slaves, old friends and children.

PRE-CHRISTIAN DEVELOPMENTS (580–510 B.C.)

Gradually, medicine freed itself from the domination of the religious. Pythagoras, a Greek philosopher, and his pupil, Alcmaeon, established the Pythagorean School in Crotona, Italy, based upon the Greek spirit of intellectual inquiry which was developing. These men were pioneers in experimental investigation. Alcmaeon dissected animals and perhaps human bodies. Metempsychosis was one of the chief subjects of the school curriculum.

Pythagoras is credited with being the first to regard the brain as the central organ of intellectual activity and mental disorder as an illness of that organ. He advocated that reason, intelligence, and passion were elements of the brain and that all mentally ill patients were accessible to reason.

Pythagoras traveled to Egypt where he observed such therapeutic measures as cold baths, amusements, reading, and other innovations. He had his own system of dietetics and approved of music as a remedial approach. He recommended a moral life and a useful occupation for the mentally ill.

Although Hippocrates (460-370 B.C.), who emphasized the natural causes of diseases, is known as the "father of medicine," it should be pointed out that medicine was known long before his time. He was given the distinction probably because of the many innovations which he introduced and the school of followers who used his ideas for centuries.

Hippocrates believed that certain combinations of heat, cold, dryness, and moisture constituted the pathology of disease. The prevailing idea was that when the brain was too hot, too cold, too moist, or too dry, the person became mentally ill. According to Hippocrates, different climates influenced the composition of the body, the disposition of the mind, and racial characteristics. He also mentioned predispositions to mental disorders and stated that injuries to the head caused motor and sensory disorders.

Hippocrates was in doubt as to the actual structure of the brain, but he thought that it might be a gland which secreted fluid to other parts of the body. He advanced the idea that fluid retained in the brain produced apoplexy, epilepsy, and delirium.

Hippocrates classified mental disorders as phrenitis, mania and melancholia. He believed that if red bile was in abundance and putrefied during melancholia, the patient developed mania. This postulation represents one of the earliest recognitions of a relationship between elation and depression.

Hippocrates' writings also contain an excellent description of a patient in alcoholic delirium. One of his most unusual theories, however, was that hysteria was caused by a wandering of the uterus, the clinical symptoms being dependent upon the location assumed by that organ in the body. Patients were advised to marry and become pregnant. Immediate attacks were treated by giving the individual substances of unpleasant taste or smell as well as purgatives.

The writings of Hippocrates contain descriptions of depressed states in which patients expressed suicidal ideas. Psychoneurotic symptoms recorded were typical of those observed today and included pressure in the head and chest, digestive complaints, and worry. Hippocrates also stated that he did not believe epilepsy was a divine disease but thought people had developed this idea from their lack of understanding of it. Most significantly, he wrote, "For my own part, I do not believe that the human body is ever befouled by a God."

The school of physicians which followed Hippocrates carried on his teachings. They used hydrotherapy, massage, friction, gymnastics, and hypnotism. Mentally ill patients who refused to eat were placed between two patients who ate well; thus, the patient was stimulated to eat. Rooms for excitable patients were supposed to be small, cool in summer and warm in winter, with walls that were smooth and monotone in color.

Plato (427-347 B.C.) expressed the pyschosomatic viewpoint that body and mind were inseparable. He believed that mental illness could be caused by both body and moral disturbances. Prophylactic measures recommended by him stressed physical health education, strengthening the mental faculties, and proper living habits.

One of the earliest references to protection of the mentally ill was published by Plato in the *Republic:* "If anyone is insane let him not be seen openly in the city, but let the relatives of such a person watch over him at home in the best manner they know of, and if they are negligent, let them pay a fine."

There was considerable speculation concerning the location of the soul during this period. Aristotle (384-322 B.C.), the pupil of Plato, considered the heart the central organ of human affairs and sensation, and thus the soul. He believed that the brain and nervous system were associated with the intellect but not with sensation. He also emphasized the importance of the whole organism and explained the difference between acquired and congenital conditions.

Herophilus (335-280 B.C.) agreed with Hippocrates' theory of body humors. He was probably the earliest systematic anatomist and is reported to have dissected human beings. Herophilus described the meninges and certain aspects of the brain circulation. He studied the four ventricles and believed that he located the soul in one of them.

Corinth was destroyed in 146 B.C. and Greek medicine shifted to Rome. Asclepiades, born in Bithynia in 124 B.C., went to Rome well prepared in medicine, oratory, and the philosophy of his day. He has been called the Father of Psychiatry. Asclepiades' system consisted of hygienic measures which included attention to diet, baths, friction and methods of keeping the skin pores open. Emetics and blood letting were used by him.

He also advocated a pleasant environment and companions, social activities, and music. Mechanical restraints were condemned by him.

The viewpoints advanced during the pre-Christian era by these eminent philosophers were of interest and future importance. It is important to remember that while some individuals advocated humane methods, others practiced cruel approaches and continued to subscribe to the demonological theory.

EARLY CHRISTIAN PERIOD

In the early Christian era, scientific medicine was regarded as sacrilegious. Treatment based upon studies at the bedside of the patient as Hippocrates and his followers practiced was replaced by a system of healing that was full of superstition. Saint Augustine ascribed all diseases of Christians to demons. The "divine trance" (later known as hypnotism) was considered a form of witchcraft and was forbidden.

Christianity did foster a new attitude toward the sick. Previously, nursing had been performed by slaves. Now it became a Christian duty to care for the sick and distressed. The deaconesses of the early church became our first nurses, going into the home and ministering to the sick.

Three methods were used during this period to expel the demons. First, the priest placed his hands upon the patient and quoted an ecclesiastical formula; holy words were supposed to be distasteful to devils. Second, the demons were spoken to disrespectfully, thus offending their pride. Third, punishment by chaining, starving, flogging and tormenting the mentally ill was given to force patients to eat and thereby restore their memory.

Aurelius Cornelius Celsus (25 B.C. to A.D. 50), a scholar who served as recorder of medical thought in early Roman times, mentioned these widely divergent methods of treatment. He also commented favorably upon the use of music, reading, sports, swinging in a hammock, and the sound of a waterfall as therapeutic measures.

Galen (A.D. 130-200) performed many experiments upon many types of mammals, birds, fish and reptiles. He also observed the human skeletons of criminals which were exposed to vultures and the preparation of body organs which he viewed at Alexandria. Although he never dissected a human body he was considered an authority on neuroanatomy for hundreds of years. Brain structures were described by him in a manner which indicated that he considered the brain to be the center of intelligence, feelings, and memory. He left a valuable summary of the knowledge of his day, but his anatomical discoveries were his outstanding contributions. Galen was obviously familiar with many mental disorders and advocated the importance of taking family histories.

Soranus (A.D. 98-138) was very advanced in humane and therapeutic viewpoints. He wrote: "The patient should be kept quiet in moderate light and temperature—beds should be low or on the floor. If they are so violent that they can only be given a bed of straw it should be picked over and made as soft as possible. Try to check their digressions in such a way as not to excite them—not to be too lenient, but let them see that their faults have been observed, give them sometimes limited freedom. Only in rare cases bonds or ties must be used but only with great precautions, for methods of repression used without discrimination only cause the madness to start up with increased vigor."[1] Soranus also advised the giving of enemas, when necessary, and recommended pleasant sights, sounds, reading and occupational therapy. He was very much against beating, chaining, and housing of patients in dungeons, which practices were being employed by some individuals.

Caelius Aurelianus (A.D. 400) advocated the best conditions of light, temperature, food and quiet. He advised the removal of all exciting influences. Of special interest are his rules for attendants in which he recommended the use of tact, avoidance of antagonism, and limited, cautious use of selected, physical restraint. In addition to diversional activities which were in use, he favored special topics of conversation, travel and other methods of distraction. He denounced simple starvation, chains, bleeding and excessive drug therapy.

THE MIDDLE AGES

The fall of the Roman Empire in A.D. 476 was followed by a period of retrogression which retarded progress in medicine and psychiatry for many future centuries. Once again the physician surrendered his art to the priest. Science was submerged by superstition which operated under the guise of religion. Primitive theories of disease again became prominent. There was discouragement of free thinking based upon factual observation.

Three types of epidemic, psychologic mob reactions occurred in central Europe which were apparently responses to suggestion and autosuggestion. One consisted of large processions of persons who traveled across the country doing penance. Dressed in black robes marked with a red cross, they bore crosses, banners and candles. Leather whips with metal tips were carried by them with which they beat the upper portions of their bodies until they bled. The second reaction was the dance mania characterized by group dancing, laughing and other contortions which continued until the individual dropped with exhaustion. Some of the old masters, impressed with the humor of these scenes, preserved them on canvas. Devil possession was the third type of affliction, resulting in violent body movements and frothing at the mouth. Holy treatment was supposed to expel the demon. If the procedure was successful, the demon jumped out with a sudden jerk and the patient was cured. A small black devil flying from the patient's mouth can be seen in some of the paintings of this period.

There was also a notion prevalent that demons materialized into animals or became stones in the brain of the possessed. An operation was then deemed necessary, and the stone surgeons came into prominence. These so-called quacks traveled from town to town claiming the ability to cure mental disorders. Their technic consisted of making an incision in the patient's scalp, followed by a subtle but noisy dropping of a stone, which they had palmed, into a basin. The effect was astonishing to the observers who considered the operation a success.

During this same period there were some medical men who protested the backward trends and advocated the use of more rational treatments, including diets, sedatives and rest. Several also continued to give thought to the localization of mental functions. There was progress in other fields of endeavor which did result in some technological inventions and discoveries but not in medicine.

The witchcraft mania raged from the Middle Ages to the Renaissance and reached its peak during the latter part of that period. Later it broke out again. It was based upon the idea that the devil induced human beings to trade their souls to him in exchange for powers. Witches were thought to be able to work all sorts of deeds and black magic. It was believed that if the devil could not effect a bargain he stole the person. This idea created such fear that neighbor suspected neighbor, and even a family member might be denounced if he appeared to act queerly. To seek out and eliminate witches became a religious duty. Thousands of persons were executed, often by burning at the stake.

The mentally ill were better treated by the Moslems than anywhere in western Europe, where the spirit which motivated the ancient Greeks and their philosophies was dying. While the Moslems were following Hippocrates' teachings, the mentally ill in Europe were being sent to the churches and monasteries to be exorcised of demons. Ceremonial rites and often severe chastisement were administered instead of medical attention.

From the year 1000 to 1300, Arabian physicians were very interested in the mentally ill, but their contributions to psychiatry were few. They founded hospitals, libraries, academies of learning and scientific societies. The mentally ill were considered by them to be divinely inspired, which prompted their humane methods of treatment.

THE RENAISSANCE (1300-1500)

In spite of advancement in the arts and other branches of learning which occurred during this period, psychiatry and medicine did not progress very much. Witches, alchemy, and the signs of the zodiac determined the diagnosis and treatment. However, several hospitals were built for the mentally ill, the first of which was established in Valencia, Spain, in 1408. Because epilepsy was thought to be contagious, an isolation hospital was built for epileptics at Rufah in Alsace in 1486.

THE REFORMATION (1500-1660)

During the reformation there was a marked increase in intellectual activity. Thinking men with scientific inclinations were attempting to grope through the shroud of ignorance, fear and superstition which surrounded mental disease.

Paracelsus (1493-1541) is important in this group because he repudiated Galen's theories and the humoral pathology of disease which had dominated medical practice for many centuries. He also ridiculed the notion of demoniacal possessions.

Paracelsus conceived of man as a miniature of the cosmos, inseparably related to it. He was attempting to interpret man in relation to the world. Thus, he forecast our biological and social concepts of man's relationship to his environment. He advocated body magnetism which later became mesmerism and then hypnotism. Starting with this period, scientific discussions were numerous and a body of scientific knowledge proceeded to develop. The organic approach was stressed, but the intangible aspects of feeling, thinking and behavior did not receive attention.

Andreas Vesalius (1514-1564) challenged existing ideas with his comparative studies of neurology, psychology, and craniology. He compared the brains of men with those of animals and laid the foundation for the study of cerebral anatomy. Vesalius published drawings of cross sections of the brain and demonstrated something of nerve and muscle physiology. Other men pioneered in anatomy and physiology; their work provided a better understanding of brain structure and function which became the foundation for later physiological concepts.

Nursing was at a low ebb, owing to the lack of education and motivation in the lay attendants who were employed in secular hospitals. Even the sisters in the religious orders, in spite of their devotion and training, were restricted by antiquated routine.

In 1547 the monastery of St. Mary of Bethlehem at London was made into a mental hospital called Bethlehem Asylum. Later, it acquired the name of "Bedlam," a word which has been passed down to us to denote a chaotic condition such as that which was probably characteristic of the asylum. The attendants were allowed to exhibit the patients for the fee of a penny; the annual income from this practice reached 400 pounds. Sanitary conditions at Bedlam and other houses established for the care of the mentally ill were deplorable. Inmates slept in rags on a bit of straw on the floor. Treatment consisted of whirling the patients at a high rate of speed in a revolving machine. Patients were taken to bathe as usual and plunged through the bottom of the tub into deep cold water. Heavy iron collars, belts and anklets were used to chain them to the walls of their cells. Patients not considered violent were allowed to go out on the street and beg.

The early colonists brought to America many beliefs and superstitions from the Old World. Seeking out witches was considered a religious duty because the church believed that persons should make use of their reason and free will to denounce the devil. In 1647, Mary Johnson was hanged in Connecticut under the law which read, "If any man or woman be a witch, that is hath or consulted with a familiar spirit, they shall be put to death."

POST-REFORMATION ERA

Persecution of witches was practiced throughout the colonies at intervals and reached its peak in Salem, Massachusetts, in 1692, when 250 persons were arrested. Nineteen of these individuals were executed; 50 were condemned; two died in prison; and one died of torture. Finally, in 1693, the Governor of Massachusetts issued a proclamation releasing all persons confined in prisons on charges of witchcraft. This action was prompted by the accused who commenced to involve prominent citizens in accusations. For a few years thereafter, witchcraft trials occurred occasionally throughout the colonies, but finally ceased.

The early settlers concerned with their immediate problems of existence were too burdened to give much thought to the care of the mentally ill. The sufferings of the afflicted were regarded as the natural consequences of a stern Providence, passing judgment on the wicked and inferior. Individuals in need of care were given attention only when their behavior was considered a social danger or public nuisance. Consequently, an integrated plan of medical care was lacking. The decision in cases of mental illness was always placed in the hands of civil officers.

Occasionally, a relatively well-to-do family provided care for the patient in the home, usually in a locked attic or cellar room. There was a stigma associated with having such a member in the family and the members tended to keep these instances a well-guarded secret. Laws were passed for the protection of the patient's property long before those related to protection and medical care of the mentally ill came into existence.

Persons without finances or means of care were considered undesirable community burdens. Great care was taken to rid a town of these individuals, often by forcing or transporting them beyond local borders, and then abandoning them. In some instances the appointed town officer, charged with their responsibility, sold them at auction to a bidder. The buyer took his chattels to his farm, maintained them as cheaply as possible and worked them for profit. On other occasions these sick persons were jailed along with beggars and criminals. For many years the almshouses, workhouses, and jails provided the only available means of detention for the mentally ill.

EIGHTEENTH CENTURY

Franz Anton Mesmer (1733-1815), an Austrian, revived the age-old art of suggestive healing which is said to have been practiced as the divine trance in the ancient temples. Mesmer effected some remarkable cures with emotionally disturbed people through what he termed "animal magnetism." According to him the universe was permeated by an ethereal fluid with magnetic properties. He believed that he and other individuals had the special power to collect this magnetic force either in their own bodies or in a receptacle filled with iron filings. When the magnetic force passed from the healer's body into the patient's, the victim was cured. On accusation of practicing magic, Mesmer was ordered to leave Austria. He fled to Paris where, for a number of years, he and his followers effected cures through a sleeplike trance which they also attributed to the power of magnetic forces.

The doctors of France considered Mesmer a charlatan and imposter. Finally a commission to investigate his activities was appointed by the French government. Benjamin Franklin, then Ambassador of the United States to France, was a member of this commission. In order to discount the claims of the mesmerists, he requested that a group of patients stand under some trees which, he told them, were magnetized. His point was proved when these patients were cured. Mesmer's explanation of magnetic forces fell into disrepute and was replaced by the psychological explanation made possible by the work of James Braid, an English surgeon, who used mere suggestion to induce hypnotic trances.

In 1752, after efforts of many years, the Society of Friends of Philadelphia, of which Benjamin Franklin was a member, finally succeeded in establishing the Pennsylvania Hospital. Doctor Benjamin Rush (1745-1813), a signer of the Declaration of Independence, became the hospital's chief in 1783. He was a prolific writer and left volumes of valuable reports to future generations; among these writings was the first American treatise on psychiatry, which was considered to be an authoritative work for 70 years. Doctor Rush, known as the "father of American psychiatry," believed in two methods of treatment approaches. Physical treatments included bloodletting, purgatives and emetics. He emphasized the importance of clean, pleasant surroundings, doing little kindnesses for patients, and occupational therapy. He also believed it was good therapy to frighten some patients, and he was convinced that this approach often resulted in the restoration of their reason. Restraint in the form of the tranquilizer chair, which he invented, was based on the scientific principle that reducing motor activity reduced the patient's pulse. This was a chair to which the patient's hands and feet were strapped. Dr. Rush also used the Gyrator as a form of shock treatment. This device, invented by an Englishman, consisted of a rotating swinging board to which the patient was strapped and whirled about at great speed.

In 1771, the New York Hospital established a basement department for the mentally ill which was the forerunner of the present Bloomingdale Hospital in White Plains, New York.

The first hospital in the United States built exclusively for the care of the mentally ill was established in Williamsburg, Virginia, in 1773. It is now known as the Eastern State Hospital.

Vincenza Chiarugi (1759-1829) was appointed the first medical director of the Bonifacio Asylum in Florence, Italy, in 1788. He abolished restraint of patients and provided medical treatment. Chiarugi also attempted to classify the psychoses and is credited with initiating the first system of performing postmortem examinations of the brain.

Philippe Pinel (1745-1826) is always associated with the commencement of the humanitarian period in which what was regarded as and called "moral treatment" was initiated. Pinel, the son and grandson of medical men, was appointed medical director of the Bicetre Asylum in France during the period of the French Revolution. Being in that position made it possible for Pinel to test his conviction that the destructive behavior of mentally ill patients was due to their horrible living conditions and the cruel treatment given to them. Patients were chained, kept in dungeons, and dressed in rags; they slept on the floor, were surrounded by filth, were often starved, beaten and deprived of sunlight and fresh air. Prisoners, working out their sentences, were assigned as keepers of the patients and often beat them unmercifully. In 1793, Pinel made history when he unchained 12 men patients and proved that they were reliable and could respond well to kindness and improved treatment. This dramatic demonstration left its impact upon society and continues to be spoken of and remembered. Later, Pinel released the women patients from their chains in the Salpetriere Clinic.

Jean Etienne Dominique Esquirol (1772-1840) was Pinel's pupil and physician to the Salpetriere Clinic. He gave lectures in psychiatry and published *Maladies Mentales*. Esquirol discussed the importance of puberty as a critical period of development, and distinguished between hallucinations and illusions.

William Tuke (1732-1822), an English merchant and member of the Society of Friends, established York Retreat at York, England, in 1796. The retreat became known for its successful and kindly care of patients, and Tuke's advice was often sought in planning mental institutions. Four generations of Tukes were engaged in the care of the mentally ill. William's son, Henry, assisted him in the work of the retreat. Samuel, his grandson, worked to get Parliament to pass laws governing the care of the mentally ill. Daniel Hack Tuke, his great grandson, was a famous psychiatrist.

While a change to moral treatment was gradually proceeding in some parts of the world, the old attitudes and viewpoints regarding mental illness and the treatment of patients persisted in other areas during this period, the eighteenth century.

NINETEENTH CENTURY

A few private asylums were established during the first quarter of the nineteenth century. McLean Hospital in Waverly, Massachusetts, was founded in 1818, and the Hartford Retreat, now known as the Institute of Living, was chartered in 1822. A movement to establish state hospitals started around the year 1830. A belief in the moral causes and treatment of mental illness prevailed; this was rooted in the philosophy of Philippe Pinel.

The mentally ill were considered to be victims of social and psychological stresses. Therapy emphasized close association with the patient, allowing for intimate discussion of the afflicted person's difficulties and the daily pursuit of purposeful activity. The individual was held in high esteem.

Charles Dickens, famous English author, visited the United States and published in 1842 an account of his visit to the Boston State Hospital in which a homelike atmosphere prevailed.[2] Dickens described the comfortable setting of the institution, the many social and recreational activities being utilized, and the excellent, congenial relationships between the staff and patients. He remarked, "The irritability, which would otherwise be expended on their own flesh, clothes and furniture, is dissipated in these pursuits. They are cheerful, tranquil, and healthy."

The doctor's family, nurses and attendants took an active part in this social treatment plan, causing Dickens to comment on the immense politeness and good breeding he observed. Everyone took his tone from the doctor who, the author said, moved about among the people like "a very Chesterfield."

Although the physicians of the early nineteenth century argued for small hospitals as the basis for close human relationships, mental institutions grew rapidly in size after 1850. The increase in population brought a demand for additional beds. Psychiatric hospitals were patterned in size and management after the example set by the methods of expanding industry. As physicians decreased in numbers, attendant staffs increased. The doctor became an administrator and increasingly too busy to mingle among the patient group or to advise attendants. Moral treatment proceeded to decline.[3]

Dorothea Lynde Dix, a Massachusetts schoolteacher who ran a private school in her grandmother's mansion, commenced her career in prison reform and crusading for the mentally ill at the age of 39 years, in 1841. Some theological students requested that Miss Dix teach a group of women prisoners in the East Somerville, Massachusetts, jail. Through this work Miss Dix acquired an inside knowledge of conditions in the institution, discovering overcrowding, uncleanliness, and the herding together of the innocent, guilty and the mentally ill. These same conditions characterized the prisons and almshouses of Massachusetts, the several states and other parts of the world. Miss Dix presented her "Memorial" to the Massachusetts state legislature, an appeal to change these conditions. Public opinion raged about her, but several influential citizens, with the best of sentiments, immediately rallied to her support. Miss Dix then proceeded to persuade other states to adopt her ideals and suggestions. Twenty states responded. She so aroused the general public's conscience that millions of dollars were eventually appropriated to build psychiatric hospitals. The remainder of her life was devoted to this special cause, and she was responsible for the founding of many hospitals in the United States, Canada, and several foreign countries. During the Civil War, Miss Dix organized the nursing service of the northern armies. In 1901, the United States Congress passed a resolution which characterized her as "among the noblest examples of humanity in all history."

In October, 1844, 13 physician hospital superintendents met in Philadelphia and founded the Association of Medical Superintendents of American Institutions for the Insane, later renamed the American Psychiatric Association. Doctor Samuel B. Woodward of Torrington, Connecticut, who is said to have conceived the idea of the association, served as its first president. This original group included Doctor Thomas S. Kirkbride who achieved fame through his knowledge and publications devoted to hospital construction. Doctor Kirkbride's plans served as the pattern for many mental institutions throughout the country. Doctor Amariah Brigham founded the American Journal of Insanity, now known as the American Journal of Psychiatry. Doctor John S. Butler advocated that mental disorder be recognized as an integral part of the field of preventive medicine. Doctor Butler was the grandfather of two distinguished American nurses, Miss Annie W. Goodrich and Miss Ida F. Butler.

In 1851, the Belgian government took charge of a colony for mentally ill patients at Gheel which had become a shrine following the miraculous cure of a mentally ill person in A.D. 700. According to tradition, an Irish princess, who had dedicated her life to the care of the poor and mentally ill, was murdered at Gheel by her incestuous father, the king, several years before the occasion of the miracle. The cure inspired pilgrimages to Gheel by the mentally ill, which resulted in their taking lodgings with the families in the community. This plan of care is still in existence. Patients live in Gheel with families, work, carry on a normal life with considerable freedom, and report regularly to a supervising psychiatrist. It is said that the recovery rate is high and the cost of the plan economical. Attempts to duplicate this type of family care elsewhere have not been as successful.

Jean Martin Charcot (1825-1893) of Paris, a neurologist and teacher, is said to have initiated the first step in the growth of modern scientific psychotherapy. He discovered that a morbid or pathogenic idea could produce hysterical manifestations and that both the idea and the symptoms could be influenced by hypnosis.

Emil Kraepelin (1856-1926) of Germany devised a classification of mental disorders which provided new points of orientation from which psychiatry could advance at an accelerated pace. His observations of patients helped to shift the emphasis in psychiatric research from the pathological laboratory to the clinical area.

Sigmund Freud (1856-1939) of Vienna went to Paris on a traveling fellowship to work with Jean Martin Charcot. Freud's psychoanalytic discoveries played a large part in changing psychiatric research and treatment. Psychoanalysis is considered a method of investigation, a treatment, and a theory of personality development. In 1909, Doctor Freud came to America, at the invitation of G. Stanley Hall, to deliver a series of lectures on his new doctrines at Clark University in Worcester, Massachusetts. His visit in this country aroused tremendous interest, some individuals readily accepting his theories, others rejecting them. Although the controversy exists to this day, most people agree that Freud made an important original contribution which stimulated much thinking and research. His psychoanalytic technic provided a basis for modern psychotherapeutic technics.

The first attempt to organize training for nurses or attendants in the

United States was made at McLean Hospital in Waverly, Massachusetts, in 1880. Doctor Edward Cowles outlined a course which included both psychiatric and general nursing instruction. However, the formal date assigned to the McLean School is 1882, when the course of nursing instruction was placed under the direction of a general nursing superintendent who conducted a substantial portion of the program. This change was influenced by the example of the effective organization of nursing schools based upon the Nightingale system in general hospitals. The establishment of other schools followed the McLean experience. By 1906, there were 62 schools of nursing in mental hospitals.

TWENTIETH CENTURY

American attitudes were shifting at the turn of the twentieth century toward social viewpoints. There was more concern for human beings which was evidenced in new welfare legislation and the enactment of child labor laws.

By 1902, Doctor Adolph Meyer (1866-1950), born in Switzerland, but an American citizen, had already won wide recognition for his outstanding research work at various state hospitals. As director of the New York Pathological Institute, later renamed the Psychiatric Institute, he instituted a course of instruction for staff physicians. Attention was focused upon the individual patient in relation to his environment. Doctor Meyer insisted that it was the patient, not the disease, which had to be treated. In addition to studying physical and emotional growth changes, he advocated a thorough study of the person's whole environment in order to determine its effects upon one's total personality. Thus, he initiated the psychobiologic theory and stimulated the development of the dynamic concept of psychiatry. He was a remarkable teacher who later became Professor of Psychiatry at Johns Hopkins University and the first director of the Henry Phipps Psychiatric Clinic there.

Clifford Beers, a former mentally ill patient, published in 1908 his well known book, *A Mind That Found Itself*, now considered a classic. Mr. Beers, a Yale University graduate, described the harsh treatment he received in three mental institutions. His illness was precipitated by fears that he would inherit epilepsy with which his brother was afflicted. A social-minded group assisted him in founding the first mental hygiene association in New Haven, Connecticut, in 1908, which developed into a national organization within one year. Doctor Adolph Meyer was one of the persons who encouraged Mr. Beer's efforts to launch the mental hygiene movement.

Doctor Harry Stack Sullivan of the Washington University School of

Psychiatry postulated the interpersonal theory which has received wide acceptance. This theory, which recognizes the effects of the individual culture and social influences upon personality development as well as their relationship to mental illness, has stimulated the development of the multidisciplinarian approach in psychiatry and milieu therapy. Its influence has been strongly felt in basic nursing instruction where much emphasis is placed upon the interpersonal relationship. Doctor Sullivan believed that the social setting and type of staff member-patient relationship in effect exerted an immediate influence upon the patient's reaction to therapy and subsequent recovery. He believed that it was important for medical personnel and others relating to patients to be aware of the emotions of patients and personnel who were interacting. Emphasis was also placed upon the process of communication because he believed that the patient's ability to communicate was impaired during mental illness. The interpersonal theory is said to be the most original contribution since that of Freud's psychoanalysis. Some investigators believe it will prove to be the most important.

Metrazol, insulin and electrotherapy came into existence during the 1930's.

NATIONAL MENTAL HEALTH ACT

In 1946 congress passed the National Mental Health Act. This legislation placed emphasis upon the development of community mental health services. It marked the first major departure from the long prevailing concept that responsibility for mental illness and mental health belonged to state governments. This important legislation contained provisions for an integrated program of functions, including research into the etiology, diagnosis, prevention and treatment of mental illness. It also provided for the education of psychiatric and allied personnel. Assistance to states for the development of mental health programs was made available under the terms of the act. In 1947 the National Institute of Mental Health was created to be responsible for the administration of the provisions contained in the Mental Health Act. The main offices and laboratories of the institute are located in Bethesda, Maryland. As more appropriations have become available, personnel have been added to the institute's staff. The activities of the institute have been expanded, intensified, and accelerated.

The institute's community service division endeavors to develop and assist the states in the use of the most effective methods of prevention, diagnosis, and treatment of psychiatric disorders. This phase of the program is closely integrated with two others, research and training. Emphasis is placed upon the development of staff, education of professional groups, community education, clinic and rehabilitation services. Consultation on mental hospital administration and problems is also made available. The mental health needs of the aged, rehabilitation of the mentally ill, mental retardation, drug addiction, and juvenile delinquency have received special attention.

In 1948, a report, *Nursing for the Future,* the result of a survey financed by the Russell Sage Foundation and conducted by Doctor Esther Lucille Brown, recommended the elimination of basic schools of nursing in mental hospitals. Affiliate programs for undergraduate students and advanced courses of instruction for graduate nurse specialists in the psychiatric field were recommended as types of educational programs to be conducted in the mental hospital.[4]

In 1948, the American Psychiatric Association established the first inspection and rating system for mental hospitals under the direction of Doctor Ralph Chambers. A special committee set up desirable standards for mental institutions and made its services available to hospitals in Canada and the United States. Inspection and accreditation procedures are now carried out by the Joint Commission on Accreditation of Hospitals having representatives from the American College of Physicians, the American College of Surgeons, the American Hospital Association and the American Medical Association.

The World Federation for Mental Health was founded during the third International Congress on Mental Health in London, England, in 1948 upon the initiative of the International Committee for Mental Hygiene. Forty-six countries had delegates representing them at this meeting. The general purposes of this organization are: to promote among all peoples and nations the highest possible level of mental health in its broadest biological, medical, educational, and social aspects; to cooperate with the Economic and Social Council, UNESCO, WHO, and other agencies of the United Nations in so far as they are promoting mental health; to collaborate with governments and with intergovernmental or international voluntary organizations which are concerned with mental health; to foster the ability to live harmoniously in a changing environment; to promote and encourage research and the improvement of standards of training in professions concerned with mental health; to collect and disseminate information in the same field; to hold conferences and meetings; and in all ways to promote activities in favor of mental health.[5]

In 1952, the American Psychiatric Association published the *Diagnostic and Statistical Manual of Mental Disorders,* a new, more inclusive classification of mental disorders.

In 1952, the National League for Nursing was organized. The league organized a Mental Health and Psychiatric Advisory service under the supervision of Miss Kathleen Black, its first director. Representatives of the Mental Health and Psychiatric Advisory service traveled throughout the country upon request to consult on nursing education and service problems. The Interdivisional Council of Psychiatric Nursing, later renamed the Council on Psychiatric and Mental Health Nursing, was organized to confer on matters concerned with psychiatric and mental health nursing. Miss Lavonne Frey served as its first chairman. In addition to the national council, several of the state leagues organized councils.

The American Nurses' Association organized a psychiatric and mental health section around the year 1958. The section has concerned itself with such matters as the nursing role and program meetings that aim to promote improved nursing care through research studies.

In 1953, tranquilizing and other drugs came into prominence in the treatment of the mentally ill. These drugs assisted in reducing overactive patients' behavior, greatly decreased the amount of shock therapies administered, increased the patient discharge rate and made treatment at home possible. Patients tend to be more cooperative and amenable to treatment. It is possible to create a more homelike atmosphere in the hospital. Length of hospitalization has been reduced for most patients. Many individuals are being treated in the community. Considerable research is still in progress and it is hoped that even better drugs will become available in the future. The drugs, however, are not a specific cure.

COMMUNITY MENTAL HEALTH SERVICES

The National Mental Health Act gave impetus to the passage of the Community Mental Health Services Act by New York State in 1954. This legislation came into being through the work and recommendations of a special commission appointed in 1949 to develop a master plan for community mental health. It provided for a permanent system of state aid to communities for the establishment and operation of community mental health services. Responsibility for these services was brought to the local government level. The state is obliged to pay one-half the cost for maintaining approved community mental health facilities. The state mental hygiene commissioner is empowered to withold all or part of the state's reimbursement if there is a local failure to comply with the law or its regulations. Most of the other states now provide some financial assistance to individual communities for the establishment and operation of psychiatric services.

HEALTH AMENDMENTS ACT

The Health Amendments Act of 1956 made more appropriations available for the continuation of the efforts of the National Institute of Mental Health. Provisions were made for the advanced preparation of nurses for administrative, supervisory and teaching positions on the basis of the applicant's scholarship and need. General information and a list of approved schools may be obtained from the Training and Standards Branch, National Institute of Mental Health, Bethesda, Maryland 20014. Applications for scholarships are made directly to the university of the student's choice (see chap. 5, p. 53).

COMMUNITY MENTAL HEALTH CENTERS CONSTRUCTION ACT

The Community Mental Health Centers Construction Act of 1963 provides guidelines for establishing comprehensive mental health programs. The growing awareness of the value of treating the mentally ill patient in the community where he lives led to this legislation. Mental Health Centers are well on the way toward replacing the older traditional state hospitals as the headquarters for treating the mentally ill. These newer facilities are much smaller in size. The emphasis is upon prevention, early treatment, rehabilitation, and outpatient services (see chap. 8, p. 89).

SUGGESTED REFERENCES

American Psychiatric Association: One Hundred Years of American Psychiatry. Columbia University Press, New York, 1944.

Angrist, S.: The mental hospital: Its history and destiny. Perspect. Psychiat. Care 1: 20, 1963.

Association of Medical Superintendents of American Institutions for the Insane: Reports published in 1855. Reprinted in Ment. Hosp. Vol. 6 (May), 1955.

Beers, C.: A Mind That Found Itself. Doubleday & Co., New York. Reprinted with additions in 1953.

Bockhoven, J.: Moral Treatment in American Psychiatry. Springer Publishing Co., New York, 1963.

Bond, E.: Therapeutic forces in early American hospitals. Am. J. Psychiat. 113: 407 (Nov.), 1956.

Carty, R., and Breault, G.: Gheel: a comprehensive community mental health program. Perspect. Psychiat. Care 5: 281 (Nov.-Dec.), 1967.

Crawford, B., Dixon, D., and Rowley, C.: Mental hospitals—an obituary? Psychiat. Nurs. 9: 18 (Jul.-Aug.), 1971.

Deutsch, A.: The Mentally Ill in America. Columbia University Press, New York, 1937.

Felix, H.: Evolution of community mental health concepts. Am. J. Psychiat. 113: 673 (Feb.), 1957.

Freedman, A., and Kaplan, H.: Comprehensive Textbook of Psychiatry. Williams & Wilkins Co., Baltimore, 1967, p.2.

Gorman, M.: Every Other Bed. The World Publishing Co., New York, 1956.

Greenblatt, M., York, R., and Brown, L.: From Custodial to Therapeutic Patient Care in Mental Hospitals. Russell Sage Foundation, New York, 1955, p. 407.

Lewis, L.: A Short History of Psychiatric Achievement. W. W. Norton & Co., New York, 1941.

Marshall, H.: Dorothea Dix. The University of North Carolina Press, Chapel Hill, N. C., 1937.

Menninger, W.: Psychiatry—Its Evolution and Present Status. Cornell University Press, Ithaca, N. Y., 1948.

FOOTNOTES

1. Lewis, N.: A Short History of Psychiatric Achievement. W. W. Norton & Co., New York, 1941, p. 52.
2. Dickens, C.: American Notes for General Circulation, ed. 3. Chapman & Hall, London, 1842, Vol. 1, pp. 105-111.
3. Greenblatt, M., York, R., and Brown, E.: From Custodial to Therapeutic Patient Care in Mental Hospitals. Russell Sage Foundation, New York, 1955, p. 407.
4. Brown, E.: Nursing for the Future. Russell Sage Foundation, New York, 1948, pp. 132-136.
5. World Federation for Mental Health: Pamphlet. The Chiswick Press, New Southgate, England, N 11.

For reviewing this chapter, grateful acknowledgment is made to Miss Florence E. Newell, R.N., and Mrs. Vivian S. Bryan, R.N.

CHAPTER **5**

Orientation To Modern Developments and Psychiatric Nursing

Significant changes have taken place in psychiatric and mental health facilities, the education of nurses, and their role during the past ten years. Although changes that were talked and written about for many years previous to this era have emerged to a noticeable degree, the task of enhancing and bringing them to greater fulfillment will continue indefinitely.

DEVELOPMENTS INFLUENCING CHANGE

Perhaps the most important development that led to change on a scale larger than ever before was the enactment of state and federal legislation. The creation of the National Institute of Mental Health in 1946 and subsequent passing of community mental health laws provided the type of motivation, financing, planning, and preparation needed to implement recommendations made by the experts (see chap. 4, p. 45, 47).

Some persons view the present shift to community psychiatry as only the beginning of an integrated plan that will eventually merge into one generalized system of health care facilities. Separate mental hospitals, as they exist today, will probably gradually be eliminated as community psychiatry develops.

As the large public mental hospital ceases to be a "dumping grounds" for unwanted patients, such as alcoholics and geriatrics, the patient population will decrease. Indeed, a considerable reduction in the population of these older facilities has already taken place. The building of special hospitals for alcoholism in some localities and the organization of various types of community psychiatric services have reduced admissions to public hospitals. The transfer of geriatric patients from mental hospitals which began in California during the late fifties has influenced similar action in other states. For many years it had been recognized that thousands of aged persons were hospitalized in state and county mental hospitals simply because there was no other place for them. Families did not want to or could not care for them at home. Public health legislation has now developed in some states into a workable plan that focuses upon identifying and transferring geriatric patients to long term care facilities. These accomodations are considered to be more appropriate to meet the physical, social and psychological needs of older persons. Retirement homes, homes for the aged and nursing care facilities are being used extensively to hospitalize these persons. To effect this long needed change, state governments had to pass legislation that prohibited the admission of aged persons to mental hospitals. State departments of public health established special divisions having personnel who are primarily responsible for the screening, transferring, and follow-up of geriatric patients admitted to long term care facilities. Nurses are beginning to play an active part as members of teams that are involved in the implementation of this legislation.

EFFECTS OF OVERPOPULATION

One of the most serious problems in our health care system had its beginning during the early eighteenth century industrial revolution. With the expansion of industry, immigration, population, and commercial growth, mental illness increased. The need for hospitalizing mentally ill patients was met by adding more buildings and wards to those facilities already established. The basic idea was to centralize management and care according to the industrial growth pattern. Actually it was intended as an economy move. Ironically, it turned out to be one of the most expensive and least effective movements in American health and hospital history. Colonial period physicians had attempted to preserve the small mental hospital of 250 beds, but their legislators were not so influenced (see chap. 4, p. 42).

Recognizing the crippling effects of the large overpopulated public hospitals, psychiatrists and social scientists of the twentieth century began to call for change. Although movement in this direction did not come about easily or quickly, enough of an impression was made upon members of the allied disciplines and society to finally bring it about. This, of course, required research studies to identify the problems, to evaluate existing health facilities and the effectiveness of treatment and care, and to develop guidelines for action. The publication *Action for Mental Health* was one of the most important documents produced to lead the way. This was a report of the Joint Commission of Mental Illness and Health, a committee, having representation from 36 organizations, that was appointed by the National Institute of Mental Health as directed in the Mental Health Study Act of 1955. Its purpose was to analyze and evaluate the needs and resources of the mentally ill in the United States and to make recommendations for a national mental health program.[1]

As recently as 1960 it was not unusual for a state mental hospital to house as many as 3,000 to 7,000 patients. A few had more. By comparison, a hospital having 2,000 patients was considered small. Therefore, it is understandable that one of the major aims of persons who promoted change was to reduce and control the size of the mental hospital as well as its population. The Joint Commission recommended that not a single patient be admitted to those hospitals that already had 1,000 patients and that no money be spent to build mental hospitals that would accommodate more than 1,000 patients.

In restructuring the mental health system the aim was to establish smaller facilities, particularly mental health centers, within a relatively short distance of a patient's home and family. The value of early admission, intensive treatment, outpatient care in clinics, day and night treatment centers, and social rehabilitation was stressed. Individualized communication approaches as well as group therapy and group activities for patients were implemented. Education of the public and members of allied disciplines were prime targets aimed at to result in a better understanding of mental illness and its prevention.

NURSING EDUCATION CHANGES

The education of nurses was also affected by changes that took place in mental hospitals. After the publication of the report *Nursing for the Future* by Dr. Lucille Brown in 1947, mental hospitals began to close their three year diploma schools and replace them with affiliation programs.[2] Psychiatric nursing courses soon became mandatory in the basic curriculum. Most nursing schools sent their students to the large public psychiatric hospitals for this experience and some sent them to the few large private mental hospitals that maintained programs. The immediate objective was to educate nurses to understand mental illness, its treatment, and nursing approaches. The long range objective was to prepare them to give comprehensive nursing care to all sick persons. Unity of body and mind was stressed as the emotional aspects of illness were discussed. Incidental to this arrangement for the education of nurses was the important fact that affiliation brought increasing numbers of nurses into large public mental hospitals and direct contact with the mentally ill. Nurses were able to observe the inadequacies of old facilities, overpopulation, crowded conditions, shortage of staff, and the obvious absence of effective treatment and care. The number of nurses employed in psychiatric hospitals increased slowly, but steadily. Gradually, nurses became more active and involved in the treatment and care of the mentally ill.

LEGISLATION AFFECTING NURSING EDUCATION

The Health Amendments Act of 1956 made funds available to educate psychiatric nurses in advanced programs taking place in the university. Postgraduate courses of one year that had previously been maintained by some mental hospitals went out of existence. As more nurses were educated in the university setting they became interested in helping to bring about and create change (see chap. 4, p. 48).

Nurse educators began to promote dynamic psychiatry. Psychiatric nursing affiliation programs focused upon the observation and meaning of behavior as opposed to descriptive psychiatry. Concepts and principles of psychiatric nursing were talked and written about as the era of their identification and integration with nursing care came into being. Mental illness was recognized as a fundamental disturbance in a person's relations with other individuals. Theories of interpersonal relations were learned and implemented during nurse-patient contacts.

In 1960 most affiliation programs for undergraduate nursing students were conducted by a centralized department of education maintained by large psychiatric hospitals. The instructional staff was employed by and worked under the supervision of the department's director of education. While this had some advantages, it was also recognized that it perpetuated, to a certain extent, the lack of understanding needed by all health personnel, especially teachers, to integrate psychiatric concepts and principles. Psychiatric nursing was, more often than not, viewed as a separate instead of an integral part of all nursing. Home schools were only too willing to permit the affiliation hospital staff to plan and take responsibility for the entire course. This was mostly because many of the home school teachers had not taken a course in psychiatric nursing. The general reaction to joint curriculum planning with the mental hospital staff was that the basic school of nursing faculty did not know enough about the subject matter and management of patient care to participate. This situation was changed when collegiate nursing programs began to send their students on affiliation with their own instructors employed by the college. As more teachers were prepared under the provisions of the Health Amendments Act, the number of instructors coming into the psychiatric hospital with affiliate students increased. Collegiate faculty members were often required to teach medical-surgical nursing as well as psychiatric nursing, depending upon the arrangement of the curriculum and the number of students needing clinical experience. This helped to strengthen and reinforce the integration of psychiatric concepts and principles.

The Nurse Training Act of 1964 provided support grants to all types of basic nursing schools that were able to qualify their applications for funds with National League for Nursing accreditation status. Many schools, including diploma programs, were able to employ qualified psychiatric nursing instructors for the purpose of having them accompany students on affiliation or to establish a course in psychiatric nursing in the home school if clinical facilities were available to provide experience in the community. Funding of faculty was not made available to the centralized department of affiliation instruction maintained by mental hospitals. This led to a gradual decline in the number of affiliation programs maintained by these institutions. Although some programs are still in existence, the trend toward having the basic school of nursing conduct the psychiatric nursing program continues to grow. As community mental health facilities and college programs increase in number we may expect to observe more of this pattern of nursing education.

THE PSYCHIATRIC NURSING PROGRAM

A nursing student enrolled in a psychiatric nursing course may have a primary, sustained clinical experience in a large public hospital, a community mental health center, or a psychiatric service in a general hospital. During the program, visits to other types of psychiatric facilities and services may be made for the purpose of gaining a greater perspective on the various types of facilities, services, and differences in treatment programs and approaches.

Any new undertaking has its moments of uncertainty and stress. This applies to the student who enters a program in psychiatric nursing. Of all the courses in the basic curriculum, psychiatric nursing appears to be the one that most students are curious about. So much has been written and said about mental illness and the mentally ill that students are, understandably, sometimes hesitant about taking the initiative to relate and communicate with patients.

INTERACTING WITH PATIENTS

Many differences in the patients' behavior will be observed as the nurse interacts with the patients. Some patients will extend a pleasant and cordial greeting. There will be some who will enjoy the presence of new nurses and try to make them feel welcome. Other patients will be sitting idle, appearing apathetic, fatigued, and low in spirits. Some individuals may not acknowledge the nurse's presence when approached. Others may actually move away or tell the nurse to leave. Contrasted with the behavior of these persons will be that of some patients who will be obviously energetic, active, and talkative.

The nurse will find it helpful to remain objective when evaluating patients' behavior. This will help to avoid developing negative emotional reactions as contacts with patients, particularly those who appear to be rejecting, are experienced. To remain objective and receptive in one's approach toward patients it is important to recognize that the chief disturbance during mental illness is in the interpersonal relationship.

Many patients are unable to verbalize their true feelings and communicate adequately with others. The roots of these difficulties may be very deep and probably have a significant heritage in the individual's family relationships and social environment. Patients who fear strangers have often experienced so much rejection during their lives that they develop fear of new acquaintances and come to anticipate them as additional sources of rejection. Thus, when meeting patients for the first time, it is helpful to remember that the patient regards the nurse as a stranger. Gradual, continuous daily approaches can be made toward the rejecting patient until the nurse has succeeded in instilling the necessary confidence and trust in the patient that leads to the establishment of a relationship.

As the nurse becomes better acquainted with the mentally ill, it will become apparent that their behavior is not as unusual as it is emotionally accentuated. Whatever the behavior, it is important to realize that it is meaningful and motivated by deeper feelings and thoughts seeking some form of expression which will bring relief from inner tension, anxiety, and fears being felt by the person.

Increasingly, it will become obvious that many of the conflicts acted out or verbalized by patients are experienced daily by other human beings who are able to resolve them. Failures in personal ambitions and careers or over-reaching toward a life goal may precipitate a person's illness. The nurse will probably meet other patients who have been deprived of or had education, careers, or social aspirations forced upon them. Patients will be observed who have been unable to free themselves from strong family attachments to develop normal social contacts. There will probably be men and women who have been unable to adjust to and sustain a healthy marital relationship. Victims of broken homes or of discordant, hostile family environments may be among those observed in a mental health facility. Intuitively, the sensitive nurse will recognize that these patients often still feel deeply the physical and emotional deprivations experienced in their former environments and relationships. Many patients crave warmth and affection, but fear to accept it owing to their deeply felt anticipation of being rejected, abandoned, and deprived again.

PSYCHIATRIC NURSING SKILLS

The skill of psychiatric nursing is demonstrated in the nurse's ability to be sensitive to the patient's feelings and thinking. A skillful nurse knows instinctively when a patient needs companionship as well as when the individual should be left alone. A capable nurse understands a patient's inability to verbalize or the need to verbalize freely. Skillful nursing is being alert to the deeper underlying feelings beneath communications and knowing when a patient does not mean what he says or actually may mean the opposite of what he said. It involves the ability to recognize the meaning of voice tones, gestures, and other expressions of behavior. Being skillful sometimes requires an ability to modify one's rate of activity in social and recreational activities so that the patient's need to achieve may be met. Sitting beside an unresponsive person or talking or listening to patients is what is known as making therapeutic use of the nurse's self in providing emotional support for others. These seemingly simple activities can be demanding for some nurses who love the tempo of general hospital nursing with its usual hustle and bustle and administration of bedside nursing procedures. To change the tenor and tempo of one's daily pattern of nursing is a real challenge to the nurse who enters the environment of a psychiatric hospital. Visiting with patients, listening to their problems, encouraging them to communicate, participating in group meetings and social-recreational activities constitute a major portion of daily nursing directed toward a therapeutic goal. The tempo is different, but the goal of care, the patient's recovery, remain the same.

PLANNING PATIENT CARE

The general hospital nurse is accustomed to following doctor's written orders and nursing care plans. Psychiatrists do write orders for medications and the few treatments administered in the mental hospital, but most of the nursing care is unwritten. The effectiveness of nursing care is dependent upon the individual nurse's ability to observe, evaluate, and make independent judgments. The skill of psychiatric nursing revolves around this chief difference in providing nursing care. The ingenuity of the nurse is challenged constantly. How well the nurse plans the patient's care depends upon how sensitive and alert she is to the patient's immediate and long range needs. Patients are dependent upon the skill of nurses and therapists who know what to do to provide care and have the ability to initiate it.

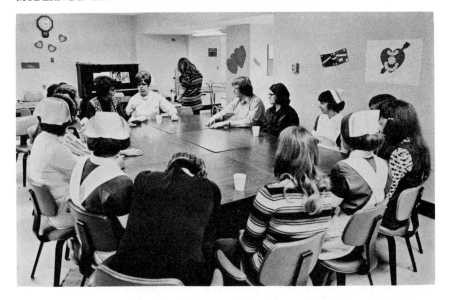

Fig. 1. Participating in a group meeting led by the nurse. (Courtesy of Swedish-American Hospital, Rockford, Ill.)

Every nurse can function as a social therapist and utilize the principles of psychotherapy in the nurse-patient relationship. Anything which the nurse can do to normalize the patient's social environment and daily existence, as well as to provide some measure of consideration toward individual patients contributes to better nursing of the mentally ill.

NURSING OBSERVATIONS

It is possible to be alert to patients' whereabouts and actions without resorting to obvious direct methods of scrutiny that cause patients to feel uncomfortable and angry. Indirect observations can be made when on the ward and when nurses are escorting patients to other locations and activities in the hospital.

PERSONNEL

There is a shortage of psychiatrists, psychologists, social workers, and nurses in mental hospitals, especially the large public ones. Misconceptions about mental illness, the location in isolated country districts of many hospitals, inadequate financing, low salaries, poor communications with society, and unsatisfactory living accomodations all contribute to this situation. In addition, some nurses find it difficult to implement the skills of

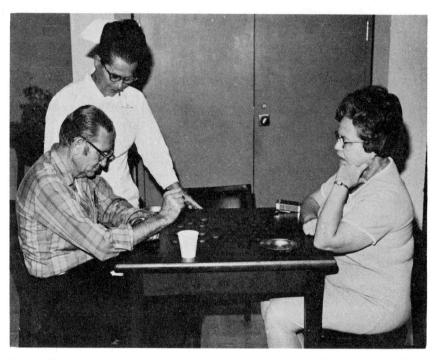

Fig. 2. Every nurse can function as a social therapist and initiate diversional activity between patients. (Courtesy of Arkansas State Hospital, Little Rock, Ark.)

psychiatric nursing in the environment of the big hospital ward. For these reasons, large numbers of psychiatric aides and technicians supplement the professional staff. Many of these persons have devoted their entire lives to the care of the mentally ill and are of real therapeutic assistance to the patients. Nurses coming from general hospitals to affiliate are often surprised to observe the amount of responsibility assumed by some psychiatric aides. Continuous education of all personnel, including aides, is proving to be a necessary and important step in achieving improved care of the mentally ill. Doctors, psychologists, social workers, nurses, and aides hold team meetings regularly for the purpose of sharing information, discussing their observations and carrying out a unified treatment approach.

There are many other personnel in the various departments of the hospital contributing to the patient's welfare, and it is imperative for nursing personnel to maintain good working relationships with these individuals. Men and women volunteers who come into the hospital from the community are nonsalaried part-time personnel who contribute their time and interest by lending companionship and emotional support to patients. Volunteers give what is often referred to as "plus" services. Parties, picnics, theatre trips, literary discussions, gardening brigades, and a great variety of other social activities are planned and conducted by volunteers. These staff members function as social therapists in providing services which patients might not be able to receive. The interest of many volunteers in the improvement of mental hospital and mental health services makes them an important link between the hospital and community.

THE NURSE AS A CITIZEN

Every nurse, in her citizen role, has an opportunity to contribute to the improvement of mental health facilities and the care of the mentally ill. What legislation can do for the mentally ill has already been demonstrated. More can be done if every citizen takes an active interest in legislation that affects the hospitalization and care of these patients.

SUGGESTED REFERENCES

Brown, L.: Nursing Reconsidered—a Study of Change, part 2. J. B. Lippincott Co., Philadelphia, 1971, p. 285.

Crawford, B., Dixon, D., and Rowley, C.: Mental hospitals—an obituary? J. Psychiat. Nurs. 9:18 (Jul.-Aug.), 1971.

Greenblatt, M., York, R., and Brown, L.: From Custodial to Therapeutic Patient Care in Mental Hospitals. Russell Sage Foundation, New York, 1955.

Joint Commission on Mental Illness and Health: Action for Mental Health. Basic Books, Inc., New York, 1961.

Mertz, H.: How the nurse helps the patient in his experience with psychiatric care. Perspect. Psychiat. Care 6: 260 (6), 1968.

Pope, J.: The changing scene of psychiatric nursing in a state hospital. Perspect. Psychiat. Care 5: 163 (Jul.-Aug.), 1967.

Stevens, R.: The treatment of the aged in state hospitals. J. Psychiat. Nurs. 9: 31 (Jan.-Feb.), 1971.

Boucher, M.: Personal space and chronicity in the mental hospital. Perspect. Psychiat. Care 9: 206 (Sept.-Oct.), 1971.

Leninger, M.: Community psychiatric nursing: trends, issues and problems. Perspect. Psychiat. Care 7: 10 (Jan.-Feb.), 1969.

FOOTNOTES

1. Joint Commission on Mental Illness and Health: Action for Mental Health. Basic Books, Inc., New York, 1961.
2. Brown, E.: Nursing for the Future. Russell Sage Foundation, New York, 1947.

For reviewing this chapter, grateful acknowledgement is made to Mrs. Marie Babrick, R.N., Mrs. Jeanette Wade, R.N., Miss Marilyn Miller, R.N., Mrs. Manolia Schult, RN., Mrs. Diane Sworm, R.N., and Mrs. Lucilla Warren, R.N.

CHAPTER 6

The Changing Role of the Nurse

Establishing and maintaining mental health facilities and care as a part of the community with its network of health agencies has influenced changes in the role of the nurse. The shift from the traditional role of supervisor, head nurse, and staff nurse with their technical management identifications has been obvious during recent years. As nurses have become more directly involved with patient care in their daily relationships the change has promoted some individuals to ask, "What is the contemporary role of the nurse?"

ROLE CHANGES OBSERVED

The shift in the nurse's role has been apparent in general hospital settings as well as psychiatric facilities. This is profoundly documented in Dr. Esther Lucille Brown's publication, *Nursing Reconsidered—a Study of Change.* Dr. Brown, who is well known for her interest in and studies of nursing, traces the changes taking place in the nurse's role in all types of health facilities. Noticeable in these observations and reports is a demonstrated ability of nurses to act more independently in developing plans for and performing new tasks that are contributing to improvement in the delivery of health care. Nurses are being challenged to analyze old ways of participating in the health care system and to develop new approaches. Included among the reports are accounts of nurses who have gone into rural areas and developed mental health services with the aid of citizen groups. One of the developments has been the successful use that mental health consultant nurses have made of persons having no previous experience in working with the mentally ill in medically and economically deprived areas of the country.[1]

ROLE MISCONCEPTIONS

The concern about the role of the nurse has caused Doctor Eleanor Lambertson to say, "One of the primary misconceptions about the nurse practitioner is that there is a universal model one can examine or that all who nurse can or should function equally effective within the entire spectrum of health care services. I subscribe to the evidence of need for a universal base for the practice of nursing, but I also hypothesize that there is a universal base of knowledge and competence for all practitioners in the health service occupations and professions, including the physician."[2]

I believe that a universal body of knowledge is the source of concepts and principles learned by professionals and applied to their practice. It should account for the reasons underlying observations made, conclusions reached, and actions taken to diagnose and meet the nursing needs of patients. Thus, there is no one nursing role. The role is determined by the individuality of the particular health agency, its purpose for existing, and the needs of people who rely upon it to prevent as well as treat and sustain the patient during all stages of an illness.

THERAPEUTIC ELEMENTS IN THE ROLE

As the nurse interacts with patients there are some elements in the role relationship that can be identified as generally therapeutic. These are the manner of showing acceptance of the person and a genuine interest in trying to be helpful. In trying to be helpful, the nurse listens well and utilizes techniques that provide an opportunity for the patient to express feelings during their communication exchanges. As the nurse gathers data about the individual's problems, the nurse may clarify some of it with the patient in order to make interpretations that may be useful in making responses and approaches. Being helpful may require the nurse to discuss some of the data with the patient in an effort to influence more rational thinking in learning how to avoid, or reduce, and react to emotional stress in the patient's life situation. Giving support to the patient, as he makes changes in his ways of adapting to stress or tries to conquer some overwhelming emotion or to achieve some goal, is a process of encouraging and strengthening the individual's attempts to succeed with feelings of confidence. These elements of nurse-patient interaction may be generally useful in all types of health facilities, especially psychiatric and mental health facilities.

ROLE ACTIVITIES

Because the activities or functions associated with a role are always of interest, it seems appropriate to mention that activities are determined by the type of service provided by the individual agency as well as the organizations' expectations and job description requirements for nurses. The changes that have been observed in role functions are primarily the result of improvement in communications among all levels of personnel. There is more interaction between nurses, patients, and staff. There has been improvement in the nurse-physician relationship. Nurses are making decisions at the work level and are planning for patient care, including plans and follow-up for the patient after discharge from the facility. Functions that were previously assigned only to physicians, psychologists, and social workers are now being assigned to and shared with nurses as team members. There has been recognition that a well prepared nurse can, indeed, be more involved in the therapeutic process. We may expect this trend to continue into the future.

The role activities that have been implemented at the Fort Logan Mental Health Center in Denver by Miss Helen Huber provide insight into the changing, more collaborative role of the psychiatric nurse. In addition to those functions carried out by nurses as listed below, nurses also administer physical care, give medications, teach patients and families specific aspects of care, refer patients to the internist, supervise the psychiatric technicians, and so forth.[1]

Nurses: *Participate with the patient in his daily living and assist him to use the events of the day as a remedial learning experience. "Events" may include occupational or recreational therapy, psychodrama, helping the patient with personal hygiene or the housewife patient in planning her day and organizing her work, helping with table behavior at meals, and so on. Nurses use support, problem-solving, confrontation, and interpretation skills in the context of a developing relationship.*

Act as individual or group therapist, with the depth of therapy dependent on the needs of the patient or patients and the skill of the nurse.

Work with patients and family members in informal situations in the home, hospital, or clinic and in informal group therapy sessions to resolve problems of communication and conflicts in the relationship.

Take the patient's social history.

Evaluate patients for various services, placement, change in program, or discharge.

Assist the patient and his family to use the resources that are available and appropriate to his needs.

Act as a change agent in assisting patients and their families to translate insights and motivation into altered behavior that is more effective and gratifying.

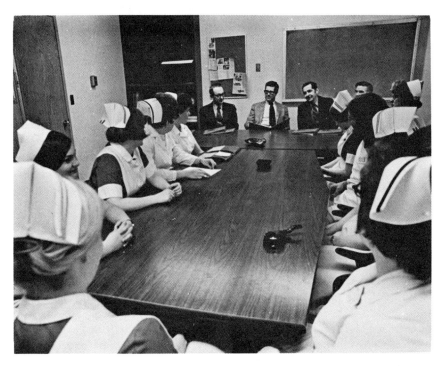

Fig. 1. Nursing students attend a multidisciplinary staff conference led by the psychiatrist. (Courtesy of Swedish-American Hospital, Rockford, Ill.)

Help non-professional workers, family members, and others to recognize the therapeutic potential of interaction with patients, and to realize that such persons can implement the patient's treatment goals through interaction.

Follow up the psychiatric care of patients in family-care homes, nursing homes, boarding homes, and sheltered workshops.

Contribute observations and suggestions concerning patients to the members of the treatment team.

Interpret to the non-medically oriented treatment staff pertinent information about the medical or physical needs of patient or family members.

Participate actively in planning overall team programs, as well as planning for the individualized care of the patient.

Serve as the liaison between their team of the Center and other community agencies (including the several new community mental health centers with which various exchanges of service are now developing).

Serve as consultant in psychiatric nursing or in a particular skill, such as psychodrama or group process.

Participate with other organizations in planning services.

This list of functions is an indication of a greatly expanded role for the nurse. As more psychiatric facilities adopt programs which emphasize interpersonal interaction in patient care and the milieu program of a therapeutic community, we may expect to see this concept of the psychiatric nursing role implemented and strengthened. It is true that other members of the team may perform some of these functions. This development has come about through deliberate action taken in modern mental health centers to place emphasis upon the blurring of roles. Its purpose was to reduce the sharp distinction between what each professional group claimed as its role prerogative. Such distinctions lead to conflict. They may actually influence some members of the younger professional group having a less prestigious identification to pattern themselves after status groups. As a consequence, patients' needs may not always be met.

SUBROLES

In the role relationship the nurse may relate with the patient through subroles that are therapeutically affective for the individual. Six subroles have been identified in connection with nursing role activities. Owing to the multiplicity of patient needs, there may be a merging of one or more subroles as the nurse performs activities which necessitates their joint implementation.

MOTHER

Mothering is a subrole that is closely linked to the fundamental concept of the nurse as a person who nurtures and assists in restoring individuals to health. Nursing activities that may be carried out by the nurse as a mother figure include bathing, feeding, dressing, reassuring, soothing, and comforting the patient. Mothering activities are considered to be natural approaches which provide the opportunity for the nurse to establish relationships and communicate with patients. The nurse will, however, discover that some patients have a greater need for mothering activities and attentions than do others. This will depend upon the degree to which mothering relationships were experienced and found to be satisfactory during earlier life periods of existence. Mothering approaches convey acceptance, warmth, closeness, tenderness and protection. Skillful practice of the mothering relationship is dependent upon the nurse's ability to recognize those patients who may need and welcome this type of relationship as well as those who have been "smothered" with mothering. The patient who has experienced excessive mothering would not appreciate or benefit from such a relationship as would the person who has suffered maternal deprivation.

TECHNICIAN

The skillful performance of technical activities requires that the nurse be as sensitive to the emotional reactions and needs of the individual patient as to the scientific principles underlying their acceptable practice. Giving a bed bath, serving food or other nutrients, and administering various types of medications and treatments are activities associated with the technician subrole. The performance of these procedures requires attention to accuracy, economy of effort, and material supplies as well as to efficient performance insuring safety to the patient. Attributes and attitudes inherent in other role activities may be shown as the technical activity is initiated and carried out to achieve certain anticipated therapeutic results.

TEACHER

It is said that every nurse is a teacher. The teaching function may or may not require an initial, specific approach. Observation of many performances of the nurse would reveal that teaching is often automatically integrated as the nurse carries out other role activities, such as those of the technician and counselor. Teaching may be practiced as the nurse communicates knowledge which may be helpful to the patient. The patient may make an unexpected inquiry to which the nurse responds with health information. Teaching may also be implemented through example-setting by the nurse. The nurse's tone of voice or an attitude shown may be an activity associated with teaching. The nurse's behavior, in such an instance, may be influential in motivating a favorable change in the patient's behavior. When the nurse orients the patient to the ward environment she is implementing the teaching function. Teaching, on other occasions may be planned. For instance, the nurse may teach a patient how and when to take a medication. In mental health facilities, nurses often teach patients how to play various games and to participate in recreational and social activities. There are many instances, undoubtedly, when nurses teach without being aware that what they are doing actually constitutes teaching. Information conveyed or behavior shown by the nurse may be teaching which results in learning for the patient. It is difficult to measure how much teaching is done in the nurse-patient relationship. We can speculate, however, that much more is done than is ever identified as such.

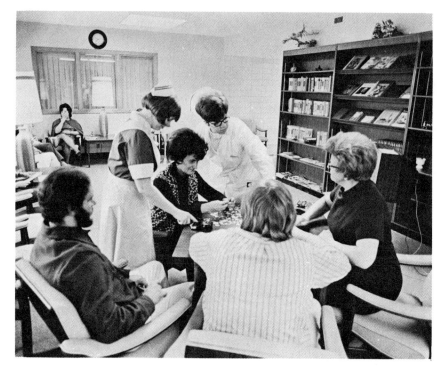

Fig. 2. Socializing in the living room. (Courtesy of Swedish-American Hospital, Rockford, Ill.)

SOCIALIZING AGENT

This is a very important subrole, the practice of which is encouraged in nursing mentally ill patients. It may be practiced when the nurse is caring for patients afflicted with illnesses other than mental ones. Through socializing activities implemented, as well as sometimes participated in, by the nurse, patients divert the focus of their often distressing, anxiety-producing thoughts. Social activities serve as energy and anxiety releasing outlets. The socializing function may be a very active or a passive nursing performance. The active socializing function is obvious as the nurse converses with patients or engages in activities with them. The nurse who sits beside the uncommunicative patient, however, is often as therapeutic a socializing agent as is the nurse who implements the more obviously active socializing relationships.

COUNSELOR

This subrole involves a psychotherapeutic relationship in which special attention is paid to the communications exchanged between the patient and nurse. The nurse as a counselor must be adept in recognizing and interpreting verbal as well as nonverbal communications. The skillful implementation of counseling requires that the nurse develop a degree of self-awareness of her own behavior and its effect upon the patient's behavior. Therapeutic counseling is dependent upon the nurse's ability to discover elements of disturbance in the patient's relationships with others and to respond with approaches which do not threaten the individual. Underlying the art of counseling are principles which, when utilized in approaches, can result in helping patients to resolve distressing problems. Listening to the patient is important, but the quality of listening is more important. Thus, the nurse counselor listens as well as observes the patient's manifestations of communications. Counseling also requires that the nurse have ability to utilize interviewing techniques which help the patient to verbalize with clarity as well as to express associated feelings. The skillful counselor knows how to help the patient to focus upon a topic, to accept feelings shown by the individual, and to delay or withhold nursing responses until their release is therapeutic for the patient. The nurse recognizes anxiety, can help the patient to release it, learn to identify its relationship to its producer, and to devise ways to cope with it so that therapeutic effects are achieved.

MANAGER

The implementation of management subrole activities involves manipulation of the patient's environment to the degree that it favors the patient's recovery. Technical functions may be merged with the managerial ones as the nurse carries on activities concerned with the care of the ward as well as the patient's personal property. Attention may be given to such concerns as housekeeping, appearance of the physical environment, preparation of food, need for repairs, purchasing of supplies, and care of patient's clothing and personal possessions. Managing requires an ability to survey needs, to organize, to record, to plan for and evaluate patient care in relation to needs, and to delegate responsibility, when indicated, to other personnel.

SUGGESTED REFERENCES

Brown, E.: Nursing Reconsidered—a Study of Change. J. B. Lippincott Co., Philadelphia, 1971, p. 285.

Coe, W., Curry, A., and Huels, M.: A method of group therapy training for nurses in psychiatric hospitals. Perspect. Psychiat. Care 5: 231 (5), 1967.

Crown, N.: The multifaceted role of the community mental health nurse. J. Psychiat. Nurs. 9: (May-Jun.), 1971.

DePaul, A.: The nurse as a central figure in a mental health center. Perspect. Psychiat. Care 6: 17 (Jan.-Feb.), 1968.

Donelson, L.: The nurse as a sanctioned representative of the healing arts. Perspect. Psychiat. Care 5: 214 (Sept.-Oct.), 1967.

Eddy, F., O'Neill, E., and Astrachan, B.: Group work on a long term psychiatric service. Perspect. Psychiat. Care 6: 9 (Jan.-Feb.), 1968.

Evans, F.: The Role of the Nurse in Community Mental Health. The MacMillan Co., New York, 1968.

Flynn, G.: The nurse's role: interference or intervention. Perspect. Psychiat. Care 7: 170 (Jul.-Aug.), 1969.

Holmes, M., and Werner, J.: Psychiatric Nursing in a Therapeutic Community. The Mac-Millan Co., New York, 1966.

Ledney, D.: Psychiatric nursing: breakthrough to independence. R.N. 34: 29 (Aug.), 1971.

Mistr, V.: Community nursing service for psychiatric patients. Perspect. Psychiat. Care 6: 37 (Jan.-Feb.), 1968.

Moore, M.: An account of a nurse's role and functions in an alcoholic treatment program. J. Psychiat. Nurs. 8: 21 (May-Jun.), 1970.

Ostendorf, M.: The public health nurses role in helping a family to cope with mental health problems. Perspect. Psychiat. Care 5: 208 (Sept.-Oct.), 1967.

Robinson, L.: Liaison psychiatric nursing, Perspect. Psychiat. Care 6: 87 (Mar.-Apr.), 1968.

Ruiz, R., Smith, C., and Harris, R.: An observed role model in psychiatric nursing. Perspect. Psychiat. Care 6: 70 (Mar.-Apr.), 1968.

Sheldon, A., and Hope, P.: The developing role of the nurse in a community mental health program. Perspect. Psychiat. Care 5: 272 (Nov.-Dec.), 1967.

Stockwell, M., and Nishikawa, H.: The third hand: a theory of support. J. Psychiat. Nurs. 8: 7 (May-Jun.), 1970.

FOOTNOTES

1. Brown, E.: Nursing Reconsidered—a Study of Change, vol. 2. J. B. Lippincott Co., Philadelphia, 1971, pp. 285, 313-314.
2. Lambertson, E.: Preparation of the Nurse Practitioner. Illinois Nurses' Association, March 1971, p. 71.

For reviewing this chapter, grateful acknowledgment is made to Miss Marilyn Miller, R.N., Mrs. Diane Sworm, R.N., Mrs. Jeanette Wade, R.N., and Mrs. Manolia Schult, R.N.

UNIT 3

The Influence of
Social Psychiatry

CHAPTER 7

Social Influences Related to
Mental Illness

There is an increasing recognition and interest in the relationship between the social influences of the patient's environment and mental illness. Various social, psychiatric aspects may be conceived of as possible, contributory, etiologic factors interwoven in the patient's personality development, affecting his pattern of behavior and reaction to conflict.

Contributory, etiologic influences may be discovered in the patient's history, especially in the data compiled by the hospital social service department staff, or during team conferences with members of allied disciplines. Clues to social factors may be detected through interpersonal relations with the patient, family members, or during visits to the individual's home. It is most unfortunate, however, that home visits by nurses and psychiatric social workers are frequently impossible, owing to the well-known shortage of trained staff in the majority of psychiatric hospitals. Therefore, the nurse will find it helpful to be aware of some of the possible contributory, social, psychiatric factors. Such knowledge will assist her in identifying and understanding the elements of environmental stress and strain which influence the patient's feelings, thinking and behavior, and which may be viewed in their totality as the individual's attempts to meet unsatisfied emotional needs. Having such knowledge will enable the nurse to give effective, emotional support to the patient and to aid in planning for care and the eventual rehabilitation of the person.

THE FAMILY ENVIRONMENT

It is said that the individual perceives and reacts toward society and its members as he perceives the influences in his family environment and responds to them.

As the basic unit of society and the primary source of mutual, emotional support, we conceive of the family as the institution for instilling and strengthening in the offspring desirable feelings of acceptance, belonging and security. Out of the family relationship grow the feeling responses observed in one's human relations. Whether or not desirable feeling reactions are acquired by the person depends to a large extent upon the stability of family relationships, the pattern of control and family attitudes.

FAMILY DISORGANIZATION

Stability in the home may be threatened by divorce, desertion, separation, illness, or death of a parent. A broken home may result in the placement of children in institutions, foster homes or the residence of relatives. Such changes alter the feeling tones experienced by the child and necessitate the need for adaptation and adjustment to a new environment with its attendant changes in family roles and relationships. Patients from broken homes often develop and go through life harboring feelings of rejection, emotional deprivation, inferiority and insecurity. These feelings may expand later into stronger responses of mistrust and hostility associated with a sense of abandonment. Owing to a lack of mutual emotional support, their self-esteem and self-confidence are often reduced whenever new challenges or changes present themselves.

Persons reared in broken homes may experience difficulty in relating to other individuals and engaging in normal social activities. Some submit passively, accepting their lot outwardly, but often carrying within them intense feelings of bitterness which they are unable to verbalize. Their pattern of reaction is to withdraw from human contacts to an isolated or removed type of existence where social distance protects them from further psychic trauma.

Other persons may react to a broken home in an openly hostile manner, resisting any form of control and manifesting a chronic, defensive reaction pattern toward others. Children of divorced or separated parents often will express feelings of hatred, abandonment and resentment toward their parents. They may be unable to maintain satisfactory marital relationships and stable family environments of their own.

FAMILY CONTROL PATTERN

The pattern of family control appears to influence the individual's feeling responses, patterns of reacting to conflict, and social disorganization.

A mutual, supportive pattern of family control with parents in complete agreement and support of each other's actions is desirable because it contributes to consistency, feelings of confidence, security, and effective interpersonal relationships. Emotional warmth in such a pattern of control is a positive influence upon the maintenance of mental health. There is, however, a passive type of mutual support pattern which is quiet and lacking in emotional warmth which produces a cold, unfeeling response in the child.

The *authoritarian* pattern of control is one in which a parent dominates other family members. Quite often the father is observed to be the dominant figure, although some mothers do assume the authoritarian family influence role. This pattern of control is observed more commonly in European and some Oriental cultures but has exerted its influence upon the American scene.

The authoritarian figure is considered to be a basically insecure person who attempts to meet his security need by projecting his feelings of insecurity upon others through the exercise of authority. In some instances this pattern of control reaches the point of excessive, selfish demands and cruelty visited upon the offspring. The other parent (usually the mother) remains submissive toward the spouse in a martyr-like manner, but is gentle and protecting toward the children. Children reared in this type of family environment withhold their intense feelings of fear and hostility, while inwardly resenting submission to authority. They frequently perceive the gentle parent's submissive response as a weakness which they associate with all women and often come to develop strong feelings of contempt towards women in general. These individuals grow into adulthood harboring feelings of mistrust and of being threatened in peer relationships. They resist all authority figures. Unfortunately, it has been observed by some investigators that the authoritarian family pattern of control is acquired and often perpetuated from generation to generation.

An *ambivalent, protective* pattern of control may be observed in some family environments. Authorities have described one parent, often the mother, as being immature, worrisome and neurotic in character. Such an individual cannot bear emotionally to observe even the most minor slight, deprivation or obstacle placed in the child's path. Criticism of the child is painful. Everything must be sacrificed or changed, if necessary, to gratify the offspring's wishes and needs. An acceptable explanation is always rationalized for the child's actions and never is there an attempt on the one parent's part to teach Junior to withhold gratification, assume responsibility, or solve conflict. When the other parent attempts to place some curbs upon the child's behavior and desires, the overprotective parent proceeds to cross these restrictions, thus shutting out reality. As a result, the child fails to recognize and learn how to solve the inevitable frustrations of life or to develop self-confidence and independence. He conceives of himself as helpless. The ambivalence of the parental relationship contributes to the individual's development of a wavering sense of insecurity. Later in life, these persons may react to disappointment and responsibility with fear, withdrawn behavior, neurotic traits, and a strong need for dependency.

There is another type of ambivalent, protective pattern of control wherein the child plays one parent against the other, seeking from one what he cannot attain from the other, and always experiencing satisfaction of the pleasure principle. These children are often found in middle-class families and constitute a group manifesting delinquent behavior.

The *overly permissive* pattern of control observed, but not acceptable according to the mores of our own culture, may develop from what might be considered a gross neglect of the family environment. Parents may be employed outside of the home or indulge frequently in entertainment and social recreation, while failing to provide a normal family atmosphere and relationship. In some instances, there is an obvious lack of mutual respect between parents, a disregard for the child's needs of affection and companionship, and disrespect for society and its behavior codes. Open, illicit relationships and low moral standards may prevail in the home. Thus, the child perceives a genuine lack of concern for social inhibitions and other human beings. A person reared in such a family environment may come to perceive of society as a cold, unfeeling, hostile world. Lacking in inhibitions, these individuals frequently lash out at society, manifesting maladjusted or delinquent behavior which constitutes a real source of concern to the social order. Their behavior knows no bounds for they are lacking in inner controls. They have strong needs for acceptance, affection and security.

In the *multiple pattern* of family control, sometimes observed in institutions or in a family environment where many persons or members of more than one family reside together, the child may be subjected to the attentions of several persons who minister unto his needs. Social contacts are brief and rare. Investigators suggest that such a child may fail to develop a warm feeling relationship toward any one specific mothering or mother substitute figure in the earliest primary relationship. Another hypothesis is that the infant is subjected to the close social acts of ministering adults, who are predominantly opposed in their actions toward the child. The child might experience both types of these early relationships at once. These persons develop a social behavior to the extent that they never experience the normal feeling responses or obligations toward other human beings. They do not conceive of other individuals as being endowed with a reservoir of human needs, feelings, and a sensitivity toward the behavior of others. Never experiencing early, sustained human warmth and love, these persons cannot give in return what they have failed to receive. They become self-centered, pleasure seeking, selfish, and are often the cause of much human distress and social violations. Rash promises are made only to be broken without concern for the possible consequences. Their behavior is considered sociopathic.

FAMILY PLACEMENT AND ROLES

The placement and role of the person in the family constellation may affect his feeling responses, self conception and pattern of behavior. It would seem reasonable to conclude, however, that additional social influences such as illness, economic status, education of the parents, and parents' attitudes toward rearing children and the size of the family would affect the attitudes expressed towards family placement and roles. In fact, roles might be changed with certain crucial events, such as illness or death, and such changes do have their accompanying feeling responses.

Dependent upon the cultural concept of family placement, an oldest child might be regarded as the subsequent head of the family and/or entitled to certain privileges, such as inheritance rights. In another family environment, the oldest child might be given unusual responsibilities for helping to care for younger children or to support the family. An oldest child might be given continual and undue affection in one family, while in another he might actually come to experience emotional deprivation.

The youngest child might be looked upon as helpless and be pampered and given affection to a considerable degree from both parents and other children. Social participation with peer family members may be denied to the youngest child, so that family placement may determine the degree of socialization. For particular reasons associated with the individual's family placement, a person might be envied, rejected or pitied. Both the oldest and youngest sibling, while possibly enjoying family placement status under certain conditions, may manifest obvious hostile feelings under other circumstances. Therefore, the interpretation placed upon family placement and the attitudes expressed toward it may initiate certain feeling tones and behavior patterns.

In addition to the oldest and youngest, there may be a number of roles assigned to members of a family constellation. The handsomest, dullest, most artistic or musical, friendliest, sickliest, favorite, most intelligent child, etc., are often identified. These roles affect expressed attitudes from others. Thus, the person develops a self concept as he perceives himself through the eyes and emotions of others. This self concept, in turn, affects the individual's reactions towards others and may determine his success or failure in interpersonal relations. A person's family role may actually lead to the selection of a career. If the role has been emphasized, the child may overreach beyond his ability, with subsequent effects upon his mental health. Family roles may also initiate sibling rivalry, the effects of which are often serious and emotionally disturbing.

Some investigators of family structures describe the entire family as a total field of emotional forces with which the patient interacts. The larger the family, the more complex the interaction system. These forces may include, beside the parent-child and sibling relationships, grandparents and other close living relatives and persons. Each one relates individualistically to the patient, affecting his identifications, emotional responses, personality development and ability to resolve conflict. Some common as well as different factors may be observed in each of the patterns of interaction making up the various systems of relationships. Thus, the family emotional structure constitutes a cross current of interpersonal relationships. The patient is exposed to the differing, sometimes contradictory mores of parents, grandparents, and others, all of whom may have been raised in different cultural settings. There are differences in the family systems comparable to that of individual cultures. This concept of the broader, all-inclusive family emotional structure and complexity of the interaction systems makes it desirable to know and consider the entire field of family forces instead of just the immediate family-patient relationships in working through problems during analysis. It is helpful for the nurse to be aware of this phenomenon in evaluating the patient's possible identifications and various types of relationships with each of several personnel.

FAMILY HEALTH ENVIRONMENT

The family health environment includes the physical and mental social influences. Socioeconomic conditions may determine the location of the home, the sanitary conditions, and provisions for heat, ventilation, sunlight, comfort, space and other physical aspects, the inadequacy of which may contribute to the development of mental illness. In other instances, there is a deliberate curtailment of expenditures which amounts to frugality with imposed deprivations in the family health environment.

Crowded living arrangements may be emotionally distressing and disturbing and deny the certain amount of quiet required at some time or other by the average human being. Pressures of close interactions between family members may initiate many negative feelings and patterns of behavior. Children may take to the streets and other locations to excape hostile relations and the negative social influences of their daily existence.

An impoverished family health environment may lead to feelings of deprivation, low self-esteem, inferiority, reactions of hostility toward the more privileged groups, and, sometimes, expansive delusions of persecution by society. A distorted sense of loyalty may be developed and extended toward individuals who can supply the material needs and emotional support of an adequate family health environment. That environment may even determine the extent to which the person may be accepted socially.

In other homes the family environment may be materialistically comfortable, even luxurious in some instances, but a negative emotional atmosphere growing out of the many aspects of the family's existence may adversely affect the mental health of individuals.

FAMILY ATTITUDES

Attitudes may be as cultural as they are personal. Constituting an integral part of one's personality, attitudes determine largely the individual's ability to adapt and adjust to changes in the social environment.

The individual develops attitudes as he perceives them in his environment. Family attitudes may cast lasting reflections which often play a part in the patient's regression during illness or therapeutic recovery. As the person widens his social range, his attitudes may be reinforced or changed, dependent upon circumstances of cultural lag and change.

The family attitude towards the acceptance of mental illness may be culturally determined. It is important for the nurse to appreciate that, unless there is recognition and understanding of this fact, the patient's recovery may be seriously affected. Some families consider mental illness to be an indication that there is an unhealthy hereditary structure in the family which constitutes a threat to the group's integrity. Others may conceive of mental disorder as retribution for sin and may actually come to feel guilty in viewing their relationships with the patient as an etiologic factor. Visiting the mentally ill, therefore, may be emotionally traumatizing to some family members, as well as to the patients who are often unusually sensitive to the family's reactions.

In some closely knit societies, it is obvious that the entire family group becomes emotionally concerned when a member becomes ill. Separation is difficult, and nursing personnel may discover that several members of one family may accompany a patient to the hospital or come to visit in larger numbers than are ordinarily permitted. Group support may be the most potent therapeutic force for some individuals when they are ill. Sometimes the only way to get the patient's cooperation in treatment is to recognize his need for the presence and emotional support of the family.

Eaton and Weil, who studied the effects of modern civilization upon the incidence of, and treatment approaches to, mental disorders in a religious sect known as the Hutterites, living a four-hundred-year-old type of communal existence in the American and Canadian West, point out the positive effects of emotional support from the group during illness.

Certain behavior was viewed as emotionally disturbing according to the group's interpretation and evaluation of behavior symptoms; this obviously affected the treatment and rehabilitation approach. Persons who were considered to be mentally ill often received emotional support from the entire community as well as from the family. In one instance, a schizophrenic patient was helped to maintain his much needed social distance with the provision of separate quarters. Food was brought to him by his sister. The patient was allowed to go to and from his residence as he chose. In another instance, five sons took turns sleeping with their senile father who expressed great fear of being alone. Sympathy was extended toward the depressed, defective, and epileptic. In contrast, a small group of persons who demonstrated certain psychotic traits, such as delusions, aggression, resistance, profanity, and symptoms of personality disorders, were excommunicated from the colony because of the inability of the group to distinguish mental illness from asocial behavior. Neurotic individuals were approached, either through humor or admonitions, to recognize their complaints as chiefly imaginary. If these approaches failed, the patient's inadequacy and need for dependency were recognized and respected. There was no change in attitudes toward individuals who had recovered from mental illness, and job opportunities were available as previously. The Hutterite attitude toward recovery was optimistic, even though the investigators recognized that many of this group conceived of mental illness as retribution for sin. These people believed strongly that through religious faith the mentally ill could overcome their temptations and subsequently be free of illness. In most instances, group support made it unnecessary to hospitalize the emotionally disturbed.[1]

In some family environments, a pathological attitude toward physical illness may be reinforced when a member who is actually in good health is conceived of, and related to, as being sickly, weak, or in need of special attention.

Parental attitudes toward increased social experiences may limit the adolescent's range of social interaction. Conflicts of emancipation and heterosexual relationships may have their roots in such attitudes. When investigated, these situations are sometimes found to be imposed through a parent's fears, lack of self-confidence to assume responsibility for the adolescent's increasing social experience, or a need to be protective. There are also parents who have deep, unconscious needs to have their children continue dependence upon them.

Family attitudes toward religious practices, such as prayer, the marriage ceremony and implications of the vows, divorce, confession, birth control, and other requirements of one's religion, may create serious conflicts leading to guilt feelings and emotional disturbance.

Stress, strain and mental conflict are often related to the influence of one's attitude toward the family social status. Feelings of superiority or inferiority may affect the person's ability to relate successfully to others. Attempts at mobility into a higher social stratum may present traumatizing events. One's attitude toward the family's social status may initiate certain social inhibitions and even limit the range of community interaction.

Attitudes toward education may be culturally determined. In some cultures, a higher education is considered more important for men than for women because of men's anticipated role as head of the family. Women are thought of as homemakers, primarily. Americans place a high value upon education. Laws have been enacted to insure the education of citizens until a legally determined, chronological age has been reached. The family attitude toward education may provide the impetus which forces a person toward higher education, regardless of his innate capacities or desires. In other instances, a low value placed upon education or economic circumstances may curtail education at an early age. It is not uncommon to discover that persons experience conflicts over education. Some have known the stress and strain of struggling to comply with the family's demands and expectations for higher education. Others have felt intellectually deprived and cheated.

Social values are attached to occupations according to the individual's personal values. Some may value monetary gains; others may seek the social status and prestige of a vocation. Also, there are certain index (favored, superior) roles within vocational institutions. For instance, the president of a bank occupies an index role in his organization. Pressure on the individual to enter an occupation from family attitudes may precipitate mental illness. In addition, there are parents who unconsciously attempt to soothe their own feelings of deprivation by forcing the offspring into higher education or a career which was unobtainable by the parent. Thus, the individual is often made to live out the unfilled life goals of the parent, instead of following his own inclinations.

Cultural attitudes towards foods may create psychic distress, sometimes to an extreme degree. In India, the cow is considered sacred, and this belief automatically excludes the possibility of beef and milk in the diet. From the time of Moses, the great sanitarian who led the Jews out of Egypt, pork has been banned from the Hebrew diet as unclean. In some cultures, fried caterpillar grubs, chocolate covered grasshoppers and beetles are considered delicacies. Such foods and others have been eaten with obvious enjoyment by persons who later, upon being informed of the true identity of the food became violently ill. Many individuals are culturally conditioned toward foods and find it most difficult to adapt readily to hospital diets.

Certain behavioral attitudes may be considered normal in one culture but abnormal in another. For instance, suspicious behavior is thought of as a paranoid trend in our culture, while in some primitive cultures the group members are trained from childhood to protect themselves by always viewing the actions of others with suspicion.

An Ozark man received a revelation from God and a call to preach it to his neighbors. After gaining considerable acceptance and success in his own and neighboring communities, he responded to a request to preach in the city. Shortly after arriving in St. Louis he was arrested for preaching on the streets during the rush hour. Subsequently a psychiatrist made the diagnosis of paranoid schizophrenia.

Suicide is considered honorable as well as the behavior of a martyr in some cultures. In others it is viewed as sinful, unlawful and the act of a coward.

Investigators believe there is a relationship between culture and inhibited drives. Some authorities mention the repression of sexual drives in the middle-class subsociety of western culture. Others report that among some Indian tribes social aggression and opposition are forbidden, while group solidarity and cooperation are stressed. Observations have been reported on the deviant behavior which has apparently erupted when the individual was unable to channel constructively these repressed drives.

Cultural attitudes may reinforce the use of specific defense mechanisms for resolving conflict. Suppression and repression may be more commonly practiced in some cultures. Persons who reveal fear and guilt as a result of sexual indiscretions and feelings of hatred toward close relatives are sometimes advised to forget about such behavior. In other cultures, the individual would be encouraged to verbalize freely to someone, or to a group, so that, through the mechanism of projection, guilt feelings would be relieved. In still another culture, the person might be advised to confess and perform some act of atonement to utilize the mechanism of undoing.

SOCIAL CLASS DIFFERENCES

Some investigators support the hypothesis that variations in the practices of rearing children in the lower, middle and upper classes of society affect personality development and mental health. Specific differences observed are concerned with the patterns of feeding, training, rewarding and punishing, as well as the methods of extending and withholding affection. In addition, there are variations in the patterns of reaction to impulsive, aggressive, and other unacceptable behavior of the growing child. Breast feeding is more common among the lower class and may continue beyond the twelfth month. Weaning and toilet training are commenced earlier among middle-class children. There is a closer father-child relationship among the middle class, involving sharing of educational and recreational activities. Lower-class children are expected to leave school earlier in order to go to work. Middle-class boys and girls are expected to help with certain household chores and the care of younger children in the family, at an earlier age.

There are differences in the social classes in types of interactions between family members and the performance of roles. Mutual support given to individual member's needs and wants, as well as reactions toward such life crises as illness, incapacitation, and death, are obviously different in each of the social classes.

It has been observed that with the aging process, persons in different social classes vary in their behavioral standards, life values and goal expectations. There is also a difference in their concepts of the definitions applied to these aspects of living and the kinds of examples presented to them as models.

EPIDEMIOLOGICAL INDICATIONS

Studies have indicated that the highest rate of mental illness is found in the lower class. Opportunities and finances for adequate psychiatric treatment are the poorest in the lower class. There is considerable evidence to the effect that a higher incidence of psychoneurotic conditions exists in the upper strata of society in contrast with a prevalence of psychotic disorders in the lower classes. Social class appears to determine the type of treatment the patient receives. More persons in the higher strata of society seek psychiatric treatment; many of these individuals receive psychotherapy. Mentally ill persons in the lower class may fail to receive medical assistance. Some may lack insight into the existence of a mental disorder. Others may be unable to pay for competent psychiatric treatment, or they remain ignorant of available community mental health facilities. Members of the lower classes who do consult a physician often receive somatic therapy. This may be owing to their lack of finances or the inability to spend a longer period of time in treatment as is usually required with psychotherapy. Additional financial hardships might be created.

Passamanick and others who studied infant growth concluded that there are positive and probably etiologic relationships between low socioeconomic status and prenatal and paranatal abnormalities which may serve as precusors to retarded behavior and certain neuropsychiatric disorders of childhood, such as cerebral palsy, epilepsy, mental deficiency, and behavior disorder.[2]

The importance of the above conclusions is in the trends developing in the area of prevention and in influencing society to make more preventive and therapeutic services available to the general public. These studies also indicate the need for the nurse to be able to identify the symptoms of mental illness in the community and to have a knowledge of available community resources.

The prevalence of certain mental disorders in particular social environments has also been studied. There appear to be more persons afflicted with schizophrenia living in heavily populated, central areas of large cities. It is thought that this excess is due to the schizoid individual's tendency to avoid close personal relations by moving away from his family to the lodging-house area. Many of the individuals studied were unmarried and had difficulties in their family relationships. It was also observed that there was considerable movement of these persons from one residence in the area to another.[3]

Eaton and Weil reported an exceedingly small percentage of mental disorder due to organic conditions in their epidemiological survey of the Hutterites. In this culture, older people enjoy a high prestige in the community, and there is protection from exposure to drugs and unlimited amounts of alcohol and from syphilis. These factors are considered as possibly prophylactic. There was, however, a youthful character about the poupulation, which the investigators recognized in pointing out that many organic psychoses are conditions of middle and old age.[1]

SEGREGATION

Segregation perpetuates social distance. Two types of segregation, legal and tacit, are recognized as social restraints which may incite intense feeling reactions leading to severe personal, emotional stress, and strain in the environment. It has been said that tacit segregation practices, such as are carried out in the northern states, are oftentimes more damaging to the personality than was legal segregation. Legal segregation sets for the individual definite social limits which are unambiguous and consistent. It is claimed that the southern Negro was able to structure social reality with less inner anxiety than the northern Negro. By contrast, the unwritten, undefined, subtle practices of social segregation one may find in the North produce fresh anxiety in many situations.

Community organizations, sororities, fraternities and social cliques may initiate some very emotionally traumatizing situations for the individual who is rejected from membership. Thus, social distance is maintained subtly.

Problems may be created when an individual fails to be "rushed" during sorority week. Students may actually fear "rush" week. There may be increasing psychic stress as other friends are accepted into sororities of their choice. There are also occasions when some students are not invited to join, and membership may be available to them only in certain less-desired groups on the campus. Such situations may produce greater personal emotional impact than is realized by most people. There have been instances when students' parents have stressed the importance of preference for a particular group. When a student fails to gain an invitation from this group, the emotional reactions may be severe.

SOCIAL CHANGE

Various types of social change may create stress and strain in the environment which leads to obviously abnormal behavior.

Cultural concepts, attitudes and restrictions appear to influence the mental health of the aged. Many capable individuals are forced to retire at the age of sixty-five years. There is an increasing recognition that the American culture, with its concept of youth and vigor as typical of the nation, fails to provide enough satisfying roles and leisure-time activities for elderly persons.

Medical discoveries leading to the cure of many formerly fatal illnesses have resulted in an increase in the life expectancy of human beings. With few opportunities available to the aged in most communities for social contacts, productivity and recreation, many elderly people have developed feelings of loneliness, uselessness and rejection. Our mental institutions care for a large number of senile persons who have deteriorated sufficiently to require medical and nursing care.

Social Security and Old Age Assistance laws have been enacted to help provide financially for this group. The great need, however, is for more adequate social planning which will prevent mental deterioration. Some provisions for new types of housing, foster home care, and social recreation centers have been developed to help solve the problems of old age (see p. 386). Several authorities have written and talked about the desirability of abandoning compulsory retirement. There are many difficulties, however, associated with accomplishing this action. Chiefly, organizations providing workmen's compensation plans still consider the aged as an occupational risk.

Psychic stress may develop during the process of assimilation when there is a merging of cultures. Some aspects of a culture may be abandoned, new ones adopted, and others blended. Voluntary immigrants are usually hopeful and enthusiastic to commence a new life. For these persons, adaptation and adjustment to the environment is not particularly difficult. Displaced persons and prisoners of war, however, often feel under considerable stress. They may manifest anxiety and other defense reactions, dependent upon the individual's former personality and degree of adjustment. Depression, psychosomatic complaints, and paranoid trends, without disorganization of the personality, may be observed. These reactions are motivated by dissociation from one's former environment, relatives and language. Poverty of finances and other personal resources contribute to the displaced person's need for dependence upon individuals who are often of short acquaintance. A sense of degradation, frustration, and fear of some vaguely defined, overwhelming situation is experienced. Fear and hostility may be projected onto those in the environment, through complaints about housing, climate, food, and differences in the manners, customs, and mores of the people. Some displaced persons sense a resistance toward them by individuals in the new culture who appear to give evidence that they anticipate competition and the possibility of losing a job to an immigrant. Prisoners of war may develop ideas of reference, mistrust, and suspicion toward others. They may become aggressive and project persecutory ideas. It is believed that their inability to speak, or understand readily, the new language may be a causative factor in the production of the behavior observed. Many of these individuals improve when returned to the security of their former environments.

War creates social change and may precipitate severe emotional disturbances. Young men in our culture were not prepared, formerly, for military assignment and often found it difficult to adjust to the quick necessity of a military career. This was especially true when World War II commenced. According to reports, about two million Americans were found to be mentally unsuited for military service. Some men found it difficult to adjust to the rigors and demands of army life. Many of these young persons experienced psychic distress when it became necessary to learn to kill in self-defense. The thought of military encounter and the sound of bombs bursting in the distance frequently precipitated an emotional disorder before the individual was involved in actual combat. A number of men who participated actively in the service developed mental illness following some emotionally distressing incident.

War creates many changes in the civilian population, including separation and changes in family roles. Women work outside of the home, and children are left in the part-time care of other persons. Many older children in the teenage group are frequently without adequate supervision in the home and made to rely upon their own personal resources. There was considerable increase in juvenile delinquency following World War II, which increase many authorities attributed partly to the changes in family roles. Rumors also have a way of getting started and spread among the civilian population. Unless people in general are kept well informed, they may become emotional victims of rumors producing fear and anxiety. When the conqueror assumes control of new territory, cultural change is often accelerated, but not completely without emotional distress for some individuals.

New inventions and discoveries may also influence the development of emotional disturbance. Mechanical inventions which replace manpower frequently produce feelings of insecurity. Labor leaders have suggested a shorter work week as a solution to unemployment. This proposal, in turn, creates the need for social planning which will help the individual to utilize his leisure time constructively; it is recognized that too much leisure can be unhealthful for the emotions.

Gunpowder, cannons, bombs, airplanes and other inventions of warfare have created, in their time, tremendous fear in persons. Eventually, counterweapons or methods have proved to be effective in preserving mankind. To cite a more recent incident involving mass and individual reactions to new inventions, one might refer to the launching of the Russian satellite. The entire world appeared to react emotionally to this event with fears of annihilation. In one midwestern city, newspapers carried an account of a woman who believed she was personally affected. She complained of receiving the satellite's signals through her metal hair curlers and was obviously disturbed emotionally.

PHYSICAL SOCIAL HANDICAPS

Congenital and acquired physical defects such as harelip, cleft palate, facial birthmarks, scoliosis, clubfoot, strabismus, saddle nose and other deformities may contribute to the development of mental illness. During childhood some very traumatizing incidents may occur. Playmates are often naturally curious, attracted to the peculiar and different, socially uninhibited, and lacking in understanding of human beings and their sensitivities. Ridicule, taunting, and name-calling related to the particular physical handicap may inflict serious psychological damage upon a child's personality.

Increasing sensitivity and feelings of rejection may lead to the development of overcompensatory behavior in attempts to divert attention from the defect and overcome the tendency of associates to conceive of the person as abnormal and undesirable. Being forced into an inferior social position may produce feelings of frustration and despair. Some individuals with physical handicaps accept the negative reactions of others and withdraw from social contacts. Some develop hostile behavior and paranoid trends. Blaming other persons for failure may develop to such a serious degree that the physically handicapped individual may be the victim of poor adjustment to friends, occupation, and marriage. Owing to lack of acceptance, some of these persons have become extremely frustrated and resorted to criminal activities.

CULTURAL CONFLICTS

Some persons believe that conflicts within the culture may possibly become conflicts within the individual. For instance, the child is expected to conform and also develop independence. We glorify the Golden Rule, but at the same time encourage competition and say, "All is fair in love and war." We praise initiative but view aggression with concern. But the question may well be asked, can initiative be achieved without some element of aggression in the personality? We believe in self-expression, but also stress the importance of group conformity for acceptance of the person. It is not too difficult to understand, from some of the above examples, how an individual may become ambivalent, indecisive, withdrawn, lacking in self-confidence, or hostile toward others.

SOCIAL STRUCTURE OF HOSPITAL

There are many negative social influences in our mental hospitals, primarily in our larger, older institutions. They are a product of the industrial revolution and patterned upon the same expansion principles used by industry of that period. Although some colonial physicians cautioned against enlarging hospitals and recommended that smaller institutions would provide better care for the mentally ill, they were unable to receive support for their opinions. As admissions to mental hospitals increased, more buildings and wards were placed under the supervision and responsibility of one superintendent. In spite of changes that have been made to reduce patient population, we still have psychiatric hospitals that house 1,000 to 2,000 patients. Some wards domicile large groups of patients under the same roof. Overcrowding has limited the freedom of movement so necessary for patient expression and comfort.

Shortage of all categories of personnel, especially professional and well-trained groups, has made it impossible to give individualized, understanding attention and care to the sick. The person admitted to this type of social environment soon loses his personal identity among a large group. Personnel are so busy that some patients may not be able to communicate readily with any member of the staff. Thus, the morale of the environment may be low. Studies sponsored by the Russell Sage Foundation pointed out the negative social influences in the traditional mental hospital environment and its effects upon both personnel and patients.[4,5]

Experiments are described demonstrating the positive results in patient improvement when changes were introduced into the ward environment. All staff members were trained to function and participate more intimately with patients as social therapists. The team approach was utilized in planning and giving care. Individualized attention, interpretation of the patient's behavior and needs, and socialization of the patient were stressed as important fundamentals. As a result, it became recognized that the social structure of the majority of our older psychiatric institutions was a real detriment to the improvement of patient care.

NURSE'S SOCIAL ATTITUDE

The nurse's social attitude is of importance to the progress and development of improved care for the mentally ill. To be helpful, the nurse must be a student of the humanities who possesses a keen sensitivity to the feelings of others. She must be able to visualize the totality of the patient's environment, viewing with understanding the background of the home, school, occupation, and all of the other social influences in the community which are related to the development of the patient's illness. A social consciousness developed through the identification and understanding of the entire constellation of influences can help the nurse to give emotional support to the patient which is the most important aspect of all nursing care.

SUGGESTED REFERENCES

Backscheider, J.: The influence of sociocultural factors in the mentally ill patient. Perspect. Psychiat. Care 3: 12, 1965.

Brockbank, R., and Gibson, D.: Mental Health in a Changing Community. Grune & Stratton, New York, 1966, p. 34.

Cumming, J., and Cumming, E.: Ego and Millieu. Atherton Press, New York, 1962, p. 89.

Freedman, A., and Kaplan, H. (eds.): Comprehensive Textbook of Psychiatry. Williams & Wilkins Co., Baltimore, 1967, p. 201.

Hayes, W., and Gazaway, R.: Human Relations in Nursing. W. B. Saunders Co., Philadelphia, 1964.

Hollingshead, A. B., and Redlich, F.: Social Class and Mental Illness. John Wiley & Sons, New York, 1958.

Jackson, J.: The role of the patient's family in illness. Nurs. Forum 1: 118 (Summer), 1962.

King, S.: Perceptions of Illness and Medical Care. Russell Sage Foundation, New York, 1962.

Miller, W.: A study in family dynamics. Perspect. Psychiat. Care 2: 9 (Mar.-Apr.), 1963.

Murphy, G.: Social psychology in The American Handbook of Psychiatry, Vol. II. Basic Books, Inc., New York, 1959, p. 1733.

Watts, W.: Social class, ethnic background and patient care. Nurs. Forum 6: 155 (Spring), 1967.

FOOTNOTES

1. Eaton, J., and Weil, R.: Culture and Mental Disorders. The Free Press, Glencoe, Ill., 1953, pp. 108, 163.
2. Passamanick, B., Knobloch, H., et al.: Socioeconomic status and some precursors of neuropsychiatric disorder. Am. J. Orthopsychiat. 26: 594 (July), 1956.
3. Hare, E.: Family setting and the urban distribution of schizophrenia. J. Ment. Sc. 102: 753 (Oct.), 1956.
4. Greenblatt, M., York, R., and Brown, L.: From Custodial to Therapeutic Patient Care in Mental Hospitals. Russell Sage Foundation, New York, 1955.
5. Von Mering, O., and King, S.: Remotivating the Mental Patient. Russell Sage Foundation, New York, 1957.

CHAPTER **8**

Nursing in Community Mental Health Centers

The community mental health center was the logical development of the observation that mentally ill patients should have treatment and care available in close proximity to their residential communities. This is a new type of facility where people with emotional problems can get comprehensive and continuing treatment in their own communities. Although many general hospitals had established psychiatric wards in their institutions, these facilities could not provide the more extensive types of psychiatric services that were envisioned to launch a full scale community psychiatric approach. Those persons who believed in and promoted the concept of community psychiatry were convinced that the sources of deviant behavior lie in the environment and in disturbed interactional processes. In accordance with this viewpoint, they believed that we have the knowledge to correct mental disturbances and that the way to extend these insights is through a diversified community approach.

DEVELOPMENT OF MENTAL HEALTH CENTERS

The late President John F. Kennedy's message to Congress in 1963 is credited for having led to the development and growth of community mental health centers. In July 1969, 185 of the 376 centers provided for in legislative actions were in operation. It is expected that there will be 2,000 community mental health centers by the year 1980.[1] This indicates that the trend is definitely away from the large state operated mental hospital.

FINANCES AND SERVICES

The centers are financed in proportionate amounts by federal, state, and community funds. To qualify for financial assistance, they must provide five essential services: (1) inpatient care, (2) outpatient care, (3) partial hospitalization, (4) emergency care, and (5) education and consultation. Those centers that are well established in their operations may offer additional services. Diagnostic services, rehabilitation programs that include vocational and educational programs, precare and aftercare services, placement of patients in half way houses and foster homes, and home visits may be conducted by the staff. Research, evaluation, and training programs may also be provided. These services are available for persons who are residents of a circumscribed area. This may be a county, suburban community, specific neighborhood, or some arbitrarily defined geographic area. In Illinois the areas are known as zones. Within the center the patient care areas may be divided into units that service the residents of a particular geographic area, such as one or more counties. Units may also be organized to care for specific types of patients, such as alcoholics, drug addicts, and mentally retarded persons who are residents of the circumscribed area or zone in which the mental health center is located.

PHILOSOPHY UNDERLYING TREATMENT AND GOALS

Social scientists were largely responsible for conducting the studies that pointed out the defects in the environment and treatment of patients in large public mental hospitals. Their efforts led to the subsequent interest in and establishment of mental health centers. Criticisms were aimed at the managerial operations carried on continuously in these institutions in behalf of the patient that caused his own control and personality functioning to atrophy. This constituted an attack upon the rules, regulations, routinized schedules, activities and ways of living in the public mental hospital that led, in their view, to desocialization of the patient. Living in such a custodial setting was considered an impoverished way of life that provided little, if any, incentive to regain one's health and become self-sufficient. It was their belief that the individual deserved a chance to try for something better, and that the professional staff had an obligation to provide that opportunity. Consequently, the environment, treatment approaches, staffing plan, services offered, aims and objectives, and ways of operating in a mental health center are a radical departure from those of the traditional mental hospital. Indeed, persons who have worked in the traditional hospitals often find it very difficult to adjust to the change of a mental health center.

Social scientists support the concept that successful rehabilitation of the patient is more likely when the individual is treated in his own cultural setting. Thus, the major goal of the community mental health center is to treat patients in their residential environments, close to the family and other social systems of the culture. This results in reduced admissions to state mental hospitals. The inpatient treatment plan is designed to limit the length of hospitalization. A variety of outpatient services and programs are offered to make it possible for the individual to live at home or somewhere in the community, work, socialize, and keep in contact with others. The rationale for this approach is that non-institutional living prevents chronic mental illness and patterns of maintaining it from developing. The inherent aim of treatment approaches is to (1) repair deficiencies in the self-concept and identity, (2) reverse the process of gradual induction into the sick role and convert it into the healthy competent role, and (3) reactivate social and job skills.

The patient population of the mental health center is small in comparison to that of the traditional mental hospital. A typical center may have between 100 and 250 inpatients. The general atmosphere is more permissive and flexible. The staffing pattern is that of a multidisciplinarian team, including psychiatrists, psychologists, professional mental health specialists, social workers, nurses, and psychiatric technicians. Unlike the traditional mental hospital, the authority is decentralized so that there is an absence of a hierarchial system. Patients are often called by their first names and nurses dress in civilian clothes. Reality therapy and confrontation may be used in group sessions with patients. These are some of the features of the mental health center that make adjustment to this type of facility difficult for the traditionally oriented staff. This accounts for the observation that the center staff is usually of the younger generation that has been indoctrinated very early in contemporary concepts of psychiatric approach.

IMPLEMENTATION OF CURRENT TRENDS

The community mental health center staff implements many of the treatment approaches and services that constitute current trends in community psychiatry. These trends have been well identified by Solomon and Patch.

TRENDS—A BASIS FOR ASSESSMENT[2]

A listing of recent trends in community psychiatric services provides a basis for judging the adequacy of such services—or at least their conformity to certain current views. These trends are toward the following goals:

(1) Treating many diagnostic categories of patients rather than just a few.

(2) Serving all age groups rather than principally children.

(3) Treating people of low socioeconomic status rather than predominantly the middle class.

(4) Working with families or others who are in close touch with patients rather than only with persons who have been defined as patients.

(5) Intervening promptly, at the critical period when help is sought, rather than imposing a waiting period.

(6) Beginning treatment at the initial contact rather than first requiring prolonged intake and diagnostic procedures.

(7) Providing brief therapy whenever possible rather than expecting long-term psychotherapy to be the technic of choice.

(8) Encouraging diversified and flexible approaches to patient care, including treatment in the patient's home, rather than holding strictly to any one model of treatment.

(9) Giving attention to primary prevention and to rehabilitative and aftercare services as well as to the actual treatment process.

(10) Ensuring maximum continuity of care rather than requiring transfers and referrals that sever therapeutically significant relationships.

(11) Broadening, rather than narrowing, the range of professional mental health skills.

(12) Cultivating close ties with resources that provide various medical and health care services rather than remaining aloof from other branches of medicine.

(13) Broadening the concept of the "psychiatric team" to include others besides the traditional psychiatrist, psychologist, and social worker.

(14) Accepting members of other professions as colleagues of the psychiatrist rather than as his subordinates; also, accepting nonprofessional and volunteer personnel as colleagues or potential colleagues.

(15) Working to enable both patients and others in the community to assume as much responsibility as possible, rather than "taking over" in ways that deprive them of responsibility.

(16) Encouraging resourcefulness and effectiveness on the part of others through appropriate decentralization and through the fostering of democratic processes rather than seeking to maximize central authority and control.

(17) Developing contractual and other working relationships among public, private, and nonprofit resources in the community in order to enhance patients' freedom of choice rather than permitting a single bureaucratized "empire" to be formed.

(18) Accepting guidance from community representatives regarding policy decisions relating to mental health rather than serving merely as a source of such guidance.

(19) Relying on cost-benefit or cost-effectiveness accounting and systems analysis as a means of allocating resources and evaluating performance.

(20) Carrying out community-wide studies of mental disorders and disabilities rather than keeping track only of currently treated cases.

(21) Consulting and collaborating with members and leaders of organized community groups from the standpoint of their interests and concerns rather than focusing simply on issues of patient care.

(22) Taking all possible steps to overcome the stigmatizing, degrading, or abusive handling of any groups or individuals within the community who are targets of hostile or punitive reactions rather than intervening only to secure greater respect and acceptance for psychiatric patients.

The use of tranquilizers and antidepressant drugs has been a distinct advantage in promoting community psychiatry, making it possible for patients to live outside of institutions. These medications help to reduce a person's feelings of fear and anxiety. Living in the community is less threatening.

INPATIENT SERVICE

The average length of stay in a mental health center is about three weeks. A well-planned daily schedule may involve nurses in joint meetings of staff with patients, family therapy sessions, psychodrama, role playing, discussion groups, occupational, social, and recreational therapies. Nurses are participants or leaders in group meetings. They function as co-therapists during group psychotherapy and family therapy. Nurses also have responsibility for giving medications, treatments, and other procedures for which they are considered to be the staff person best prepared to assume such a responsibility. There has been considerable protest about nurses not being permitted to function as independent therapists in individual as well as group psychotherapy. Psychologists and social workers are allowed to practice independently, but very few nurses are permitted to do so.[3] However, we may expect this number to increase as nurses become more vocal on the subject of role discrimination. Many nurses believe that modern, master degree-level university-prepared psychiatric nurses are highly skilled in the art of relating with, interviewing, and counseling mentally ill patients. The diversity and scope of services provided by the mental health center staff reaches into many community social systems and organizations. Because of this extended, far-reaching approach, nurses may discover a growing need for their independent services as the establishment of community mental health centers and their services increase.

OUTPATIENT SERVICES

Nurses assist with the reception and interviewing of patients who come to the center's outpatient clinic for initial evaluation and treatment of emotional distress. They also conduct follow-up interviews of patients who return to the clinic for progress evaluation, observation of medication effects, adjustment to families, occupation, and community life. Nurses also make home visits to observe discharged patients in their family settings. These visits may be made alone or in the company of a senior therapist from the center. The nurse may serve as a co-therapist when a family therapy session is conducted in the home. Nurses make observations of the home environment, sanitation, family nutrition, and interpersonal relations. They do health teaching, assist the patient and family in organizing a daily activity schedule, and help to plan budgets. Home visits may lead to follow-up contacts with other welfare and social agencies. Observations in the home may be helpful in understanding the conditions and relationships in the family environment that are influencing the course of the patient's illness. Reports of these observations may be of assistance in planning treatment approaches and counseling the patient and family. Nurses from the center help to organize and assist with outpatient clinics that are held on specific days in a neighborhood facility, such as a church, school, social club, or youth center.

PARTIAL HOSPITALIZATION

A day or night treatment service or both may be provided in the mental health center. Patients may spend the day or night in one of the inpatient wards or a special unit. The plan enables day patients to maintain contact with their families in the evenings, early morning, and on weekends. They may perform necessary functions in the home as they maintain family relationships and social contacts in the community. Nurses participate in the treatment plan which may include individual, group psychotherapy, meetings with staff, family therapy sessions, social recreation, and education programs. Patients usually return home for the evening meal with their families. There are occasions when a day patient may remain overnight in the center one or two evenings a week. The night service is provided for patients who come to the center after working in the community during the day. They usually partake of the evening meal which provides an opportunity to socialize with others before participating in group meetings or individual therapy sessions planned for them. They remain overnight, have breakfast and then return to their jobs in the community. Weekends are spent at home and in community activities.

EMERGENCY SERVICE

Mental health centers, like other inpatient psychiatric facilities, provide emergency service. Patients may be brought to the center by family members, police, health officers, and other authorized individuals with or without advance notice. All states have laws that provide for the admission of persons in need of emergency psychiatric admission, observation, examination, and treatment. Nurses often help to admit these patients, carry out treatment orders, and make observations that may assist in evaluating the person's behavior and mental status. Suicidal observation may be required. Establishing a relationship, acquainting the patient with the center environment and plan of treatment, and providing emotional support are nursing approaches during such periods of emotional stress.

The mental health center may also provide consultation for a community organization or group that establishes a telephone service for emotionally distressed persons. In some communities these "people to people" lines are kept open for 24 hours. Volunteers or paid personnel may provide this service. Callers may be given emotional support during conversations or assisted with making a contact that will initiate emergency admission or an appointment for psychiatric care. These services have been widely publicized and have been quite successful in a considerable number of communities.

CONSULTATION AND EDUCATION

Within the mental health center consultation and evaluation may be carried on between members of the various disciplines, including nurses. They confer about the dynamics of specific behaviors observed, approaches used during therapy sessions, and vocational and rehabilitation plans. Community consultation may be extended to general hospitals, geriatric institutions, convalescent homes, general practitioners, home visiting agencies, police officers, clergymen, courts, school authorities, public health departments, neighborhood health clinics, and other welfare agencies. Consultation may concern evaluation of emotional problems and states for the purpose of determining the need for inpatient or outpatient psychiatric treatment. It may include the making of a direct observation of specific behavior problems for the purpose of advising on psychiatric approaches. Staff members from the center may serve in advisory capacities on local mental health boards, health organization committees, and citizens' groups.

Mental health centers maintain ongoing education programs for the training of staff members at all levels. These include orientation as well as continuing education programs. They also provide clinical facilities and experiences for students of medicine, nursing, psychology, social workers and social scientists. Education programs may be scheduled in the center for patients and their families. The objective may be to help them understand mental illness, how to re-establish community contacts, and seek and obtain job opportunities after discharge. Families are helped to anticipate what to expect from patients and how to relate and cope with their behavior on home visits and after discharge. Vocational training programs are arranged for patients within commuting distance of their homes. The center's staff may help to plan and participate in programs designed to educate community groups in mental health concepts, treatment approaches, and the availability of psychiatric services.

REACTIONS TO MENTAL HEALTH CENTERS

Most authorities agree that the mental health center and community approach is a necessary movement in the direction toward providing improved mental health programs and care. Like any new system, however, the centers have had their share of criticism. We may expect this to continue until they are well established in their operations and have sufficient time to review and evaluate the effectiveness of the system. Some critics have complained that the centers overlook the chronically ill patient and give their attention to those persons who show promise of recovery.

Some complaints have been voiced that the centers discharge patients prematurely and that this results in readmissions. The conclusion is that there is no correlation between statistical discharge rates and improvement. There are also therapists who do not believe that direct confrontation aimed at getting the patient to face his problem and take the initiative to do something about it should be used as a choice approach. The responses to these criticisms are that mental health centers are an improvement over the drab, depressing, crowded atmosphere of the large state hospital. The plan of care in the center focuses on a much smaller number of patients as individuals. In the densely populated wards of public mental hospitals patients are often neglected and lose their personal identity in the crowd. The patient in the mental health center is said to be stimulated to actively participate in his treatment and rehabilitation. This is in contrast with the inactive patients who become institutionalized in the public mental hospitals. Even though patients discharged from the centers may return to be readmitted, their improvement is shown in being able to live in the community between the period of discharge and readmission instead of requiring custodial care that leads to chronic mental illness. Thus, the mental health center is a facility that, with the passing of time and more experience, appears to be the treatment center of the future for the mentally ill.

SUGGESTED REFERENCES

Boucher, M.: Personal space and chronicity in the mental hospital. Perspec. Psychiat. Care: 206 (Sept.-Oct.), 1971.

Brown, F.: Social Linkability. Am. J. Nurs. 71: 516 (March), 1971.

Bulbulyan, A., Davidites, R., and Williams, F.: Nurses in a community mental health center. Am. J. Nurs. 69: 328 (Feb.), 1969.

Butler, H.: Comprehensive community mental health centers: a progress report 1969. J. Psychiat. Nurs. 7: 245 (Nov.-Dec.), 1969.

Crow, N.: The multifaceted role of the community mental health nurse. J. Psychiat. Nurs. 9: 28 (May-Jun.), 1971.

DePaul, A.: The nurse as a central figure in a mental health center. Perspect. Psychiat. Care 6: 17 (Jan.-Feb.), 1968.

DeYoung, C., and Tower, M.: The Nurse's Role in Community Mental Health Centers. C. V. Mosby Co., St. Louis, 1971.

Evans, F.: The Role of the Nurse in Community Mental Health. The MacMillan Co., New York, 1968.

Fagin, C.: Family-Centered Nursing in Community Psychiatry. F. A. Davis Co., Philadelphia, Pa. 1970.

Koegler, R., and Brill, L.: Treatment of Psychiatric Outpatients. Appleton-Century-Crofts, New York, 1967.

Leninger, M.: Community psychiatric nursing: trends, issues, and problems. Perspect. Psychiat. Care 7: 10 (Jan.-Feb.), 1969.

Oltman, P.: One approach to real community involvement. J. Psychiat. Nurs. 9: 18 (Sept.-Oct.), 1971.

Solomon, P., and Patch, V.: Handbook of Psychiatry. Lange Medical Publications, Los Altos, Calif., 1969.

Ujhely, G.: The nurse in community psychiatry. Am. J. Nurs. 69: 1001 (May), 1969.

Zahourek, R.: Nurses in a community mental health center. Functions, competencies, and satisfactions. Nurs. Outlook 19: 593 (Sept.), 1971.

FOOTNOTES

1. National Association for Mental Health, Inc.: Facts about Mental Illness.
2. Solomon, P., and Patch, V.: Handbook of Psychiatry, ed. 2. Lange Medical Publications, Los Altos, Calif., 1971, pp. 602-603.
3. DeYoung, C., Tower, M., et al.: The Nurse's Role in Community Mental Health Centers. C. V. Mosby Co., St. Louis, 1971.

For reviewing this chapter, grateful acknowledgment is made to Miss Marilyn Miller, R.N., Mrs. Jeanette Wade, R.N., Mrs. Diane Sworm, R.N., and Mrs. Carol Woodworth, R.N.

CHAPTER 9

The Extending Community Nursing Role

Observations made about the changing role and future of the public health nurse have implications for psychiatric nursing. It has been said that psychiatric nurses will provide extending services to patients in the community through public health departments. This movement already appears to be well under way.

MORE INDEPENDENT JUDGMENTS

French says,

I think the community nurse will continue to provide services in health guidance, counseling, and interviewing, but, in addition, she will assume more responsibility for direct patient care. This will require a rational reorganization of the roles of the physician and the professional nurse; specific patient-care procedures that have been carried out previously by the physician will be legally transferred to the community nurse. She will have more responsibility for the coordination of care, and she will do more to help the patient through the maze of the health care system. Several demonstration projects have shown that public health nurses are capable of assuming such responsibility and providing more comprehensive care. The nurse, in turn, will delegate some of her present tasks to family health workers and aides.

There is evidence already that the community nurse of the future will work in a variety of settings—neighborhood health centers, hospital outpatient departments, group practice centers, private physicians' offices, as well as health departments. This will mean that the staff nurse will become a more independent practitioner, directly involved in decision making.[1]

THE THERAPEUTIC COMMUNITY

Much has been said and written about the positive affects of a therapeutic community in a mental hospital. There are therapists, however, who believe that the therapeutic community should be the residential community of the outside world. This viewpoint is an extension of the belief that mental disorders are psychiatric social problems that develop in one's social environment and relations, and that treatment should focus upon helping the individual to solve problems in living in the community, the natural life setting. This theory goes so far as to visualize the eventual elimination of mental hospitals. It conceives of mentally ill persons living with their own or foster families in the community, carrying on with the daily events and pursuits of living just as has been done in Gheel, Belgium, since 1851 (see p. 43). It is in this kind of setting that emotionally supportive therapy and prevention of primary mental disorders and relapses would be undertaken.

Some communities have established an interagency board for the exchange of information concerning the operation of health services maintained by several local organizations. Community general hospitals, psychiatric institutions, social welfare agencies, clinics, visiting nurse associations, schools, and other groups offering health services have representatives on the board who share information and arrange to pool their resources for the patient's and each other's benefits.

COMMUNITY MENTAL HEALTH CENTERS

The community mental health center is already considered the central agency for evaluating, treating, and following up patients. The center has become the pivotal point for establishing, maintaining, and assisting with various types of community psychiatric services, including consultation, education, and research. Services extend into homes, schools, courts, clinics, churches, social centers, welfare agencies, etc. The expansion of these services enables members of various disciplines to reach and keep in touch with many more individuals than could be assisted in the traditional state mental hospital. Furthermore, it can be done as people needing psychiatric services carry on with the requirements of everyday living and earning a livelihood (see chap. 8, p. 89).

PSYCHIATRIC SERVICES IN GENERAL HOSPITALS

Approximately 617 community general hospitals, or about one out of every ten, have separate units for treating psychiatric patients. Another 681 general hospitals admit psychiatric patients to their regular medical facilities.[2] These services have come into existence based on the philosophy that a hospital to be truly "general" must be equipped to give total and comprehensive care to all patients, as well as to manage unexpected behavior of an emergency nature. The average length of stay in these services is about three weeks. Authorities believe that having psychiatric units in general hospitals presents definite advantages. Early treatment is made available to persons in the community because people show a readier acceptance of psychiatric facilities attached to the general hospital. With few exceptions, admission is on a voluntary basis. The stigma associated with mental illness is reduced and admissions to public hospitals are decreased. Mental health teaching programs offered by the staff to citizens help individuals to adjust in society and to achieve a better understanding of mental illness and the needs of the mentally ill. Smaller groups of patients can receive individualized care. Psychiatry is integrated into the general field of medicine. Specialty barriers among professionals break down. There is consultative sharing between the medical and psychiatric staffs which results in better understanding of the emotional aspects of illness. This raises the level of care received by the patient. A better teaching center results because opportunities for learning integrated care are present throughout the medical nursing courses of study. Allied personnel attached to the hospital staff also share in the learning process. Nurse members of the psychiatric service staff participate in the treatment plan by implementing medical orders, attending interdisciplinary conferences, assisting with physical treatments, leading group discussions, initiating social and recreational activities, and relating with individual patients.

HALFWAY HOUSES

Institutional psychiatric personnel have long recognized a group of patients whose progress in the mental hospital is at a standstill. Continued hospitalization of these persons fosters dependency, loss of initiative, and neglect of potentialities for healthy living. Patients in this group are able to maintain their emotional equilibrium in the hospital, but cannot do so at home. They recognize their need to escape the inevitable stress and strain of the outside world, but in the hospital they avoid attempts to help them resolve conflict. These patients occupy a position midway between sickness and health. Halfway houses have been established for these individuals.

Health is emphasized in an optimum environment for testing and realizing the potentialities for health.

Halfway houses are maintained by laymen in cooperation with psychiatrists. Patients are prepared for this experience in living through counseling and group therapy. Employment is obtained for them in the hospital or community before they are transferred. Periodic visits are made to the home by vocational rehabilitation counselors to determine the individual patient's adjustment to the home and work.

FOSTER HOME CARE

It is well known that some persons cannot maintain healthy relationships with members of their own families. Living in the same home may lead to disturbances in the emotional climate that affect the individual's mental health. That is why psychiatrists sometimes recommend that patients having such interpersonal difficulties make arrangements to live away from their own homes with congenial companions or in a foster home after being discharged. These persons are assisted in obtaining employment before leaving the hospital. Arrangements are usually made for their return to the outpatient department for follow-up on their adjustment.

Foster home placement of patients in private families or nursing homes has also been arranged for elderly patients. Social workers and public health nurses have become increasingly active in transferring elderly patients from mental hospitals to long term care facilities. The enactment and implementation of Medicare provisions for the aged has given impetus to this movement. Public health nurses are working with mental hospital staff members to make arrangements for these transfers. Nurses involved in this service are required to visit and become acquainted with the quality of nursing care that is provided in nursing homes. Public health departments have established, in cooperation with Medicare provisions, certain standards and guidelines for judging whether or not individual nursing homes meet the standards for placement of aged persons.

NURSING IN HOMES

It is now possible for persons with mild emotional disorders to remain at home while under the care of a community physician. Tranquilizing and antidepressant medications have been largely responsible for this development. Some of these individuals may require nursing observation and emotional support from a visiting nurse. Local physicians may refer patients for follow-up care to the visiting nurse association. Psychiatric hospitals use an interagency referral form to request home nursing care from the visiting nurse association for patients being discharged. The request has information about the patient, his illness, treatment, and observations to be made by the nurse in the home. The nurse acts as a liaison between the patient, his family, and the hospital.

There are many ways in which the community psychiatric nurse can be of assistance to patients and families in their homes. Emotional reactions may develop and be detected in patients who are primarily physically ill. Family members may also manifest symptoms of emotional disorders. In addition, there may be evidence of environmental stress and strain which affect the patient's recovery. Specific reactions to drugs and treatments may be observed. A nurse's observations in the home may require her to teach family members how to organize the environment, schedule daily activities, maintain sanitary conditions, make a budget, plan a menu, perform simple nursing procedures, and give the patient emotional support. Well-prepared nurses can help families to accept a member's illness and admission to a psychiatric service or hospitals. Nurses can be helpful in explaining the hospital's admission procedures, rules, and regulations. In some instances, nurses can interpret the diagnosis and treatment procedures so that these are meaningful and acceptable to the family.

Families can also be assisted to prepare for and accept the patient for trial visits in the home and upon discharge from the hospital. Nurses can help patients and families to accept extended hospital treatment when this is recommended. They can also direct family members to community agencies offering health and financial assistance and other services which may be needed.

Through the services they provide and their community contacts, nurses can establish relationships which effect better understanding and acceptance of mental illness, the factors which contribute to its development, and available treatment. Good public relations can help to obtain adequate resources for community mental health needs. Working with local physicians, courts, schools, welfare, and other agencies can result in early diagnosis and treatment of emotionally disturbed children and adults. The community can be encouraged to develop a philosophy of acceptance for the mentally ill person upon discharge from treatment.

OUTPATIENT PSYCHIATRIC CLINICS

In 1967 there were 2,259 public and private outpatient psychiatric clinics in the United States providing services for children and adults. Many of these are part time. Most of them have long waiting lists. It is estimated that a full time clinic is needed for every 50,000 persons or twice as many as now exist.[2] These clinics are located in psychiatric and general hospitals. Others are maintained in separate facilities, such as clinics that are operated by a community or county mental health board. More recently, neighborhood mental health centers have come into existence. These services are operated in social centers, churches, schools, housing complexes and other locations that are near to and convenient to neighborhood families. Neighborhood centers were established as the result of social studies that showed that psychiatric services were not readily available to low income families and persons.

The staff is usually composed of a psychiatrist, psychologist, social worker, a receptionist, and sometimes nurses. The nurse's role is dependent upon the size of the clinic, its plan of operation, her education and experience, and patients' needs. Nurses give medications and assist with physical treatments, such as electroconvulsive therapy which is sometimes administered in private clinics. They may interview patients and take histories. Nurses also evaluate progress made by hospital discharged patients and their reactions to prescribed medications. They assist with the admission of patients to the inpatient services of hospitals to which mental health clinics are attached.

Patients are usually screened by the clinic staff as a preliminary step in order to determine the need or urgency for treatment. Referrals are made by local physicians, social agencies, clergymen, teachers, and psychologists. Patients being discharged from inpatient psychiatric services of hospitals may also be referred for follow-up by the clinic. Most clinics have a sliding scale fee to fit the ability of the patient and his family to pay for service. The clinic staff maintains contact with local referring individuals and agencies from the time of the patient's admission, through treatment to discharge.

Social workers spend considerable time interviewing patients and families and writing case histories. Psychologists test patients and evaluate their progress during the course of treatment. In some clinics, the social workers and psychologists provide psychotherapy under the assignment and direction of the supervising psychiatrist. Interviews with patients and group sessions are discussed regularly with the senior psychiatrist. Some clinics carry on an active research and educational program. Graduate and undergraduate students may receive training in these facilities.

The clinic interprets its work to the community through a mental hygiene program which may consist of a series of lectures related to mental illness and mental health. Oftentimes, staff members serve on local discussion panels for the purposes of enlightening the general public about mental illness and to obtain their cooperation in the rehabilitation of patients.

DAY AND NIGHT TREATMENT CENTERS

The primary purpose of day and night treatment centers is to provide a comprehensive psychiatric treatment program for patients who are able to remain at home part of the time. Persons coming to the day care center are able to take some responsibility for management of their homes while they live with the family. Those coming to the night care center are gainfully employed in the community. These services function as specifically planned programs within the mental hospital and mental health center while making use of the available facilities and other services.

Patients come to the day center voluntarily from the community. They usually attend five mornings a week and leave for home in the late afternoon. In the hospital, they sometimes are joined by a smaller convalescent group of inpatients who are being rehabilitated prior to their discharge. Patients are selected on the basis of their ability to function in a group society and cooperate with treatment. Those patients manifesting psychotic, persecutory, or overactive behavior are excluded from these services because their needs could not be met in these programs.

Nurses participate in the daily treatment schedule which usually commences with a morning coffee meeting. Informal group discussions, individual counseling, and group psychotherapy may be used. Tranquilizing and antidepressant medications may be prescribed for individual patients. Social, recreational activities may be included in the treatment plan.

The original motivation in establishing a night center grew out of the recognition of the need to treat individuals who could not afford to leave their employment. Persons having such financial problems were observed to continue in their jobs and struggle with their conflicts and anxieties until the breaking point was reached. Often their efficiency on the job was reduced and pathological mental disorder developed. As a result, treatment was more difficult and prolonged. The major emphasis, therefore, in treating patients in a night center is upon prevention.

Patients come to the night center about 6:00 P.M. following their daily work in the community, five nights each week. They sleep in the center. Weekends are free for visits at home and with friends.

These persons have supper in the hospital, receive prescribed medications and treatment, and participate in group discussions, individual counseling, or group psychotherapy. Because they have been doing prescribed work during the day and have maintained their own contacts in the community, they do not enjoy structured social activities after therapy. The informal social hour where they just sit, chat, smoke, and relax is enjoyed more. They retire about 10:30 P.M. In the morning, they eat breakfast and leave for work about 7:30.

There are advantages associated with day and night treatment centers. The patient is able to continue his social contacts with the family and community. Their illness period is shortened and there are fewer problems in rehabilitation. The unit serves as a valuable demonstration teaching service for professional persons. The staff working with these patients hold open house one afternoon or evening a week for patients' relatives. Sometimes a film is shown and discussed by the attending therapist. Public relations are improved with patients, relatives, and local physicians.

SCHOOL NURSING

Emphasis upon prevention has resulted in an increasing recognition of the importance of early detection of physical and emotional disorders in school children. When physical deficiencies and emotional problems are investigated and treated early, pathological illness can often be prevented from developing in the child.

The importance of emotional aspects related to children's physical and mental disabilities has already produced some changes in the educational process and the related roles of the school nurse and teacher. Educators and school nurses are now required to study subject matter related to the field of mental hygiene. The school nurse is expected to serve as a consultant to the teaching staff and a liaison between the school and home. She visits the homes of children presenting health problems. This enables her to discuss during consultative meetings with educators the family environment, relationships, and observations. Sharing observations and information helps the staff to work together most effectively when attempting to assist the child and family to resolve problems which are emotionally distressing and affecting the child's academic performance.

Children may have fears and phantasies related to school life, teachers, parents, and parent substitutes. Fears of failure, punishment, parental disappointment, competition, aggression, physical injury, rejection, abandonment, and other uncomfortable reactions are common in the developing child.

The capacity to achieve intellectually may be hampered, by unfavorable physical and emotional influences. Investigators stress the importance of proper nutrition and the need to perform additional, more reliable hearing and vision tests on some children. Routine examinations do not always reveal existing defects which affect the child's hearing, vision, and subsequent ability to learn. Unless reliable information is made available, the remedial approach may be inadequate and fail to resolve emotional reactions in the child and the teacher's attitude toward the problem.

A well meaning educator may have no conception of a child's underlying emotional needs and the problems which his behavior reflects. Broken homes, unstable family relationships, sibling rivalry, and unsound health practices related to diet, rest, and recreation may sometimes be detected in the home environment. These conditions may exist owing to ignorance of the effects they may produce upon the child's capacity to learn and adjust. Thus, a well prepared nurse can often establish an effective relationship with teachers and families to integrate consultation and health teaching.

Some of the problems encountered in schools cannot be solved without the assistance of other consultative and treatment services. Some schools have established child study departments which provide psychological, psychiatric, and case work services to teachers and parents. Children and parents are sometimes referred to community public health, mental health, social, and welfare agencies. Child guidance clinics have demonstrated well the effectiveness of an interdisciplinary approach to the study and treatment of the problems of children and their parents.

Mental health problems are also encountered in the teenage, high school group. In addition to poor academic performance, problems of juvenile delinquency have increased. Dislike for school, truancy, stealing, addiction, disruptive classroom behavior, and hostile aggression towards other students, teachers, and society's members have presented difficult situations in the local school system. Treatment of these problems requires competent investigation, consultation, and counseling for students and parents. The services of community agencies may be enlisted to assist in the resolution of some of these problems.

Mental health services have been established in some higher institutions of learning. Students sometimes manifest symptoms of emotional disorder or present problems in adjustment to the academic program and social life. The changes in living encountered in a university setting as well as new study and social demands may precipitate emotional reactions in some students. Loneliness, fear of scholastic failure, rejection from coveted groups, or the inability to measure up to the expectations of family and friends may be inherent in some students' problems and behavior.

INDUSTRIAL NURSING

Emotional disorders and pathological mental illness are the most common causes of human disability. Eighty-five percent of all industrial accidents are believed to have an underlying factor of mental or emotional disturbance. About seven of ten workers dismissed because of inefficiency are actually suffering emotional disorders.[3] Recognizing the symptoms of these conditions and the need for counseling or prompt psychiatric treatment is an important responsibility of the industrial nurse.

Industrial psychiatry grew out of the concept that the combined efforts of psychiatrists, psychologists, and social workers could result in better selection of personnel, job placement, and efficient production. It was believed that these results would be advantageous for employers and contribute to the personal satisfaction and happiness of the employee. Authorities maintain that accident rates are reduced when emotional problems are recognized and resolved.

Some industries maintain well organized mental health services. Psychological testing of workers and placement of employees according to their aptitudes, interests, and abilities are important parts of these services. Educational programs are also provided to acquaint administrative and supervisory personnel with an understanding of mental health concepts, emotional disorders, and their symptomatic expression. An employee counseling service is provided to assist with problems of job dissatisfaction, marital, and family problems. Close working relationships are maintained with community agencies, clinics, hospitals, and private physicians.

The industrial nurse is considered to be the eyes and ears of the medical division regardless of whether or not the plant maintains an organized mental health service. Nurses who allow employees to ventilate their problems and feelings may sometimes be able to offer helpful counsel. More obvious symptoms, however, may indicate an underlying emotional conflict which should be promptly referred to the physician. Employees may be seen by the company doctor or encouraged to visit their family physician. The nurse can also direct employees to community agencies which offer the services needed by them.

Industrial nurses may be required to visit the home of an employee who is absent for a considerable period of time owing to illness. This provides an opportunity for the nurse to observe the family situation and its influence upon the person's health. The interest shown by the nurse during these visits and the manner in which she relates with the patient and family may result in improved relationships between management and employees.

OFFICE NURSING

There is increasing recognition that many emotional disorders and accompaniments of mental illness are observed by general practitioners. Much emphasis has been placed upon the preventive role of the family physician. It is said that local doctors examine and treat a large number of obviously psychoneurotic persons and individuals afflicted with psychosomatic conditions. In addition, the general practitioner is often acquainted with the home environment and other family members. This is considered advantageous from the diagnostic and treatment standpoint.

Nurses employed in doctors' offices may assist in compiling preliminary and follow-up information which can be helpful in determining the diagnosis, treatment, and progress. Being alert to the patient's account of the illness and the results of treatment may enable the nurse to detect significant emotional aspects related to the patient's complaint. Such information may be incorporated in the record of illness. It may indicate an underlying emotional conflict and unmet needs. An understanding nurse can frequently listen to and reassure patients concerning their fears and help them to accept treatment and hospitalization when these are prescribed.

Family members sometimes call at the doctor's office to inquire personally into the nature and extent of the patient's illness. At such times, nurses encounter persons who are in need of emotional support.

Answering telephone calls in the physician's absence can require the nurse to allow patients to talk and ventilate some of their feelings. A listening ear and understanding responses on the nurse's part can be anxiety relieving for some patients.

THE SHELTERED WORKSHOP

The sheltered workshop is a medically supervised place of remunerative employment where the physically or mentally handicapped individual, living in the community, is provided an opportunity to work in accordance with his physical and emotional resources. Persons who are reluctant to leave the hospital can be encouraged to do so when the possibility of employment in a sheltered workshop is available. Patients who are unable to fill the demands of full employment often adjust well to this type of experience. Vocational counseling, on the job training, and supportive psychiatric care are provided when necessary. Without the workshop's assistance in training and rehabilitation some patients tend to develop anxiety and procrastinate in seeking employment.

SECURITY HOSPITAL NURSING

The care of mentally ill prisoners is said to be a neglected responsibility of the medical profession. Very few nurses are employed in prison clinics or security hospitals which provide care for mentally ill persons sentenced to prison. Research studies have yielded valuable information concerning the extent of mental disorders among prisoners and repeated offenders. Prison clinics, more scientific methods of classifying prisoners, and the creation of special institutions for mentally ill legal offenders resulted from this work. Having a prison clinic with a staff prepared in the field of mental hygiene is advantageous. Persons afflicted with mental disorders and those who are mentally retarded can be identified and placed in an appropriate hospital for treatment. The objective is to reduce the incidence of repeated offenses after discharge from prison. Inmates can be helped to adjust to the prison environment and assisted in their return to the community. A clinic provides a valuable means for continuing research into the nature, causes, and treatment of certain types of illegal behavior.

Investigators have written about the lack of understanding and proper treatment of prisoners by untrained guards. Rigid restraints, security measures, and restrictions placed upon the inmates' movements and social activities are cited as causes for concern. Recommendations are made to employ better educated staffs, nurses having experience in caring for the mentally ill, modern treatment methods, and social activities.[4]

THE FUTURE IN COMMUNITY NURSING

French concludes,

The future in community nursing, as I see it, is one of more responsibility for coordination and direct patient care, carried out in a variety of settings by nurses functioning as members of interdisciplinary teams. The nurse will be expected to perform her duties in a responsible, independent fashion; and she will be directly involved in the decision making process. She will also take more responsibility for community diagnosis and bringing about appropriate community action.[1]

SUGGESTED REFERENCES

Blair, K.: It's the patient's problem and decision. Nurs. Outlook 19: 593 (Sept.), 1971.

Carye, J., and Swartz, J.: Mental health service in a community college. Am. J. Nurs. 71: 1189 (June), 1971.

Crow, L.: The multifaceted role of the community mental health nurse. J. Psychiat. Nurs. 9: 28 (May–Jun.), 1971.

Evans, F.: The Role of the Nurse in Community Mental Health. The Macmillan Co., New York, 1968.

Fagin, C.: Family-Centered Nursing Community Psychiatry. F. A. Davis Co., Philadelphia, 1970.

French, J.: This I believe—about community nursing in the future. Nurs. Outlook 19: 173 (March), 1971.

Gebbie, K., Delougery, G., and Neuman, B.: Levels of utilization: nursing specialists in community mental health. J. Psychiat. Nurs. 8: 37 (Jan.-Feb.), 1970.

Golub, S.: The new human ecology: community psychiatry. R.N. Journal 33: 36 (July), 1970.

Koegler, R., and Brill, N.: Treatment of Psychiatric Outpatients. Appleton-Century-Crofts, New York, 1967.

Leininger, M.: Community psychiatric nursing trends, issues, and problems. Perspect. Psychiat. Care 7: 10 (Jan.-Feb.), 1969.

McLaughlin, B.: Mental health in a community health program. Ment. Health Dig. 2: 22. (June), 1970.

Mistr, V.: Community nursing service for psychiatric patients. Perspect. Psychiat. Care 6: 36 (Jan.-Feb.), 1968.

Oltman, P.: One approach to real community involvement. J. Psychiat. Nurs. 9: 18 (Sept.-Oct.), 1971.

Petersen, S.: The psychiatric nurse specialist in a general hospital. Nurs. Outlook 17: 56 (Feb.), 1969.

Poswistilo, A.: Psychiatric patients reenter the community. Am. J. Nurs. 68: 2158 (Oct.), 1968.

Robinson, L.: Liaison psychiatric nursing. Perspect. Psychiat. Care 6: 87 (Mar.-Apr.), 1968.

Robison, O.: The treatment of school phobic children and their families. Perspect. Psychiat. Care 5: 219 (Sept.-Oct.), 1967.

Sheldon, A. and Hope, P.: The developing role of the nurse in a community mental health program. Perspect. Psychiat. Care 5: 272 (Nov.-Dec.), 1967.

Ujhely, G.: The nurse in community psychiatry. Am. J. Nurs. 69: 1001 (May), 1969.

FOOTNOTES

1. French, J.: This I Believe—about Community Nursing in the Future. Nurs. Outlook 19: 174, 175 (March), 1971.
2. National Association for Mental Health, Inc.: Facts about Mental Illness.
3. National Association for Mental Health, Inc.: The High Cost of Mental Illness.
4. Duval, A.: The Criminally Insane—Our Neglected Responsibility. Ment. Hosp. 8: 10 (April), 1957.

For reviewing this chapter, grateful acknowledgment is made to Miss Marilyn Miller, R.N., Mrs. Diane Sworm, R.N., Mrs. Jeanette Wade, R.N., Mrs. Marie Babrick, R.N., and Mrs. Lucilla Warren, R.N.

UNIT 4

Behavior Dynamics, Patterns, Symptoms

10

Psychodynamics of
Personality Development

EFFECTS OF GROWTH AND DEVELOPMENT

The growth and development of the human being is an individualistic process. Commencing with prenatal life the organism undergoes progressive changes in appearance as well as in its ability to adapt and adjust to the anxiety-producing stress of many external influences. What happens to the person during the growth process influences his response to life situations to the degree that the individual develops a distinctly unique personality.

When attempting to understand the behavior of a person it is necessary to have an understanding of the usual changes which occur during growth and development as well as the unique situations and circumstances of life to which the person was exposed. It is these individual situations and circumstances which are of special importance when one is endeavoring to understand why a person thinks, feels and behaves as he does. The symptoms observed during mental illness constitute both an expression of psychic conflict and the individual's defense against it.

The personality, which undergoes continuous change throughout the developmental stages of life, is the sum total of inherited and acquired features. All persons inherit certain personality traits to an individual degree through the genes or character determinants of the chromosomes in the parents' reproductive cells. Children in the same family may inherit varying degrees of these traits. The person's body physique, the color of his skin, eyes and hair, and his temperament are considered to be inherited traits. Acquired characteristics are the result of exposure to the mental and physical factors of an individual's culture and environment. These include health and the ability to communicate, relate with others, and adapt to the moral and ethical standards imposed by a person's cultural and social groups.

As will be observed in the following discussion of the historical stages of life, the individual grows from a dependent to an increasingly independent as well as interdependent person. Satisfaction of certain basic physical and emotional needs is essential for survival and healthy personality development. Whether or not these needs are met to a gratifying degree for the individual will influence his subsequent behavior and mental health.

RELATIONSHIP TO NURSING CARE

One of the prime ingredients of quality nursing involves sensitivity to and ability to meet the needs of human beings. Although the needs are the same for all people, regardless of their chronological age, it is through the study of personality development that the nurse learns to recognize behavior which is motivated by an individual's past and present living experiences as well as the needs which underlie manifest behaviors. Thus, a dynamic nursing approach is based upon an understanding of all the forces which have been influential in shaping the individual's personality. These include biological growth changes, feelings experienced during interpersonal relations, various deprivations, stress situations, and acquired defensive behaviors.

According to Erik Erikson's concept of personality development, all persons strive through the sequential stages of growth and personality development to achieve basic senses of (1) trust, (2) autonomy, (3) initiative, (4) industry, (5) identity, (6) intimacy, (7) generativity, and (8) integrity.[1] As the nurse becomes acquainted with these component strivings of personality development she may be able to visualize relationships between the strivings inherent in behaviors expressed and situations observed in the nurse-patient relationship.

PRENATAL DEVELOPMENT

Although some investigators continue to concern themselves with the genetic aspects of human development, it is generally believed that heredity is responsible for a very few of the disorders which are observed among persons who manifest psychologic disturbance. Evidence lending credence to the postulation that certain disorders, such as Huntington's chorea, Alzheimer's disease, and Pick's disease, are the result of genetic transmission has been accumulated. Some other disorders have been observed to afflict more than one member of a family. However, the possibility that these illnesses may be due to cultural and environmental influences, particularly interfamily relationships, always enters into discussions related to the findings of these studies. Hereditary postulations cannot be clearly demonstrated and continue to be disputed.

The physical and mental health of the pregnant woman has been of interest to researchers attempting to discover influential relationships between the mother's health and behavior during pregnancy upon the unborn child's development. It has been shown that if a pregnant woman is afflicted with a highly infectious disease, such as German measles, physical and mental defects may be produced in the unborn child. The growing fetus may also be adversely affected by nutritional deficiencies, certain drugs, metabolic disorders, heart conditions, and other illnesses experienced by the mother during pregnancy.

Whether or not the mother is subjected to psychologic distress, has receptive attitudes towards being pregnant and having a child, or feels fearful and anxious during pregnancy is also of interest. Some authorities believe that the emotional responses of the mother can affect the growing fetus. Postulations have been offered that maternal rejection and anxiety affecting embryonic existence may influence concomitant effects upon the child's subsequent adjustment and personality development.

DEVELOPMENT OF THE PSYCHE

Some of the driving, motivational aspects of behavior are conscious, but more are beyond awareness. Understanding the development, structure, and activity of the psyche provides insight into these motivational aspects of human behavior.

The psyche and soma (mind and body) develop as one structure. Although their functions can be differentiated, there is an interrelation between these two aspects of the living organism. The condition of one of them is known to influence reactions in the other. Recognition of their inseparability as a functioning unit of human existence has given impetus to the development of psychosomatic medicine as well as the "whole" or "complete" concept of medical treatment and nursing care. Modern nursing approaches are based upon the emotional and the physical reactions and needs of patients.

STRUCTURE OF THE PSYCHE

The structure and functions of the psyche have been of great interest to contemporary investigators. Sigmund Freud conceived of the psyche as being divided into three portions—the conscious, preconscious, and unconscious.

THE CONSCIOUS

The conscious portion of the mind is that part which functions when the person is awake, causing the individual to be aware of himself, his thoughts, feelings, perceptions, and what is going on in the environment.

THE PRECONSCIOUS

The preconscious, sometimes referred to as the subconscious mind, may be thought of as being situated between the conscious and unconscious portions of the psyche. It contains some partly remembered, partly forgotten experiences of living which can usually be recalled spontaneously and voluntarily.

THE UNCONSCIOUS

The unconscious is said to be the largest portion of the psyche. It contains the memories of one's past life, particularly those experiences which have been unpleasant and emotionally painful, stored away from conscious awareness and difficult to recall except under certain circumstances.

The unconscious level of the psyche is considered to be the area of the mind in which a great deal of independent activity, of which the individual is not aware but which can produce effects upon one's thoughts and actions, takes place. It is believed to function when the person is asleep as well as when awake.

EVIDENCE OF UNCONSCIOUS ACTIVITY

Evidence of behavior motivated by unconscious activity has been demonstrated in various ways. Perhaps the easiest example to understand are those which provide some insight into the influence of unconscious motivation. The everyday slips of the tongue and pen which are elicited without apparent conscious control are experiences familiar to almost everyone. Forgetting well-known names, telephone numbers, appointments, to mail letters, or to commence or complete some task is often associated with unconscious activity which appears to be motivated by opposing wishes and thoughts.

Behaving in a way which is contrary to one's conscious wishes and knowledge of what is appropriate and safe in specific situations and circumstances has also been designated as unconscious activity—for example, the sarcastic remark made by an individual to a person upon whom the speaker may be dependent for some kind of support. There are persons who often alienate themselves from others owing to their inability to control behavior motivated by thoughts and feelings stored in the unconscious.

Another example of unconscious motivation may be demonstrated in the analysis of a situation which produces an overwhelming feeling reaction in a person responding to the specific situation. The feeling perceived may be recognized as being equated with the feeling which was experienced during a similar situation occurring at an earlier level of growth and development. For instance, the feeling perceived when one anticipates rejection may be equated with earlier responses to fear of rejection.

People who are accident prone or who habitually drop or break articles are said to be behaving under the unfluence of the unconscious mind.

Evidence of unconscious mental activity has also been demonstrated during hypnosis, narcotherapy, psychoanalysis, analyses of dreams, amnesic episodes, and fugues. It is said that behind every dream there are unconscious thoughts and desires. Sometimes the dream produces a satisfying effect upon the dreamer which cannot be achieved during conscious awareness because of drives and impulses. The relaxation occurring with sleep permits some unconscious thoughts, ideas, and wishes to be expressed. Analysis of dreams requires special skills owing to the disguised forms through which the content of the unconscious is often expressed. What appears to be a jumble of mixed events and happenings in some dreams is thought to be due to the influence of the unconscious mind which cannot accept pure expressions of some unconscious thoughts, feelings, and impulses. Investigators believe that meaningful connections, which can be discovered by one who is skilled in making analyses of them, exist between the content of such dreams.

Unconscious motivation has also been recognized in art and other creative productions. Analysis of abstract paintings, interpretive dancing, and literature have evoked considerable interest and speculation concerning their underlying creative force and meanings.

Evidence of the unconscious may be associated with the behavior of neurotic as well as psychotic patients. Phobias, compulsive actions, symbolic manifestations, delusions, hallucinations, and other irrational as well as bizarre behaviors can be understood when one attempts to determine their meanings in relation to unconscious motivation inherent in repressed thoughts, wishes, feelings and impulses of the individual.

Observations of the psychologic effect of hypnotic suggestion are also evidence of unconscious mental activity. Therapists have demonstrated the effect of psychologic suggestion in the treatment of hysterical conditions, such as hysterical paralysis of an extremity. Suggestion has also been utilized in the preparation of women for painless birth-giving experience.

ID, EGO, SUPEREGO DEVELOPMENT

Freud distinguished three functionally related aspects of the psyche which he called the id, ego, and superego. Psychoanalysts often refer to these structures of the psyche. The id, composed of the untamed, uncultured primitive drives and impulses of the individual, is assumed to comprise the entire psychic apparatus at birth. The ego and superego, originally parts of the id, are considered to be separate, later developments which evolve as growth and development proceed. The ego is regarded as the conscious self which tests and deals with reality as one interacts with the environment. The superego is considered to be that critical, censoring portion of one's personality, referred to often as the conscience, which tends to check the expression of socially unacceptable id drives and impulses. Thus, the ego may be thought of as that part of the personality which acts as the moderator of the external struggle between the id and superego. If the person does not develop a strong enough ego to effect a compromise between id impulses and superego control, he will experience interpersonal and intrapersonal conflict.

BODY AND TEMPERAMENT TYPES

Observations have been made by investigators which are not strictly relevant to personality development, but which are usually mentioned in a discussion of the subject. Kretschmer described types of body physique and Jung discussed temperament types which some investigators have attempted to correlate with the development of specific mental disorders in individuals. Although these observations are of interest many psychiatrists do not consider them to be significant.

Pyknic Type

Usually short stature. Stocky, round-body figure. Barrel-shaped chest and abdomen. Short, but large extremities. Round facial features. Ruddy complexion. A tendency to accumulate fat.

Asthenic Type

Height usually normal. A few are short. Slender, thin-boned body figure. Thin, sunken-appearing chest and abdomen. Poor muscular development. Oval facial features. Pale or sallow complexion.

Athletic Type

Strong muscular development, especially around the neck, shoulders, legs, and arms. Broad shoulders. Narrow hips. Square facial features with bony prominences.

Dysplastic Type

Variations in physique are composed of combinations of the three main body types. A tendency to accumulate fat in some particular part of the body, such as around hips or shoulders.

Owing to the absence of fatty tissue in both the asthenic and athletic types, Kretschmer referred to these two types under one main group which he called "leptosomics," a term meaning lean-bodied.

A large percentage of persons of the dysplastic type are afflicted with endocrine disorders. Some psychiatrists believe the incidence of manic depressive psychosis is higher in individuals of the pyknic type than in those of the other types. Schizophrenia is said to be more commonly observed in the asthenic and sometimes in the other two types. This correlation, however, is disputed.

The three main temperament types described by Jung are the extrovert, introvert, and ambivert. The manner of investing life energy distinguishes each type.

Extrovert

Actively aggressive, ambitious, enthusiastic, uninhibited; expresses feeling and relates to other persons readily. Inclined to engage in organization, political, business activities. This type has been linked to the pyknic body physique and manic depressive disorders.

Introvert

Reserved, quiet, shy, contemplative, serious, studious, sensitive; limits social relations and feeling expressions; interests and attention are subjectively directed. Inclined to engage in scientific pursuits and the creative arts. The introvert has been linked to the leptosomic body physique, especially the asthenic type, and schizophrenic reactions.

Ambivert

Possesses characteristics of both the extrovert and introvert, but does not lean too heavily in either direction. Most persons manifest this middle type of personality temperament.

AGE OF COMPLETE DEPENDENCE (BIRTH TO ONE YEAR)

Infancy is known as the age of complete dependency because the baby's survival is dependent upon the ministrations of the mother or mother substitute. All of the basic needs essential for existence (food, warmth, comfort, love, and so on) must be supplied by the mothering figure because the infant is physically incapable of obtaining them or giving anything in return.

The external environment has its conditions for breathing, temperature, maintenance of body circulation, obtaining nourishment and support of body position which are not comparable to those conditions experienced by the infant during embryonic life. The mother's provision of protection, warmth, nourishment, proper support and positioning of the infant's body, and affection given through body contact transfers satisfaction feelings which help the baby to adjust to extrauterine life. Erikson believes that the first demonstration of social trust in the baby is the ease of his feeding, depth of sleep, and relaxation of his bowels.[1]

Because the mother meets the basic needs for existence she becomes the most important figure in the infant's life. At this early stage of life the mother becomes associated with the pleasurable things, also she is the provider of the basic elements of security. This early feeling of pleasurable association may extend into later life. Under threatening circumstances the grown child as well as the adult may appeal to the mother for protection and assistance when security feelings are threatened. The strong desire to be dependent, often observed in the physically mature person, is said to originate from the period of complete dependence. The adult who seeks assistance from the mother when confronted with making decisions and the individual who tends to rely upon and achieve attention and security feelings from a superior are examples of persons who retain such feelings of dependence. There are individuals who are unable to emancipate themselves from parental dependency to a degree that interferes with their emotional growth and development. In the mental hospital we sometimes observe patients who curl up into the fetal position or who become physically inert to the point of requiring attention to their physical needs, such as bathing, dressing, and feeding. Dependency needs may also be shown by individuals in various types of situations and treatment facilities. Nurses may be requested to give attentions, appearing to be unnecessary, which are actually nursing actions which meet dependency needs. When these needs are recognized for what they really are and met by the nurse it often helps to make the patient feel accepted and secure in the nurse-patient relationship. As needs are met and security feelings strengthened the patient can gradually be encouraged to become more self-reliant. Some deprivations are so severe that it may be possible to help an individual meet needs produced by them only in part.

The first year of life is frequently referred to as the "oral stage" of development because the infant's earliest experiences occur through the mouth. The sucking reflex is developed at birth, enabling the child to nurse. The infant cries when hungry or uncomfortable, is fed through the oral route, and explores all new objects within his grasp with the mouth. This early exploration is a manifestation of environmental testing.

Thumb-sucking, a substitute mechanism, develops during this period. The infant will suck his thumb, even when well fed, to achieve oral gratification. The need for oral gratification may extend into later life. Gum-chewing, kissing, drinking, and eating are all pleasurable tension-relieving oral traits. Some persons, even those who have successfully passed through the oral stage of development and are regarded as well-adjusted individuals, resort to oral, tension-relieving actions when confronted with emotional conflict. Observations may be made of emotionally distressed persons who overeat, chain-smoke, and chew. And it is said that the alcoholic patient is as dependent upon the bottle as is the infant.

An infant knows only two sensations—pleasure and discomfort. The baby will cry when hungry or wet until discomfort feelings are replaced with comfort feelings. This early tendency to be concerned only with gratification of self needs is often referred to by psychoanalysts as primary narcissism. It constitutes the utilization of the libidinal drive, the massive force of energy with which the individual is endowed at birth. Narcissism is a term derived from the Greek legend of the youth, Narcissus, who fell in love with his own image and was unable to love anyone but himself. As the infant grows and externalizes his energy the libido is invested in relationships with other significant persons, including the mothering figure, family members, friends, partners in courtship and marriage. Thus, the term "libido" does not mean sexual love only.

Formerly it was believed that it was advisable to prolong responding to the infant's cries. Immediate attention-giving was thought to interfere with the infant's learning to withhold gratification, a requirement for adjusting to life situations. Contemporary authorities believe that an infant's needs should be met as soon as possible in order to strengthen feelings of trust, confidence in others, and security. These feelings facilitate the ability to adjust to life situations which cannot be resolved immediately.

The first six months of life are sometimes referred to as the symbiotic phase of development. During this period the infant's special senses are not developed sufficiently for the child to distinguish himself as a separate being from the mothering figure or other individuals. The mother's breast and body and the infant's body are all one and the same. Around the sixth month of life, or a little earlier in some instances, the infant's special senses are developed to a degree that the baby commences to conceive of himself as a separate being. This development can be observed as the child responds to the mother's coming and going, is sensitive to her presence or absence, follows her movements by focusing vision in her direction, and favors the mother's ministrations and contact to those of other individuals. It is regarded as the beginning of ego development, or the self concept, the ability to distinguish the "I" from the "not I."

The child's interest in the mother's presence and preference for her is considered to be an apparent striving for trust. If the mother responds with actions which engender trust the child is soothed and relaxes. Gradually, the infant learns to anticipate the mother's going and coming and is able to adjust to her normal periods of absence owing to the sense of trust which has been transferred through the mother's responses. It is through conditions of trust perceived by the child that security feelings are achieved which have an important effect upon the child's ability to adjust to more difficult situations and requirements throughout the successive stages of growth and development. If the infant develops feelings of mistrust to a pathological degree, they will influence his subsequent adjustment as well as relationships with other persons. Separation of the child from the mother for a prolonged period, for any reason, after the infant recognizes his separateness as a being can be so traumatic that the child's health and development will be affected. Children subjected to maternal deprivation with its loss of body contact and love have been known to lose weight, become listless, and fail to respond appropriately to their environment. Testing for trust in situations is a behavior which nurses may observe in their relationships with patients and other human beings. Trust is one of the major ingredients of rapport when it is established during health and illness situations. The symbiotic phase of development is of special interest to investigators. Some schizophrenic children who have reached a later chronological age of development appear to be unable to distinguish themselves as separate from other beings.

Weaning is commenced early in our culture, a practice considered to be a deprivation which reduces achievement of oral gratification through sucking. In some cultures, children are weaned much later and may feed at the mother's breast until the age of three years or older. It is believed that replacements of value to the child should accompany deprivations. The infant's taking of nourishment from a cup may be supplemented by allowance to regress to the bottle on occasions and to be spoonfed by the mother.

The infant learns to respond and communicate through perceptions of the mother's actions and voice. Sounds, such as gurgling and cooing, made by the infant, are attempts to emulate the language heard. It is important for the mother to talk to the infant so that verbal communication may be learned. Generally speaking, it is believed that if the mother is a warm, accepting, loving person toward the infant that the child will learn to react toward and relate well with individuals. The child who develops an early sense of trust and security feelings will be better able to adapt and adjust to later social requirements than will the child who has not developed such feelings.

EARLY CHILDHOOD (ONE TO THREE YEARS)

This phase of life is also known as the "habit-training" and "anal" period because the child is toilet trained during this time. Investigators believe that the child who has incorporated feelings of trust, of security, of being wanted and loved will not feel so threatened with the demands of toilet training as will the insecure child. Habit-training represents the first "giving" of the child who has previously received.

The child begins to develop an increasing awareness of himself in relation to other people and environmental objects as he perceives the reactions shown towards him in his attempts to manipulate and control the environment. His sense of self-identification is a product of people's behavior toward him and the roles which they assign to him in relationships. Dependent upon whom he interacts with, the child may be related to as a sibling, playmate, an offspring of parents, a stranger, and so on. Thus, he sees himself in terms of the images other people have of him.

The sense of continuing self-identity is closely allied with the development of the self-esteem. There is a strong urge to explore the environment, to learn how things operate and what can be done with them. When testing actions are forbidden or thwarted, feelings of humiliation, anger, and lowered self-esteem may be experienced by the child. Insistent and resistant actions may be observed in the child's responses. This behavior may be so conspicious that many investigators consider the need for autonomy the outstanding mark of selfhood in the second and third year of life.[1,2]

The striving for autonomy is also apparent during the habit-training process. The child recognizes attitudes of acceptance and rejection in the mother by observations of her facial expressions and gestures when he conforms or fails to conform with the demands of toilet training. When the child conforms by moving his bowels at the appointed time, the mother will smile and be in a complimentary, affectionate mood. When the child does not conform, the mother may scold and admonish him. The child does not want to lose his mother's love. Through reality-testing he eventually learns that conformance will gain her approval and affection. Giving in return for mother's affection will not be so difficult for a child who has felt loved during infancy. But the child who has failed to emerge from the first year of life with such feelings will feel frightened and threatened with greater loss.

As the responses of the mother are perceived, feelings of doubt and shame increase the need to test the mother's trust and love as well as what is socially acceptable and unacceptable. The superego or conscience is an integral aspect of the child's reactions. Shame is an emotion which causes one to feel literally small in relation to others in measures of size and power and prompts the use of face-saving devices. Much of our social life is influenced by the self-esteem. Awareness of this motivates us to use tact in order to avoid offending and injuring another's pride.

A child of this age is aware that he is physically unable to retaliate toward the demands of toilet training. He has not developed physically to the degree of being able to resist such demands with outward physical force. Thus, feelings of anger and hostility are internalized. But the child soon learns that one silent weapon is within his complete control. No one can force him to move his bowels at an appointed time unless he alone is willing. To retaliate toward the demands for conformance, the child may withhold bowel action—a passive-aggressive response. Thus, the striving for autonomy is inherent in decisive action and self-assertion as opposed to the actions of another. The child who continues to experience the need to act out hostility feelings by withholding actions may develop an extreme pattern of negativistic behavior whenever he feels threatened in later life. Persons who withhold information from others in later life may be demonstrating a personality trait carried over from this period of life. Catatonic patients manifest extreme negativistic behavior—a nonverbal expression of "no."

Nurses may observe lesser degrees of negativistic responses in their relationships. Withholding may be observed in passive-aggressive responses, such as procrastination, devious delaying or blocking tactics, making oneself personally inaccessible to other people's company, and the like. The childish trait of negativism may be so well preserved in some adults that they become chronically countersuggestible. Resistance is offered to every proposal and counterargument to every argument. The patient who appears to want things his own way or to tell the nurse how to perform some service may be expressing a residual of the striving for autonomy. On the other hand, one may observe individuals who have so repressed a need for autonomy that helping them to sense with trust the freedom of decision-making and self-expression may be a therapeutic approach which promotes personal growth.

The guilt feelings which arise in persons who harbor hostile thoughts or who project hostility onto others in later life may be turned back upon the self through the mechanism of introjection. Depreciatory estimates of the self may be verbalized as manifestations of a punishment need. Hostility and guilt may be physically introjected through self-mutilation and suicidal actions.

The elimination of feces is a pleasurable act which permits "letting go," reduces tension, and brings feelings of comfort. But the responses of the mother may instill shame feelings. As the child attempts to collect and use feces in play activities, the mother disposes of them and substitutes sand and water. This early tendency to collect and create is extended into later life. We observe individuals who derive satisfaction from stamp, coin, art, and other forms of collection. We also observe an overt manner of collecting and creating in patients who habitually collect and hoard all sorts of odds and ends, such as old newspapers, rags, and strings. These actions may be distressing to psychiatric nurses and aides who have in mind only the health-hazard aspects rather than the motivating underlying-need dynamics. The ingenious nurse or aide who can recognize such needs may draw upon some of the hobbies and crafts taught in mental hospitals to replace these undesirable actions of patients.

The mother who succeeds in toilet training her child at the expense of his developing feelings of rejection, insecurity, lowered self-esteem, hostility, guilt, and anxiety is undoubtedly unaware that these feelings may emerge and develop into later overt behavior responses. The flexible, patient mother who can overlook lack of continuous cooperation from the child with an encouraging, willing-to-wait attitude can do much to foster more favorable feeling responses and behavior. It is said that a mother who emphasizes cleanliness and conformance, who is disapproving and anxious during the habit-training period may rear an anxious child who seeks approval by being overly meticulous and conforming.

LATER CHILDHOOD (THREE TO SIX YEARS)

This is the age when the child becomes sexually aware—another aspect of the developing self concept and sexual identification. Differences in the parents' physiques become apparent and the child behaves curiously about his or her own body. This natural curiosity causes the child to touch and explore his body. Parents may become overly concerned, interpret the child's action as masturbation, and develop threatening attitudes. The boy child may be threatened with loss of his penis and the girl with loss of her hands. Feelings of fear of loss may emerge into what Freud termed the "castration complex"—a sense of being "cut off." When threatened in later life with some great loss, such as the loss of financial security, the death of a family member, or divorce from a loved person, the castration-complex reaction of fear, tension, and anxiety may be reactivated.

In later childhood there develops an awareness that there is an attraction between the parents. A child of this age begins to resent the attention paid by the parent of the opposite sex toward the parent of the child's sex. Still wanting all of the attention and affection, the child develops feelings of hostility and rivalry toward the parent of the same sex. Studying the attributes of the parent of the same sex, he attempts to identify and imitate that parent's mannerisms and dress in order to attract the parent of the opposite sex. Erikson speaks of this behavior as a striving for initiative. In a colloquial sense he calls it being "on the make." This rivalry is termed the "Oedipus complex." (The term has its origin in a Greek legend. Oedipus, a son of the King and Queen of Thebes, separated from his parents in early childhood, met and killed a stranger who was actually his father. Later, he met and married his unrecognized mother.) According to psychoanalytic theory the Oedipus attachment develops into identification with a love object ideal. Frequently a young person chooses a love and marriage partner who possesses personality traits in common with the parent of the opposite sex. In some instances the attachment to the opposite-sex parent becomes so strong that parental fixation develops. The individual may be unable to make a successful adult heterosexual adjustment. There are parents who derive such satisfaction from this strong attachment that they unwittingly encourage it to the detriment of the child's personality adjustment. In some instances we observe adult patients having emotional conflicts involving parental fixation. These persons require psychiatric assistance to gain insight into their problem.

Beginning and subsequent initiative strivings are said to be fraught with guilt feeling reactions, the result of gnawings at the conscience due to having transgressed the parental relationship. Testing for trust extends with the growing realization that the envied relationship between the parents continues. Psychoanalysts speak of the child's unconscious wish to possess the parent of the opposite sex, an incestual longing. Boys and girls who have stated intentions to marry their mothers and fathers have lent credence to these postulations. Rejection feelings emerge as the binding parental relationship, not understood in its totality by the child, remains unchanged. Repression of incestual longings due to guilt has been offered as a dynamic explanation for adult sexual impotence and other deviations. Fetish acts, such as the stealing and possession of garments of a member of the opposite sex, have been analyzed as deviate sexual gratification behaviors. But the castration and Oedipus complex theories continue to be disputed by some investigators who do not believe that they are universal phenomena of human growth and development. According to those who dispute Freud's postulations, not all persons encounter infantile sexual conflicts.

Initiative strivings may be observed in persons who compete—try to impress or conquer—for the sake of winning approval. Some initiative strivings have been interpreted as a drive to prove one's sexual identification. Observations have been made of individuals who repeatedly pursue love objects, the conquest of which strengthens their own sexual identification; but in these individuals there results instead a restlessness and anxiety which never appear to be alleviated. The psychic elements and feelings inherent in a deeply perceived, lasting love relationship are not achieved in conquests motivated by a need to prove one's sexual self.

In the nurse-patient relationship one may observe the striving for initiative in patients who express a need for approval by being overly helpful. Initiative strivings may also be healthy manifestations of a stage of illness which follows regression to a level of behavior where dependency needs must be met by the nurse.

If the parent of the same sex with whom the child identifies is a dominating or poor physical specimen, the child may develop the traits associated with the opposite-sex parent. This process may become the core of severe maladjustment, particularly in the sexual sphere in later life.

When another child is born into the family, the older child, if not prepared for the event, may develop feelings of neglect and jealousy. Parents have been advised to be alert to these possibilities and to show by their words and actions of affection that the older child is still loved.

The older child may develop a competitive type of behavior toward the new child to maintain parental favor. Such behavior is known as "sibling rivalry" and may continue on into adult life. The life histories of many patients reveal varying degrees of sibling rivalry within families. This trait may also be observed as a "carry-over" manifestation when one is interpreting the behavior of individuals who are experiencing difficulty in their relationships with co-workers and associates.

The later childhood period is also referred to by some investigators as the phallic phase of personality development owing to the individual's focus upon genital organ development with its associated reactions.

LATENCY PERIOD (SIX TO TWELVE YEARS)

When the latency stage is reached the child has mastered organ and ambulatory control. However, biological endowment and control are not sufficient for the child to become self-sustaining or a family producer or provider. These abilities require the learning and mastery of more complex tasks through the use of tools available in the environment and interpersonal skills. Strength in one's personal sexual identification is another requirement for normal adult relationships. Endeavoring to be accepted as a member of the peer group and to accomplish the tasks performed in group associations are considered to be industrious strivings. Inferiority feelings may be perceived as the child observes and tries to master new tasks and to overcome interpersonal conflicts which may be threatening to the self-esteem and personal integrity. The need to be accepted and achieve as a member of a productive unit becomes a driving, motivating force.

Attendance at school during this period of life requires that the child leave the intimate family circle for the first time. The interpersonal field is enlarged. Sexual curiosity diminishes and is replaced by the child's absorbing interest in new task experiences and personalities. Redirection of sexual energy into play activity and intellectual curiosity utilizes the sex impulse at this level of personality development. The latent potentiality for normal sexual attraction and activity does not emerge until puberty.

The schoolteacher supplements the mother's role to a degree. From her, the child absorbs ideals, standards, philosophies, and personality traits which may be introjected. It is not unusual to observe children of this age group playing school and enacting the teacher's role. Thus, the continuing development of the self concept may be influenced through new observations and learnings associated with the latency period.

Inferiority feelings may motivate industrious striving towards the mastery of new tasks performed. Much energy is expended in group play—climbing trees, rolling hoops, playing house or cowboys, tossing ball, and so on. The basic need for group acceptance causes the child to make adaptations and adjustments in behavior.

Interpersonal relations with members of the same sex increase. Boys associate with boys mostly, and girls form friendships with other girls. The opposite sex is frequently ridiculed and obviously bypassed as companion ties with members of the same sex are strengthened. This tendency to prefer the companionship of one's own sex is considered a normal homosexual phase of development which aids in establishing personal sexual identification. It is usually outgrown during adolescence. Conflicts in sexual identification which indicate that such identification has been weakened or arrested at the latency level homosexual phase are observed in adult life.

Conflicts in interpersonal relations in adult life are sometimes traced to the difficulties experienced in group association during the latency period. The adult who fears group contacts, maintains social distance from others, and refrains from competitive activities may have strong inferiority and inadequacy feelings originating in the latency period.

The need to learn higher-level and new tasks is essential for being self-sustaining in the community, a principle which underlies the rehabilitation of patients. Motivation of industrious strivings may be necessary to help patients to overcome inadequacy feelings in order to make adaptations required for learning new ways to cope with physical infirmities and interpersonal disturbance accompaniments of mental illness.

Generally speaking, the latency period provides the early conditions and experiences for development of independence and self-sustenance. Removed from constant parental influence and protection, the child frequently finds it necessary to defend himself physically, adjust to others, and make compromises if he wishes to be accepted and approved on his own merit.

PUBERTY AND ADOLESCENCE (12 TO 21 YEARS)

Childhood comes to an end with the advent of puberty, a period of two to three years which precedes adolescence. Secondary sexual characteristics develop with the emergence of the sex impulse and body physical changes. Physical development is an individualistic process. Girls usually commence to develop earlier than do boys. Climate may influence the time when physical changes occur. In warm climates these changes have been observed as early as the tenth year of life. In cold climates it may not commence until the child has reached the age of 16 years.

Boys manifest change in the voice tone and growth of pubic and axillary hair and a beard. Erotic dreams accompanied by nocturnal emissions may be a disturbing experience for some boys. Girls commence to develop changes in body contours; their breasts enlarge—pubic and axillary hair appears and menstruation begins.

Menstruation may be welcomed as a sign of approaching womanhood by girls who are well informed. Its onset may be psychologically disturbing to some adolescent girls who may fear or resent it or harbor hostile attitudes toward it—the attitudes directed toward the mother, as if the mother had imposed a burden which must be endured. Other conflicts may involve fear of social relations with men or envy of the masculine role. Some girls may refuse to discuss the menses as if attempting to deny their occurrence and their own femininity.

This is a period in life when the emotions are heightened. It is a very insecure phase of development. The adolescent realizes that he is neither child nor adult. The outstanding conflicts of this stage of growth concern role identifications. There is a striving to identify with and be accepted into the adult group as well as to identify with an occupational role. Lack of definite status produces feelings of inferiority and inadequacy which the person may attempt to compensate for with behavior which can be very trying for both the adolescent and those in his environment. The teenager who is trying to gain acceptance and social status may exhibit loud, boisterous behavior, demanding attitudes, exhibitionistic dress, show of material possessions, and expressions of strong opinions in current world and home affairs.

The adolescent boy may associate with the gang and the adolescent girl with her clique. These friendly ties help to strengthen the adolescents' sexual identification and provide opportunities for social activities and discussions of mutual interest. In some instances the gang and clique associations have resulted in delinquent behavior and difficulties with the law. It is generally believed that much of this might be prevented if parents had better insight into the needs of adolescents and devoted more time to the development of constructive activities and learning experiences for them. The many youth organizations which have developed in American communities help adolescents to socialize in planned, supervised activities, which utilize their energies constructively and achieve satisfactions for them.

Wanting independence from parents and other adults who represent control, teenagers may talk a language which only they understand. Slang excludes the adults, permitting, at the same time, the expression of hostility, which cannot be vented through direct criticism.

The problems associated with adolescence in the American culture are not observed in some primitive cultures which have been studied by anthropologists. In these societies, ceremonies, known as rites of passage, to admit the youth into adult society are performed when puberty is reached. Special privileges denoting adult status are conferred. Preparation for responsibility, including occupational task learning, family life, and perpetuation of customs, and mores is commenced.

With the reawakening of the sex impulse the conflicts of later childhood may be reactivated. There may be a renewal of the attraction between the adolescent and the parent of the sex opposite to that of the adolescent. Unconscious guilt feelings may motivate the adolescent to do something which rejects and alienates the parent of the opposite sex. At the same time there develop rebellious attitudes toward the influence and control of the parent of the same sex as that of the adolescent.

Normal heterosexual attraction helps to resolve the Oedipus conflict, to achieve emancipation from parents, and to weaken ties with the gang or clique. Erikson considers "falling in love" during this stage an attempt to clarify one's sexual identification through the eyes and reflections of the opposite sex rather than an urge for intimate sexual relations. Thus, adolescents often prefer to discuss and settle matters of mutual identification and interest than to embrace.

If the Oedipus complex is not resolved or if sexual identification is not well established, the associated conflicts may extend into adult life.

YOUNG ADULTHOOD

In young adulthood there is a striving for a basic sense of intimacy which can be achieved only if the individual has emerged successfully from the earlier struggles of establishing personal identification. When one is free from identification conflicts there is an ability to relate well with others, form friendships, and engage in a normal heterosexual relationship. There is a desire, ability, and willingness to share a mutual trust and to regulate work, procreation, and recreation to a satisfying degree essential for harmonious integration of the personality with the environment. Feeling certain about one's personal identification instills confidence feelings which foster success in relations with others. Persons who do not have a strong sense of self-identification may avoid normal social contacts, develop feelings of isolation from others, and become preoccupied in self-absorbing activity. Disturbances in interpersonal relations may be observed, some of which are more obvious and profound than others. The striving for intimate, satisfying experiences in work, love, and play may be observed in overtures made to relate to others and attempts to participate by the individual who continues the struggle to achieve harmonious emotional integration. Recognizing these behaviors and responding to them appropriately are nursing functions which can aid in strengthening the individual's self concept and the capacity to integrate.

ADULTHOOD

Establishing and guiding the next generation are the primary responsibilities of adulthood. If one's generative energy is not invested in family relationships and guidance it may be directed constructively into some creation which absorbs the intellect and interest and results in some socially useful contribution. An individual who cannot achieve a basic sense of useful generativity may experience instead an aura of personal stagnation and interpersonal impoverishment. There are adults who experience conflicts fraught with a pervading sense of not having made the best, fullest contribution or achieved to their satisfaction. Helping such individuals to invest themselves in activities which utilize their energies constructively for their own as well as other persons' benefit produces feeling responses which aid in strengthening personality development.

MATURITY

Maturity is considered to represent the complete physical and emotional development of the individual. Although most persons attain complete physical development by the age of 21 years, it is generally believed that the majority do not attain complete emotional development until much later. Perhaps the largest number of individuals reach maturity sometime during the fourth decade of life. Usually they have undergone many necessary adjustments and, in the light of their own experiences, have by this time a greater appreciation for the inevitable frustrations which are experienced by human beings in a constantly changing economic and social structure. Some persons never reach maturity and may be observed manifesting immature behavior. Through a thorough study of these individuals' physical and emotional development, the level of their manifest behavior may be recognized. An important step in the medical treatment of these persons consists in helping to reeducate and rehabilitate them toward a mature level of behavior.

Erikson speaks of the mature individual as one who has achieved a sense of integrity. According to him, the mature person has achieved harmonious emotional integration which enables him to participate in the social systems of the culture (religion, politics, science, arts, etc.) as well as to accept the responsibility of leadership. One who has integrity is able to accept the happenings of the past and to defend one's way of living as well as the culture. When the past cannot be accepted, there develops a sense of despair that it is too late to try out new routes toward the achievement of integrity. Death is feared. Erikson views Webster's definition of trust, "the assured reliance on another's integrity," as significant. Visualizing a relationship between infantile trust and integrity, he concludes that healthy children will not fear life if their parents have integrity not to fear death.

SUGGESTED REFERENCES

Allport, G.: Pattern and Growth in Personality Development. Holt, Rinehart & Winston, New York, 1961.
Breckenridge, M., and Vincent, E.: Child Development. W. B. Saunders Co., Philadelphia, 1965.
Bueker, K.: Adolescents need attention. Am. J. Nurs. 60: 372 (March), 1960.
English, O.: Emotional Problems of Living. W. W. Norton & Co., New York, 1964.

Erikson, E.: Childhood and Society. W. W. Norton & Co., New York, 1963, p. 247.

Hurlock, E.: Child Development. McGraw-Hill Book Co., New York, 1964.

Kalkman, M.: Psychiatric Nursing. McGraw-Hill Book Co., New York, 1967, p. 15.

Kolb, L.: Noyes' Modern Clinical Psychiatry, ed. 7. W. B. Saunders Co., Philadelphia, 1968, p. 34.

Leavitt, S., Gofman, H., et al.: A guide to normal development in the child. Nurs. Outlook 13: 56 (Sept.), 1965.

Martin, M.: The development of the conscience. J. Psychiat. Nurs. 2: 62 (Jan.), 1964.

Melat, S.: The development of trust. Perspect. Psychiat. Care 3: 28, 1965.

Noyes, A., and Kolb, L.: Modern Clinical Psychiatry, ed. 7. W. B. Saunders Co., Philadelphia, 1968, p. 374.

Ribble, M.: The Rights of Infants. Columbia University Press, New York, 1965.

Rouslin, S.: Interpersonal stabilization of an intrapersonal problem. Nurs. Forum 3: 69, 1964.

Stastny, J.: Helping a patient learn to trust. Perspect. Psychiat. Care 7: 16, 1965.

Stringer, M.: Therapeutic nursing intervention following derogation of the nurse by the patient. Perspect. Psychiat. Care 4: 36, 1965.

Waechter, E.: Recent research in child development. Nurs. Forum 8: 374 (Fall), 1969.

FOOTNOTES

1. Erikson, E.: Childhood and Society. W. W. Norton & Co., New York, 1963, pp. 247, 253.
2. Allport, G.: Pattern and Growth in Personality. Holt, Rinehart & Winston, New York, 1961, p. 118.

For reviewing this chapter, grateful acknowledgment is made to Mrs. Leone Cox, R.N., Miss Elizabeth Maloney, R.N., Mrs. Gloria Matulis, R.N., and Mrs. Jeanette Van Orden, R.N.

CHAPTER 11

Concepts of Anxiety,
Frustration, and Conflict

ANXIETY IN MENTAL ILLNESS

The concept that mental illness can be understood as an individual's reaction to unbearable anxiety has been widely recognized. Mentally disturbed people attempt to alleviate anxiety through mental symptoms which are expressions of unbearable anxiety. Thus, mental illness and mental symptoms are regarded as products of anxiety as well as defenses against it.

ANXIETY RESPONSES

Anxiety is a phenomenon of human existence which every individual experiences at times to a lesser or greater degree. It is a subjective or feeling experience which is not confined to the mentally disturbed.

As a manifestation of human behavior, anxiety is an invisible form of energy, the presence of which is perceived subjectively by the person experiencing its effects. Affectively, it is an unpleasant, diffuse, vague and frequently unexplainable feeling of apprehension, uncertainty and helplessness which interferes with an individual's thinking and concentration.

Mild anxiety may serve as a normal response to alert the person experiencing it to protect the self against anything which may threaten the person's manifested attitude or a way of behaving which has been acquired in the process of attempting to resolve problematical life situations. Moderate and more severe degrees of anxiety may be perceived as an all-pervasive distressing feeling response to a threat perceived, motivating defensive behaviors which are consciously or unconsciously aimed to reduce or alleviate anxiety's associated discomfort.

OBSERVATION OF ANXIETY

Varying degrees of anxiety may be detected in numerous behavior manifestations, such as changes in voice tone, rate of speech, preoccupation with thoughts, increased talking about a particular topic, avoidance of a conversation topic, or blocking of communication. Anxiety may also be observed as an inherent aspect of restlessness, perspiration, fatigue, palpitation, increased respiration and pulse rate, frequent urination, anorexia, insomnia, tremor, sensation of a lump in the throat, vomiting, diarrhea, changes in abdominal sensations, pupillary reactions, and the like. When anxiety is severe the person may feel helpless to the extent of being immobilized in thought and action. In rare instances, when defenses against anxiety fail to bring relief the person may experience a state of panic or terror. During these times the person concentrates all attention and energy upon a goal of escape from unbearable anxiety. If these attempts to relieve anxiety fail, there results a temporary disintegration of the personality with random destructive tendencies against the self or others. Fortunately, panic and terror states are short-lived conditions owing to the human organism's quick defenses for overcoming effects which prolonged duration of panic or terror would exert.

THEORIES OF ANXIETY

Various theories have been offered concerning the dynamics which give rise to anxiety as a subjective experience. Anxiety has been discussed as a consequence of separation from the mother at birth. Rank viewed this as the earliest emotionally traumatic, threatening experience. From the period of infancy, anxiety's subsequent increase in power as a perceptual response has been linked to additional separation experiences at various phases of personality development and individuation. This hypothesis includes separation at the time of weaning to separation from people at death.

The most commonly shared hypothesis concerning the dynamics of anxiety is that which originated with Freud but which Sullivan incorporated later into his interpersonal theory, with a different explanation from that of Freud. Sullivan's concept views anxiety as a perceptual response aroused by the emerging power of formerly repressed unacceptable thoughts, feelings, drives, wishes, and action. Sullivan considered these forbidden inner experiences to be interpersonal ones whereas Freud viewed them as repressed instinctual or innate drives.

According to the interpersonal theory, anxiety is experienced as the anticipated disapproval or loss of love from the significant people of an individual's early life relationships from whom the anxious person learned to discriminate between acceptable and unacceptable drives, attitudes, and actions. Later on in life this anticipation of disapproval may be transferred from the original significant people who educated the individual to persons having emotional significance with whom the individual interacts. Disapproval by significant people is thought to be vital enough to account for severe anxiety reactions. The origin of these responses has been linked to the infant's needs for dependency upon the earliest mothering persons for fulfillment of basic needs.

According to Sullivan, the child's need for love and approval, as well as the anxiety associated with rejection and disapproval, is utilized by the significant adults during the early processes of educating the child for interpersonal adjustment, socialization, and acculturalization.

Horney envisions a central relatedness between anxiety and hostility. Hostility is anticipated by others during interaction and sensed by the anxious person himself. Anxiety is thought of as being related to a fear of disruption of one's interpersonal relationships. Considered together these viewpoints imply acceptance of the concept that anxiety is connected with anticipated fear of disapproval and punishment, withdrawal of love, disruption of interpersonal relationships, isolation, or separation. Frieda Fromm Reichmann connects all of these explanations of anxiety to her conclusion that anxiety has a close psychological affinity to loneliness. She believes that the emotional states referred to as anxiety by theorists are actually states of loneliness or fear of loneliness.[1]

CONFLICTS CAUSING ANXIETY

The conflicts most likely to cause anxiety are those concerning a person's social relations with other individuals which involve ethical standards maintained by one's cultural or social group for the purposes of exerting controls over behavior influencing personality development. Through verbal and nonverbal communications people form relationships with other individuals and become a part of their social environment. Owing to the need to be dependent upon others for survival it becomes necessary to accommodate one's self to seemingly stronger and superior persons in an individual's surroundings. As physical, emotional, and intellectual growth lead to various stages of individual emancipation, the person gains a certain amount of independence. During the process of maturation, certain demands are made upon the growing person; these demands are gradually incorporated into the developing personality. As a result of this process, the person always carries within himself the memory of his experiences with the significant persons of his past (mother, father, siblings, and others). Although there is a tendency to prolong the pleasant experiences, the agreeable, as well as the distressing, events of the past continue to be remembered owing to the person's capacity for selective memory.

CLARIFICATION OF ANXIETY

The concept of anxiety may be clarified by pointing out the differences between it and fear, with which it is closely associated. Fear is a response to an objective threat. The threatening stimulus is an external danger which the person and others recognize. For instance, the person may fear dogs. All dogs, even those who are friendly and held by a leash, are feared for what they symbolize. Thus, the specific danger perceived is on a conscious, discriminating level. Fear tends to be an acute, temporary response to some localized danger which subsides when the danger has passed. Anxiety is a response to a subjective or internal danger. The experience is often on an unconscious, undiscriminating level. The distress is usually not recognized for what it is and is often said to be unexplainable. Anxiety tends to be a chronic reaction, an all-pervasive feeling, a more fluid response which is sometimes described as being "free floating" and unattached to a specific, identifiable threat. When it is unidentifiable an anxious person may say, "I feel jittery, as if something terrible is going to happen, but I don't know why. I can't think of anything that should make me feel this way." There is no clear-cut object or circumstance to which the individual can attribute the feeling stated. The person's capacity to utilize the mechanism of repression may have dissociated emotionally traumatic experience from the affective response.

NORMAL ANXIETY

Generally speaking, normal anxiety is not out of proportion to the threat perceived. The person is on the alert, sees, hears and grasps more than previously. An individual experiencing it does not have to manage anxiety by using defenses (mechanisms) which force it out of conscious awareness. Instead, its existence is recognized and faced realistically by attempting to alter or resolve the situational circumstances recognized as causative or motivating forces.

ABNORMAL ANXIETY

Abnormal anxiety responses seen in the neuroses and psychoses are out of proportion to the actual threat perceived. The person's perceptual sphere of awareness is narrowed as the focus of attention, thinking and communication is drawn toward the anxiety-producing conflict. The anxious person hears, sees and grasps less of what is going on outside of the sphere of awareness but can be directed toward movement away from the immediate focus through the intervention of other individuals. When anxiety is severe, the person's perceptual field is greatly reduced. The focus is upon detail or many scattered details associated with conflictual elements. In states of panic the detail previously focused upon is elaborated upon and becomes an exclusive interest.

FRUSTRATION AND CONFLICT

Anxiety is said to be a product of frustration. Anything that interferes with or blocks one's drive to attain a need or a desired goal which would achieve feelings of satisfaction and security is considered an obstacle or barrier constituting a frustration. Obstacles may be active or passive, animate or inanimate, personal or impersonal. Intense interference with one's desires and needs arouses in the individual feelings of helplessness, disappointment, inadequacy and anxiety. The source of frustrations may be external, such as active or passive actions of interfering individuals who seek to thwart another's progress toward a desired goal. A person may set goals which are not realistic in terms of achievement or another individual, such as a parent, may set goals for the person which are not desired nor possible.

When frustration is experienced repeatedly, owing to obstacles which prevent attainment of the goal, anxiety is felt. This uncomfortable state of tension is perceived as a personal threat to one's security and motivates defensive behavior in the individual. Three possible responses to frustration may be observed: (1) the person may change the goal to one which he has a better chance of attaining, (2) the goal may be abandoned so that one simply withdraws and dissociates the feelings experienced with its frustration, such as aggression, as well as those needs for satisfaction and security which were not achieved, and (3) the individual may try to work around the goal and achieve it through the use of a fixed response or mental mechanisms which had been used successfully in similar past situations. When mechanisms fail, the person resorts to pathological behavior which may be observed in the aggression, withdrawal, apathy, and somatizing behavior of the mentally ill.

Frustrations of all kinds which increase the anxiety and tension under which we live are experienced in our complex society. Every social regulation, world crisis, cold war maneuver, and act of racial strife increases frustrations and tensions. Each person must learn to cope effectively with them or suffer the discomfort of stresses which develop when we are unable to adapt to the prevailing conditions. Technological advances have helped to overcome the frustrations experienced by our ancestors as they attempted to solve problems related to the improvement of living and health conditions. There has been much less progress in solving the frustrations which occur during interpersonal relationships. No completely satisfactory way of living in harmony with other persons has been discovered.

Mental conflict is an internal source of frustration having one feature similar to frustration. In both frustration and mental conflict the individual is prevented, at least temporarily, from attaining the goal. Here the similarity ends. In conflict there are two opposing or incompatible drives or action systems. The person is required to make a choice between the possible responses, both of which have either a negative or positive value to him. The conscious difficulty experienced in making the choice constitutes the conflict which causes the person to hesitate, vacillate or be unable to decide upon a course of action to reach the goal. Most conflict situations are of relatively short duration. Resolution is effected when one action is inhibited and the other freed. When both operate the individual is unable to act, and confusion or inability to make an adjustment occurs. This may happen in the following types of conflict situations:

When both choices have value for the person so that making a choice is difficult.

Both choices may be unpleasant alternatives, causing the individual to vacillate and weigh one against the other for the lesser of two evils.

Realization that attainment of the valued goal is overshadowed by negative, threatening consequences.

PSYCHOTIC AND NEUROTIC BEHAVIOR

From a quantitative point of view a person is considered to be psychotic when the anxiety indicative of conflict results in a marked disturbance of personality functioning which temporarily or permanently affects the whole person to the extent that the individual is unable to take care of himself and requires the assistance and support of others. The neurotic reaction is a partial disturbance in personality functioning which never totally incapacitates the individual. The terms "psychotic" and "neurotic" do not describe causal factors. Neither do they imply which mental functions are primarily impaired. The following changes in personality functioning are considered to be cardinal characteristics of a psychotic reaction:

Distortion of interpretation of reality

Deviation from culture and logic of environment
Disorder in mood of a severe degree
Reversion to primitive biologic behavior patterns
Personality disintegration
Temporary or permanent reduction in level of awareness[2]

FEELING COMPONENTS OF ANXIETY

The feeling components of anxiety may be more obvious and identifiable by both the anxious person and observers than is the anxiety state of which feelings are an integral aspect. The anxious person may be completely unaware that his feelings actually constitute an anxiety state unless he has some insight into the phenomenon. What is talked about or acted out are the predominant feeling components experienced by the individual.

The feeling of fear may be very intense. The anxious person will make references to the specific object feared when the object is recognized (example, phobia). When anxiety is "free floating" and unattached, the person will usually talk about the fear element perceived, but state that its specific attachment is unexplainable.

Degrees of feelings of anger may be expressed through various behaviors, such as irritation, exasperation, resentment, flare of temper, and show or talk of hate and rage. Anger may be expressed not because the outer provocation is great, but because some thwarting or blocking experience touches off the displacement of inner feeling. The underlying motivation for expressions of anger may be rooted in entirely different sources or former experiences unrelated to the happening in which the feeling is released.

In the hospital, patients sometimes displace hostility formerly felt, but repressed, toward significant persons in their natural environment onto authority figures or other patients. The internalization of hostility is deep rooted in the early education for socialization process with its rewards for acceptable behavior. The social environment of the hospital serves as an acting-out, hostility-release setting.

Depression is a feeling involving an element of sadness and helplessness. There is little drive for socialization or communication. Although depression is the predominant, outward feeling shown, the fear, anger, and guilt components of anxiety are internalized or turned inward upon the self. The fear of unleashing anger or hostility, or exposing to others guilt-producing unacceptable thoughts and wishes, reinforces the learning of the internalization of anxiety. The individual has learned during the socialization process to anticipate rejection, disapproval and loss of love leading to disruption in interpersonal relations.

Another accompaniment of anxiety is, curiously enough, what appears on the surface to be an absence of feeling. The patient may say, "I feel dead," "I feel numb all over," or "I feel empty." In some instances the patient does not communicate. It is as if the individual has internalized the component feelings of anxiety so well that they have been deposited into a freezing compartment of the self system from which their emergence with emotionally painful accompaniments is blocked. Freezing of feelings may be observed in catatonic stupor and deep depression. I believe this reaction to be different than immobilization of thought and action which may occur in severe anxiety.

Ambivalent feelings may also be components of anxiety. The coexistence of love and hate feelings toward another individual, such as is sometimes expressed toward a parent figure, is sometimes obvious in a person's communications and acting-out behavior.

Masked feelings may be components of anxiety. The anxiety associated with showing open hostility may produce a superficial show of love which masks the underlying hostility. For instance, there are men and women who feel basically hostile toward the opposite sex owing to earlier rejection experiences. The presence of the opposite sex is a threatening experience which triggers anxiety so that the person is alerted to avoid the anticipated rejection. The action is often at the unconscious level of behavior.

THREATS PRODUCING ANXIETY

The kinds of threats which produce anxiety vary widely with different people as does the ability to tolerate degrees of anxiety. Generally speaking, anything which threatens the self security of the individual may produce anxiety. When there is anticipation that the basic needs for human existence may be withdrawn (examples: acceptance, love, dependence, self esteem) the self system is threatened.

COPING WITH ANXIETY

Horney views attempts to cope with anxiety as being learned during the early years of personality development. Controls and restrictions which block or thwart the child's attempts to be a person in his own right and express energy freely produce anxiety. Linked to this is a feeling of helplessness. A child in such circumstances, unable to show open resistance, feels frustrated. Blocking of the child's attempts to achieve self realization may be the behavior of elders who actually love the child. Their actions may be due to problems and anxieties which they experience and which interfere with their ability to notice, accept and help the child to develop behaviors which permit free expression. To cope with the inner uncomfortable response to outer threat, the growing child develops defenses which may become strongly entrenched, acquired personality traits. When these ways of coping with inner discomfort are threatened, as happens when they conflict with the demands and expectations of reality, anxiety arises. Three major defense patterns may be acquired to dispel anxiety. They seldom appear in pure form. The person using them may use different ones in different circumstances. These ways of coping with anxiety are not considered to be signs of disturbance in themselves.

1. Moving against: The person becomes aggressive, competitive, seeks to rise above others, to control others, and may attack in various ways.

2. Moving away: The individual remains emotionally uninvolved by withdrawing, remaining aloof and detached from a situation.

3. Moving forward: The person may conform to the situation, accept substitutes or practice appeasement towards others.

SECURITY OPERATIONS

These behaviors are so named because they are an individual's way of protecting the self and maintaining interpersonal security. Compulsive actions, such as frequent handwashing or precise ways of performing some activity in a ritual-like manner, are behaviors which prevent the emergence of unacceptable, anxiety-threatening thoughts, wishes and feelings.

ANXIETY IS A NURSING PROBLEM

Anxiety is one of the basic problems associated with nursing care. During illness, there may be many anxiety-creating situations. There are greater opportunities for anxiety to threaten the patient when the illness is prolonged and serious, but minor and short-term illness experiences may also produce anxiety. Being human, the nurse may also perceive anxiety which may be sensed by and communicated to patients. Thus, it is important for nurses to have some insight into the phenomenon of anxiety.

USING ANXIETY FOR LEARNING IN NURSING

The nurse can learn to recognize anxiety in herself when it is perceived, understand its motivation, and how to manage it. Sometimes this learning is acquired by talking over anxiety-creating situations with another person who can view them more objectively. Self awareness, developed through personal experiences with anxiety, can lead to learning how to make help-giving approaches to anxious patients. Using anxiety to learn requires enduring the anxiety while searching out causes and developing a successful response to replace the former unsuccessful approach. Helping patients to alleviate anxiety is a skill. The nurse's ability to detect anxiety and respond in ways which help the patient to clarify the nurse's observations so that subsequent nursing approaches lead to learning for the patient requires a willingness to listen, careful observation, and the making of thoughtful responses which lead to learning. A nurse who has unmet needs of her own, however, will not be able to give attention to the cues in situations which lead to the identification of anxiety in patients.

Helping the patient to cope with anxiety requires that the nurse first learn to recognize anxiety in the patient. When anxiety is observed the nurse may help the patient to develop an awareness of its presence by making an inquiry, such as, "Is something bothering you?" or "Are you uncomfortable?" or "Are you upset about something?" The patient may or may not say "yes" immediately. Additional interaction and communication may lead to the patient's acknowledgement of discomfort feelings. The nurse may then try to get the patient to connect the present discomfort with similar past discomfort experienced and to recall what actions produced relief. For instance, the nurse might ask, "What do you do when you feel like this to feel more comfortable?" The next step in the process of helping patients to identify and cope with anxiety is to try to get the patient to identify and describe situations and interactions which go on immediately before the episode of anxiety is experienced. This approach helps the patient to connect cause with effect. It helps the individual to improve his ability to make connections between remote past experiences and immediate situations as well as the more inclusive pathology of the disorder he is experiencing. Hopefully, the patient will, as a result of this learning, be able to participate with greater self awareness in counseling sessions with therapists.[3]

SUGGESTED REFERENCES

Aasterud, M.: Defenses against anxiety. Nurs. Forum 1: 35 (Summer), 1962.
Berblinger, K.: Psychiatric Perspectives in Medicine. Reprinted from "Psychosomatics," Vol. 2, #6, 1961, Vol. 3, #1, #2, 1962.
Garre, W.: Basic Anxiety. Philosophical Library Inc., New York, 1962.
Heckel, R., and Jordan, R.: Psychology—The Nurse and the Patient. C. V. Mosby Co., St. Louis, 1967, p. 213.
Nehren, J., and Gilliam, N.: Separation anxiety. Am. J. Nurs. 65: 109 (Jan.), 1965.
Neylan, M.: Anxiety. Am. J. Nurs. 62: 110 (May), 1962.
O'Hara, F., and Reith, H.: Frustration and adjustments. Chap. 7 in Psychology and the Nurse. W. B. Saunders Co., Philadelphia, 1966, p. 124.

Paul, L.: Crisis intervention. Ment. Hyg. 50: 141 (Jan.), 1966.
Peplau, H.: Interpersonal techniques: the crux of psychiatric nursing. Am. J. Nurs. 62: 53 (June), 1962.
Stein, M., and Vidich, A., et al.: Identity and Anxiety. The Free Press, Glencoe, Ill., 1960.
Tarnower, W.: Psychological needs of the hospitalized patient. Nurs. Outlook 13: 28 (July), 1965.

FOOTNOTES

1. Stein, M., and Vidich, A., et al.: Identity and Anxiety. The Free Press, Glencoe, Ill., 1960, chapter by Frieda Fromm Reichmann, p. 129.
2. Berblinger, K.: Psychiatric Perspectives in Medicine. Reprinted from "Psychomatics," Vol. 2, #6, 1961, Vol. 3, #1, #2, 1962, p. 8.
3. Peplau, H.: Interpersonal techniques: the crux of psychiatric nursing. Am. J. Nurs. 62: 53 (June), 1962.

For reviewing this chapter, grateful acknowledgement is made to Mrs. Ruth Connelly, R.N., Mrs. Leone Cox, R.N., Mrs. Jane Rosamilia, R.N., Miss Elizabeth Maloney, R.N., and Miss Emma Manfreda, R.N.

CHAPTER 12

Mental Mechanisms

The terms "Mental Mechanisms," "Mental Dynamisms," and "Mental Defenses" are used interchangeably in psychiatry when discussing methods used by individuals to resolve mental conflict. All human beings use mental mechanisms to alleviate the anxiety perceived during times of stress and strain. Just as our bodies have physical defenses which combat disease conditions, such as the action of white blood cells, so do they possess mental defenses which aid in the resolution of mental conflict.

Ordinarily, the rational use of a defense mechanism will help to resolve a conflict and reduce or alleviate the tension and anxiety produced by it. When mechanisms fail to resolve emotional conflict, an individual's defenses may become pathological to the extent of attracting attention and requiring treatment and sometimes hospitalization. Overt pathological manifestations of mental mechanisms represent attempts to resolve overwhelming mental conflict. Pathological defenses may be observed in the behavior of patients showing ritualistic behavior, those who deny reality and phantasize, as well as others.

It is generally believed that by the tenth year of life defense mechanisms are well established. These mechanisms are characteristic ways of behaving in response to situations which threaten the security of the self system. Mental mechanisms may be used consciously or unconsciously. They are seldom used alone but are more often used in combination with one another. They may be viewed as reactions to conflict which are associated with one of the three major defense patterns: moving against, moving away, and moving toward (see p. 142).

REPRESSION

This is a common mechanism which is first unconsciously used in very early life. Unpleasant, unacceptable thoughts, desires, and impulses are stored in the unconscious mind. Although the material is not admitted to conscious awareness, it is not forgotten. Some persons call the process of repression "selective forgetting." Others say it is "selective remembering." In later life, these experiences may invade conscious awareness to become the core of pathological behavior. During nurse-patient relationships, patients often unconsciously avoid discussing those repressed anxiety producing experiences which are emotionally difficult to verbalize. Repressed experiences may be recalled under certain conditions. As trust develops and anxiety is reduced in the nurse-patient relationship, the patient may be able to discuss emotionally painful repressed experiences. Narcotherapy and hypnotism may also be used to bring repressed material to the conscious level. The development of self-awareness by the nurse is a process which recognizes the influence of repressed experience upon behavior.

SUPPRESSION

Suppression resembles repression because it is also a mechanism which permits the individual to store away or forget unpleasant, emotionally painful experiences. It is the conscious, deliberate forcing of unpleasant anxiety-producing experiences into the unconscious mind. The patient avoids talking about a situation or becoming involved in facing it realistically. Some examples of the behaviors symbolizing suppression are such responses as, "I'd rather not talk about it." "I'll think about it tomorrow." "Don't talk about that." It is not uncommon for the nurse to have a patient she visits remark, "I don't feel like talking." "I've got nothing to tell you."

RATIONALIZATION *leads to delusions grandeur persecu*

Rationalization may be consciously or unconsciously used, but it is more often used on the level of awareness. It is a defense which explains and justifies an individual's ideas, actions, and feelings in a plausible light. The person states reasons which favor approval of his behavior by others. Rationalization helps to "save face" in embarrassing and anxiety producing situations. Patients have been known to rationalize their admission to the mental hospital with the explanation, "I'm really not sick. I'm just in here to get a rest." Rationalization is also used to soften the disappointments connected with unobtainable goals, such as, "John really loved me, but he married Helen because he felt sorry for her." Some of the factual reasons associated with a situation are deliberately ignored or not stated.

DENIAL

This is a mechanism used to evade or escape the unpleasant or disagreeable realities of living by ignoring or refusing to acknowledge their existence. People sometimes ignore or deny criticism expressed about them. Few individuals accept the full inevitability of death. We may turn away from unpleasant sights and cannot endure discussing them. In various ways, the aged often deny evidence of their physical decline. Schizophrenic patients may deny and withdraw from the emotionally painful aspects of the real world with its anxiety producing situations.

COMPENSATION

Compensation is used when a person attempts to overcome some inability or inferiority. This defense helps to maintain one's self-respect and raise the self-esteem. Compensatory or compromise feelings of satisfaction are achieved through successful actions or developments which make up for the lack of satisfactions in the area of the person's inabilities or inadequacies. When this mechanism is used there is some relationship between the inadequacy or inferiority and the compensating act or development. For instance, the unsuccessful actor may turn to playwriting or producing. An unattractive person may dress like a fashion plate to attract the admiration of others. A short person may compensate by talking loudly and at length on a topic as if attempting to gain acceptance and approval through intellectual stature. A person who overeats may be compensating for a lack of approval and affection.

OVERCOMPENSATION reaction formation

This mechamism is sometimes called "reaction formation." Unconscious attitudes and desires may be repressed and replaced by the adoption of conscious attitudes and behavior which are just the opposite of the unconscious ones. Essentially, it is doing the opposite to conceal a socially unacceptable desire or feeling which, if openly expressed, could lead to emotional conflict. An individual may show extreme concern for the welfare or health of someone he does not like. A person having a strong desire to drink alcohol may condemn the use of alcohol by others. It is said that some individuals who hold puritanical views toward or crusade against sexual life may be unconsciously protecting themselves against the release of their own erotic impulses. A patient who feels hostile and angry may overcompensate by withholding these feelings and instead verbalize sentiments of warmth, affection, and appreciation towards another, such as,

"Honey, you're so good to me, so wonderful and kind." Overcompensation may also be used to offset the unpleasantness and distress of failure as the individual attempts to achieve a goal which is the opposite of the first, unobtainable goal.

SUBSTITUTION

unacceptable or unattainable goal is replaced by one that is more acceptable to the ind — adopting children

This is a compromise mechanism which is used when the goal is blocked. It is the acceptance of something else in place of a desired object or need when the original cannot be obtained. The substitute is easier to obtain, socially acceptable, and helps to achieve, at least, partial gratification. A rejected suitor might utilize substitution by accepting the affection of another love object. Pathological use of this mechanism may be observed in the behavior of the alcoholic person who resorts to the bottle for the temporary relief of anxiety to the extent of incurring social disapproval. This is a mechanism which is often confused with the defense sublimation with which it has no connection unless the two are used together.

DISPLACEMENT

Displaced from orig. obj to a less threatening source.

Displacement is a transfer into another situation of an emotion felt in a previous situation where its expression would not have been socially acceptable. For instance, emotions such as anger or hostility may not be permitted open expression in some situations where they are evoked. The individual temporarily checks the feeling but releases it later in a different situation where personal security is not threatened. For example, a supervisor may not dare to resent openly a superior's criticisms but later may displace her original feelings of resentment toward her superior by reprimanding those she supervises. Patients sometimes express feelings towards doctors and nurses which were originally felt toward other persons, such as a parent. One may also displace feelings on environmental objects, such as slamming a door or pounding a table while mulling over a previous happening.

INTROJECTION

starts as identification → introjection

This mechanism derives its name from the word "introject" which literally means to take into or ingest. Individuals are constantly introjecting philosophies, ideals, knowledge, customs, mores, attitudes, and so on. For instance, feelings of persecution might be introjected by the growing child who listens to discussions filled with ideas of persecution. In later life, he might use such ideas to explain a failure. Patients sometimes make pathological use of this mechanism by introjecting their aggressive impulses through injuries inflicted upon themselves or by making suicidal attempts.

SUBLIMATION

mech. by is energy of repressed directed to useful + acceptable goals.

Sublimation is the release into a different situation of the unused energy or impulses which cannot be realized or socially approved in one situation. The unconscious mind contains strong, primitive impulses which could prove harmful to the individual or those in his environment if they were not altered or tempered to conform with socially approved and accepted behavior. For instance, strong sexual urges might be sublimated into creative arts such as writing, sculpture, or design. Hostile impulses might be sublimated into sports, debating, or business activities. The arts, crafts, music, and recreation departments of mental hospitals provide activity channels through which patients sublimate their energy and impulses.

PROJECTION

mech. in w thoughts unacceptable to self are attributed to others — ideas impulses. echoes of one's unconscious

Literally, projection means to "throw off" and is often referred to as the "blaming" or "scapegoat" mechanism. Individuals may blame others for their failures or specific happenings, such as blaming others for mistakes because it is emotionally painful and personally threatening to accept responsibility for them. People sometimes unconsciously attribute to others their own undesirable feelings, ideas, and behavior characteristics. They treat other persons as if the behavior originated in them and not in themselves. For example, the comment, "He's conceited," may actually be a projection of a behavior characteristic that is emotionally painful to accept. The student who fails a course may blame his failure on poor teaching. The patient who remarks, "I'm not sick. It's my wife who is sick," may be projecting. The suspicious patient who is secretive, carefully inspects his food, bed, and immediate living arrangements may project his scrutinizing behavior by saying, "They're spying on me."

Projection pattern patients (schiz) leads → delusions, hallucinations, paranoia — auditory hallucinations

IDENTIFICATION

mech. by is person assumes personal qualities of other - after you assume it it becomes part of you → introjection. unconscious -

Identification is a defensive process which involves affects and deep feeling tones. It is an unconscious imitation or patterning of one's mannerisms, behavior, and feelings in accordance with those of another person. Identification with a sexual image is believed to begin with the girl's identification with her mother and the boy's with his father during the Oedipal period. Children identify with their teachers, heroes, and heroines. Perhaps some of the unhealthy patterns of maladjusted and delinquent behavior have their roots in this process. The growing boy may identify himself with a ruthless gang leader or fictional character to the point of creating serious social disturbances. Or we may see the mechanism used by family members who identify so strongly with the pain and discomfort of a sick member that they are unable to give comfort or physical assistance to the patient because of their own anxiety. This is a defensive behavior which should not be confused with imitation or mimicry.

CONVERSION

Conversion is a mechanism whereby an individual converts an emotional problem into a physical symptom or outlet which provides a release for the tension and anxiety associated with the conflict. This mechanism may be used early in life when the sick child discovers that being ill is a way to obtain sympathy and attention and to escape some feared or unpleasant situation. For instance, the person who lacks the self-confidence to assume executive responsibilities may develop the symptoms of an illness which could prevent his acceptance of a promotion. Actually, the patient does suffer from his symptoms owing to the emotional turmoil within him. These symptoms do not subside until he is helped to understand and resolve his problem. Conversion is a mechanism observed in psychoneurotic patients who frequently manifest physical symptoms for which there is no demonstrable organic basis.

CONDENSATION

Condensation results from a delusional system fortified over a long period of time. It is the fusion of two or more ideas or experiences into one experience or manifestation. In a condensed form of acting out, the patient may convey ideas with associated feelings in connection with a delusion. The patient who says, "I am Clark Gable," has condensed into a few words his belief of being a famous movie star—tall, dark, and handsome. Condensation also occurs in dreams where more than one situation and persons connected with them appear in the one dream representing one experience. Upon awakening, the dreamer is usually unable to visualize any connections between the fused situations. A skillful analyst who understands, but does not personally share the patient's unconscious dream motivation, may be able to interpret connections which are usually disguised and symbolic in nature.

ISOLATION

Isolation is used when the person consciously protects himself by avoiding painful situations or separates disturbing ideas from their affects. Some persons suppress their feelings and manage to avoid taking part in a problem situation by saying, "I don't want to become involved." We observe this mechanism in various ways. Phobias and taboos are behaviors through which the patient relieves anxiety associated with unconscious experiences which are isolated from the patient's surface affect and behavior. Unconscious isolation of aspects associated with former experience often make it difficult to identify and connect underlying motivation with behavior, such as is observed in ritualistic behavior and compulsions. While expressing fear of some danger or enacting a ritual the patient does not recognize the isolated, motivating forces. Compulsive actions are isolated from unconscious forces.

SYMBOLISM

Symbolism is a mechanism whereby a person attaches significance to shapes of objects, colors, materials, slogans, words, and so on. "Green as grass," "smooth as velvet," "sturdy as an oak," are symbolically meaningful statements. It is said that man's ability to symbolize experience distinguishes him from his animal predecessors. Unconsciously, we symbolize almost constantly. An idea, feeling, quality, or object is represented by a meaningful sign. Painting, drawing, dancing, and other forms of the arts may symbolize themes. In general, symbolic communications and behaviors represent thoughts and feelings held by an individual. A patient seeking a warmer relationship with the nurse may symbolize his thoughts by communicating, "You're an iceberg." Acting out may also symbolize an emotional conflict. Analysts have said that the patient who lies curled up in the fetal position is symbolizing a longing to return to the dependency fetal period when life was nonthreatening, uncomplicated, and sustained without personal effort. Repetitive hand washing may symbolize guilt feelings. A soldier admitted to the mental hospital stood at attention and saluted the clock each morning before entering the dining room. This ritualistic behavior apparently symbolized some aspect of an emotional conflict.

UNDOING

Undoing is an unconscious, symbolic attempt by the patient to eradicate or eliminate the existence of a previous painful experience. Feelings of guilt and anxiety are relieved for the moment as the patient symbolically reversely enacts or undoes the steps of the painful experience. These reverse actions help the patient to feel more comfortable. It is a way of going back and amending or atoning for some past action. In a realistic way, we use the mechanism when we return to establish rapport with persons with whom we have broken rapport. The mechanism may be symbolic as in the patient who periodically rushed to the door in an intense welcoming gesture. Some years ago she had refused to allow her now deceased brother to enter their home.

REGRESSION

Regression is a process whereby an individual escapes the frustration and anxiety of conflict by returning to methods of adjustment that proved successful at an earlier stage of life. The behavior acted out by the person is considered reminiscent of behavior observed in an earlier stage of personality development. The adult who sulks and pouts instead of realistically facing a problem on a mature behavior level has regressed to an earlier mode of adaptation. The person who becomes ill in the face of disappointment has regressed to a form of behavior which brought about sympathy and attention as a child. Sometimes patients regress to an infantile level of behavior which was pleasurable and satisfying. They may require nursing care, including bathing, feeding, dressing, and so on. It is said that the patient who curls up in the fetal position has regressed to the embryonic level of behavior.

PHANTASY

The use of imagination or daydreaming is common behavior, especially during adolescence. When used to a discreet degree, phantasy may be beneficial in satisfying innate longings, fulfilling denied wishes, and affording solutions to and relief from the anxiety of minor emotional conflicts such as phantasizing that one is glamorous, adored, or has achieved some particular recognition or power. The phantasy of some artists may be a useful creative process through which society benefits. The story, "Alice's Adventures in Wonderland" is an example of useful creative phantasy. However, when phantasy replaces reality in the life of an individual, it is pathological behavior. Living in the imagination becomes a refuge from the realities of everyday living, such as is observed in the behavior of schizophrenic patients who escape into a world of their own making.

SUGGESTED REFERENCES

Coleman, J.: Abnormal Psychology and Modern Life, ed. 3. Scott, Foresman & Company, Chicago, 1964.

Freedman, A., and Kaplan, H. (eds.): Comprehensive Textbook of Psychiatry, ed. 1. Williams & Wilkins Co., Baltimore, 1967, p. 296.

Heckel, R., and Jordan, R.: Psychology—The Nurse and the Patient. C. V. Mosby Co., St. Louis, 1963, p. 196.

Kolb, L.: Noyes' Modern Clinical Psychiatry, ed. 7. W. B. Saunders Co., Philadelphia, 1968, p. 61.

Laughlin, H.: Mental Mechanisms. Butterworths, Washington, D. C., 1963.

O'Hara, F., and Reith, H.: Psychology and the Nurse. W. B. Saunders Co., Philadelphia, 1966, p. 133.

For reviewing this chapter, grateful acknowledgment is made to Mrs. Gloria Matulis, R.N., Mrs. Rosemary Wynn, R.N., and Miss Nancy Fell, R.N.

CHAPTER 13

Dynamics of Behavior Patterns
and Symptoms

A pattern of behavior represents an individual's typical way of responding to a threatening, anxiety-producing stimulus. During periods of
conflict, frustration, and anxiety, some patients act out a pattern of behavior having a dominant characteristic, such as withdrawal or aggression.
These ways of reacting have been learned in attempts to adapt to life
situations, but they may become grossly pathological in both their appearance and affects. When attempts to resolve mental conflict are not successful, frustration and anxiety increase. The outcome may be a neurosis,
psychosis, or character disorder during which the patient acts out a pattern
of behavior which typifies his defensive reaction.

A behavior pattern is a syndrome or complex of symptoms observed in
the actions, feelings, and thoughts of a patient's acting out. The individual
symptoms symbolize the conflictive and defensive elements of an emotional
conflict. They provide clues to what the person has been and is thinking,
feeling, and experiencing and responding to in his struggle to resolve
conflict as well as to meet his deprivations and needs.

Behavior symptoms are not as easily interpreted or understood as are
physical symptoms, such as a temperature elevation or localized pain. For
these manifestations we have clinical laboratory tests which yield specific
information and understanding upon which treatment is based.

Owing to the interrelation of bodily systems, some behaviors are
secondary reactions to physiological disturbances, such as those associated
with toxic states, brain injury, tumors, and other bodily conditions. Others
are the product of psychological processes of which the patient has little or
no awareness. They are motivated by forces in the preconscious and unconscious mind which automatically initiate their appearance during periods of stress and strain.

Although there may be similarities in patterns of behavior, particularly in the dominant behavior characteristic, no pattern syndrome is made up of a specific combination of symptoms. For instance, not all withdrawn patients hallucinate. Not all aggressive patients manifest a flight of ideas in their communications. Although a pattern may be generally typical and recognizable, one must look beyond its most striking characteristic behavior feature for the clues inherent in the symptoms making up the pattern syndrome which often represent the acting out of pathological defenses. Thus, the nurse is challenged to make astute observations of symptoms and their inherent defenses. Together, these manifestations symbolize the conflictual elements of an emotional disorder, the frustrations, feelings, attitudes, thinking, deprivations, and needs of individuals. Behavior is understood in relation to all past and present physical and emotional forces which may have imposed demands upon the personality that exceeded its capacity to adapt, thereby causing the person to act out his response to the threat perceived.

Some behavior symptoms are very subtle in appearance. Others are more profoundly bizarre and pathological. To understand and interpret their meaning requires an intellectual ability to visualize relationships between the patient's behavior, his immediate and past living experiences, interpersonal relations, attitudes, feelings, thoughts, deprivations, and needs. This constitutes the process of making dynamic interpretations upon which dynamic nursing approaches are based.

A discussion of behavior symptoms is included in this chapter to help the nurse to identify them in a pattern and trace them back to their developmental source. This is comparable to identifying the source of physical pain with its associated factors and treating and removing them. The more important function of understanding their causative motivation (the reason for the behavior and the goal toward which it is aimed) requires an ability to hypothesize in connection with what is observed and known about the patient as an individual. This is a process during which the nurse makes use of intuition and logic in relation to information gained from various sources, such as the patient's record, nurse-patient interviews, and interviews with relatives, friends, physicians, social workers, and members of other disciplines who may be involved in the patient's treatment and care. To formulate conclusions concerning the meaning of behaviors observed, quality listening and observing are essential, followed by self-directed queries regarding the appearance, motivation, and goal aimed for through the behavior, such as the following:

Is the patient reacting to any internal stress or strain produced by a toxic or organic affliction? Intellectual impairment symptoms are often associated with such conditions. (For example, disorientation, confusion, memory defects, hallucinations, delusions, illusions, incorrect identifications, etc.)

Is the individual experiencing feeling reactions to a specific situation or some conflict in living which motivates his behavior? (For example, feelings of rejection, hostility, helplessness, loneliness, fear, anxiety, guilt, inadequacy, mistrust, etc.)

Has the patient experienced any problems in his relationships with significant persons which cause him to relate with and respond as he does toward other individuals?

What attitudes does the patient show towards himself and other persons?

What is his self-image in relation to his personal, social, sexual, and vocational identifications and roles? Can he accept these or are they anxiety producing?

What deprivations in life has the person experienced and what appear to be his strivings and needs? (For example, need for trust, security, autonomy, acceptance, recognition, dependence, power, intimacy, reassurance, self-esteem, love, limitations.)

SYMPTOMS THAT MAY BE PART OF A PATTERN

Waxy Flexibility

An overt response to stimuli of a suggestive nature is observed in waxy flexibility. A body posture imposed by another is readily accepted and maintained rigidly for a prolonged period of time by a patient who may be perceiving an overwhelming emotion or threatening stimulus, such as fear or hallucinations. The joints of the individual's extremities may be flexed or extended during a catatonic episode just as one bends a soft candle into position.

Pathological Limb Rigidity

The introjection of a high level of anxiety and other emotions perceived in response to a threatening situation. It may symbolize withdrawal from emotionally painful reality with an associated need communication.

Compulsions

Ritualistic displacement of anxiety through repetitive actions carried out against the patient's conscious wishes, such as repetitive hand washing, counting, checking, and touching which have a symbolic relationship to underlying conflict.

Echopraxia

Compulsive displacement of anxiety through automatic duplication of the immediately observed movements and gestures made by another individual in the patient's presence. Echopraxia may be a security achieving operation which is stronger than one's conscious control.

Impulsiveness

Sudden, unpredictable outbursts of activity, such as striking physically at someone, without first thinking about the rationality and effects of the behavior. A fearful, hallucinating patient might project hostility upon a person who approaches and interrupts his hallucinatory behavior and to whom the patient may attribute the voices being heard.

Tics and Spasms

Involuntary jerking and twitching of some part of the body, usually localized in the neck, face, and head. This behavior appears to be of organic etiology but may be of psychic origin. Anxiety is displaced through such actions as intermittent eye blinking and spasmodic movements of the mouth or neck which are motivated by unconscious emotional conflict.

Echolalia

Repeating the speech of another, like a resounding echo, as if experiencing a compulsion to respond. Echolalia may be a security achieving operation or the pathological suppression of data which is emotionally painful to verbalize.

Punning

The injection of witty or clever remarks into a conversation, or the humorous use of a word in such a way as to suggest a different meaning, or the use of words having the same sound, but different meanings, which attract the listener's attention and gain for the patient the control of the immediate environment.

Rhyming

Rhyming of phrases or whole sentences in a lyrical poetic manner during conversation or writing which may symbolize the conflictual elements and needs associated with a mental conflict. For example, "I am knitting a halter for Walter to lead me to the altar."

Clang Association

A linkage of similar word sounds, such as seven, heaven, eleven, to compensate for defects in memory and communication which may be of psychic or organic origin.

Neologisms

The coining of new words that have symbolic meaning, or the conferring of new meanings upon words that are used commonly: Eisenhead (Eisenhower), newspulp (newspaper), "You don't *dig* me."

Blocking

Sudden stopping of speech which occurs when the trend of thought has been lost owing to anxiety producing thought associations.

Irrelevance

Verbal responses which are not pertinent to or related to the immediate communication content, giving the impression of distractibility or a defect in comprehension and thought processes.

Circumstantiality

The inclusion in conversation by a highly anxious individual of many unnecessary details, scattered thoughts and explanations. The pressure of invading thoughts and feelings tends to disorganize the communications and delays the reaching of the goal point of the conversation.

Flight of Ideas

A continuous stream of conversation with rapid shifts in topics owing to pressure of thoughts, sometimes characterized as topic jumping. An alert listener can detect connections to the fundamental topic of conversation. Often the shifts can be traced to stimulation of preceding statements as in the following:"Three ships sailed out of the harbor of Beirut. We are three brothers. I liked my older brother best. The best man in the service. Not a wedding service in the ship's sail. Three ships. He was stationed in Beirut."

Word Salad

A disconnected flow of communication made up of a mixture of words, phrases, and sentences which sound meaningless and as if the product of dissociations and the pressure of invading thoughts. For example, "This is the atomic age and I will see the light. You could be Helen of Troy. Or are you? Blue, yellow, green red is a rainbow in the sky. I am dedicated to a cause. My father was cremated in a barrel. Last night there was thunder and I was poisoned. The golden rule is broken. One, two, three, four. That fellow they said is mental. Who did it?" (Patient laughs without cause.) "It's a sure thing. You're telling me?"

Mutism

The state of being silent or voiceless. In the absence of organic etiology mutism is of psychic origin. It may be the result of early life frustrations experienced when attempts were made to use verbal language or it may symbolize a need to communicate.

Euphoria

An abnormal, exaggerated feeling of well-being which is out of proportion to environmental and interpersonal stimuli. Euphoria may represent a pathological reaction-formation (overcompensation) to an opposite feeling state. It may precede an emotionally exciting phase of illness and is revealed in statements such as "I feel great! Terrific! Absolutely Jim Dandy!"

Elation

An affective reaction extending beyoud a state of euphoria. It is characterized by increased anxiety and psychomotor activity in which the person's thinking, communications, and body movements escalate.

Apathy

A reduction or dulling of emotional response to stimuli so that one reacts with less interest, attention, and feeling than normally.

Blunting

A flattening of affect or loss of the capacity to experience and express emotion at normal intensity. It may progress to a loss of feeling of sympathy toward a relative and to a loss of such primitive emotions as fear, rage, and the sexual drive. Blunting is not considered a favorable prognostic sign. Even an unfavorable emotional response is considered more desirable because it indicates the presence of an affective capacity which can be stimulated with the hope of effecting a behavior response and change.

Ambivalence

The coexistence of two opposing drives, desires, feelings or emotions. For example, an individual may have feelings of both love and hostility toward someone. Wanting and also fearing an anticipated happening. One of the components of ambivalence is usually repressed but gives rise to feelings of guilt and anxiety which may be projected.

Lability

Sometimes characterized as emotional instability. Owing to the sharp influence of rapidly changing thoughts and feeling tones, the patient manifests quick shifts in his emotional responses, as if gliding from one into another affect. For example, pleasantness may be followed in quick succession by a show of irritability.

Irritability

Feeling emotionally out of harmony with a situation. For example, the individual may say, "I don't want to talk. Don't bother me."

Suspicion

A lack of trust in others, often accompanied by an anxiety producing anticipation of a response from others or a happening that is feared.

Insight

Being able to recognize and accept the fact that one is ill even though the dynamics of the illness are not understood.

Disorientation

Being unaware of the correct date, time, place, etc. For example, "This isn't a hospital. It's a concentration camp!" A dissociative process related to memory impairment which may be organically caused or the result of acute mental conflict with highly affective related factors involved.

Comprehension

Having an ability to understand communications as well as what is taking place in one's environment.

Distractibility

The interference of anxiety and environmental stimuli with one's ability to focus attention upon communications and occurrences. For example, the door opens, and patient turns his attention from the immediate act or conversation.

Impairment of Judgment

An inability to adequately size up a situation or recognize the logic of explanations owing to intellectual impairments caused by organic changes or psychic conflict.

Attention

Being able to focus one's special senses and intellectual responses upon communications and environmental situations for a period of time.

Suggestibility

Being readily responsive to stimuli of a suggestive nature. Examples are: accepting an imposed body posture (waxy flexibility) and carrying out a posthypnotic suggestion.

Preoccupation

Persistent introspection and inward reflection, thus internalizing instead of externalizing intellectual activity and affect. It is a manifestation of the defense mechanism introjection.

Hallucinations

Impairment of the special senses (auditory, visual, tactile, olfactory) by which the patient perceives in response to his own inner stimulation, that is, his beliefs, delusions, feelings, unfulfilled wishes, and needs.

Illusions

A misinterpretation of an external stimulus by any of the special senses. Examples are: hearing thunder and identifying it as a bomb, seeing a shadow on the wall and identifying it as an amimal.

Delusions

A false belief motivated by the affective aspect of the personality to which the patient clings. For that reason, delusions cannot be changed through intellectual appeal approaches, such as, attempts to reason with the individual. There are many types of delusions: delusions of persecution, guilt, poison, grandeur, unworthiness, infidelity, etc. Examples are: "They're out to get me." (persecution) "This food is poisoned." (poison) "I don't deserve to eat." (unworthiness) "I've done terrible things that hurt so many people." (guilt) "I live like a country squire." (grandeur) "My wife has another man." (infidelity).

Ideas of Reference

A belief held by the patient that something in the environment has a meaning especially intended for him. For example, a patient hears two night nurses whispering while making rounds and says, "They're plotting against me. I heard them." He may read a newspaper item and interpret it as a message or warning intended for him.

Alien Control

A belief held that one is under the stronger influence of another person or force. For example, a patient explains his destructive action by projecting the blame. "God told me to do it." "I'm being dictated to from another world."

Cosmic Identification

Expressing the delusion that one has abilities which may be likened to the powers of a supreme being. This is a pathological identification defense that may be used when one has experienced personal failure and feelings of helplessness.

Depersonalization

Verbalizing the belief that one no longer exists or experiences the former normal feeling reactions but is instead perceiving as if one were something inanimate or unreal and had lost the capacity to perceive as a living being. This may extend to one's perception of the world as being unreal. It symbolizes a losing of one's personal identity and escape from the reality of an emotionally intolerable situation by an insecure and self-observing personality. It may be a reaction-formation defense (over-compensation) against anxiety, rage or deprivation when other defenses have failed, such as hypomania. Examples are: "I don't feel like I used to any more." "I'm like a ghost, an empty shell." "I'm not my real self."

Transfer of Personality

The patient believes that he is someone else, and he acts like that other person. The mechanisms of denial and identification are manifested in this behavior. There is dissatisfaction with the true self and the need to be dissociated from the discomforts and anxiety of the realities of living. Repression is also part of this defensive behavior. An example is that of a patient who assumed the mannerisms of a prominent movie star, adopted her well-known style of behaving, hair fashion, and name.

Memory Impairments

Memory defects vary in degree and type and may be of organic, emotional, or mixed origin and sharply circumscribed in limits of time. Experience or recollections are split off and become consciously inaccessible. A loss of memory for recent events is known as anterograde amnesia. Forgetting events in one's past life is known as retrograde amnesia. Anterograde amnesia may be associated with a senile psychosis, as a temporary effect of electrotherapy, or an aftermath of a catastrophe, such as an earthquake, fire, or flood. Retrograde amnesia may be observed following a long interpersonal struggle which terminates in a crisis situation. It demonstrates the use of pathological repression and dissociation of the present with one's past life.

Stupor

A reduction in mental alertness and awareness which may vary in degree and depth from drowsiness to comatose states and the appearance of pathological body reflexes. In the absence of organic causes the origin may be psychic, as is observed in catatonic stupor which is a dissociative reaction to an overwhelming emotion.

Confabulation

Falsification of facts or distortion of memory which is not deliberate but the result of mental deterioration which produces gaps in memory that motivate defensive compensatory actions.

Pseudologica Fantastica

False logic of a fantastic nature that is motivated by a low self-esteem and weak superego. Impersonation of celebrities, pathological lying, and the writing of false signatures are abnormal uses of the mechanism of identification.

SUGGESTED REFERENCES

Bellak, L., and Small, L.: Emergency Psychotherapy and Brief Psychotherapy. Grune & Stratton, New York, 1965.

Burd, S., and Marshall, M.: Some Clinical Approaches to Psychiatric Nursing. The Macmillan Co., New York, 1963, pp. 168–238.

Field, W.: When a patient hallucinates. Am. J. Nurs. 63: 80 (Feb.), 1963.

Kolb, L.: Noyes' Modern Clinical Psychiatry, ed. 7. W. B. Saunders Co., Philadelphia, 1968, p. 88.

McCown, P., and Wurm, E.: Orienting the disoriented. Am. J. Nurs. 65: 118 (April), 1965.

Prange, A., and Martin, H.: Aids to understanding patients. Am. J. Nurs. 62: 98 (July), 1962.

For reviewing this chapter, grateful acknowledgment is made to Mrs. Gloria Matulis, R.N., Mrs. Rosemary Wynn, R.N., and Miss Nancy Fell, R.N.

CHAPTER 14

Patterns of Withdrawal and Aggression

Patterns of behavior, considered to be adaptive responses to stress situations producing anxiety, are syndromes or aggregates of symptoms having one distinguishing or dominant characteristic. Patients manifesting these syndromes may be characterized as withdrawn or aggressive.

As one observes behavior patterns it is apparent that there are variations of individual patterns. The dominant characteristic may be manifested to a greater or lesser degree. Symptoms appearing in the expression of one variation of a pattern may not be observed in another variation; for instance, not all patients characterized as withdrawn express delusional mental content or hallucinate. The study of why a particular patient is withdrawn or aggressive would take into consideration all of the past and present relative factors associated with experiences in living. The inquiry would include study of the individual's relationships with significant persons, and how experiences and events were interpreted unconsciously by the patient as well as the usual pattern of adaptation utilized in response to them. It is said that the pattern manifested is the individual's particular way of attempting to adapt to conflictual, anxiety-producing experiences.

PATTERNS OF WITHDRAWAL

Withdrawal may be expressed in degrees varying from the maintenance of social distance from others while being in good contact with reality to the extreme of phantasizing and being out of contact with reality. It is said to be a habitual mode of adaptation developed in response to anxiety-producing threats perceived. As anxiety increases the person moves away from the threatening stimulus. Through some manner and degree of withdrawal the patient attempts to achieve relief from anxiety and meet

some pressing inner need. Oftentimes the patient's response is on an unconscious level and made as if automatic.

Dynamically, withdrawal has been accorded as many interpretations
as its manners and degrees of expression. While these explanations are of
interest they may be of limited use in evaluating the total life experience
and response of the individual.

PATTERN VARIATIONS AND INTERPRETATIONS

Withdrawal, in some instances, has been explained as a defense
against rejection anticipated from other individuals. It has been interpreted
as avoidance of the reality aspects of an emotionally distressing situa-
tion.Withdrawal has been described as a state of existence removed from
the realm of reality in which the patient indulges in phantasy to the extent
of gratifying unfulfilled wishes and unmet needs and preserving the self-
esteem. On occasions, withdrawal has been regarded as adaptation through
self-control. The person's imposed isolation prevents the unleashing from
within of resentful, hostile feelings and impulses towards significant persons. It has been viewed as a manifestation of personal punishment—a
state of introspection imposed to introject guilt and condemnation of the
self. Withdrawal has been explained, in specific instances, as a mode of
behaving which effects punishment in significant persons, causing them to
feel, in response to the pattern, anxious, guilty, and uncomfortable. The
pattern has been interpreted as a means utilized to prevent other individuals from learning about the intimate life of a person. Withdrawal may be a
manifestation of grieving following a deep personal loss, a pattern of
behavior which favors the release of emotion as well as reintegration of the
personality. It is a pattern which has also been interpreted as behavior
which aims to adapt by control of the environment, to evoke the sympathy,
attention, and comforting approaches of significant persons.

APPROACH TO WITHDRAWN PATIENTS

Obviously, the approach to patients manifesting patterns of withdrawn
behavior requires of the nurse psychodynamic interpretations, astute observations, and a sensitivity to interpersonal factors involved. Interpretations
should include unconscious factors of which the patient may be unaware—
that is, to hypothesize how the patient may have understood or unconsciously interpreted similar events and experiences in living. For instance, if
the patient experienced rejection repeatedly during earlier life interactions
he may have interpreted it as a response to anticipate from individuals
during the socializing process.

Movements made toward the withdrawn patient to establish a relationship are often fraught with difficulties which may be challenging to the nurse. For example, a patient may become anxious when interaction with other individuals poses the possibility of being discussed personally. Communications exchanged by the nurse with the patient then would follow the patient's conversation lead. Thus, it is important to identify the threatening stimulus and to visualize connections between it, the patient's behavior, and past experiences. Interpretations made may help to guide the nurse toward making nonthreatening approaches. In some instances what the patient does not talk about, or avoids being drawn into a discussion about, may be a clue to the threatening stimulus. Eventually, the patient may be able to form a closer relationship and initiate discussion of personal topics, the communication of which may be therapeutic.

Timing of movements made toward the withdrawn person, as well as persistence coupled with patience in making attempts to reach out in some manner toward the individual, is important. Timing involves knowing when it is psychologically favorable to approach the patient and being sensitive to the individual's endurance for interaction. There may be occasions when the patient or nurse commences to show anxiety after a very brief interaction of a few minutes. The nurse's removal of her presence may or may not constitute temporary removal of the threatening stimulus. Endurance may be increased as the nurse-patient relationship progresses and leads to development in the patient of tolerance for interaction.

Rejection of the nurse by some withdrawn patients is a common response when attempts to establish a relationship are made. If the nurse recognizes the tendency to reject before being rejected as part of the pattern, she will feel more comfortable about making additional attempts in a forward-movement direction. Actually, the patient may want and need a closer relationship with other persons but cannot cope with the anxiety engendered owing to anticipation of rejections. The tendency to avoid the patient may be an automatic response in the nurse which could lead to reinforcement and strengthening of the patient's withdrawn mode of adaptation. Thus, the return of the nurse, at regular intervals, if only to recognize and show acceptance of the patient, may help to change the individual's pattern of adaptation.

Brief encounters with withdrawn patients may be helpful in eventually establishing a longer-sustained relationship. Indeed, they may lead the patient to make overtures toward the nurse which should be recognized as such and acknowledged. Brief encounters may be effected through the daily greeting given by the nurse as she acknowledges the patient's presence in the social environment. The nurse may establish brief contact with the patient by providing a magazine—a tangible offering which conveys acknowledgment. She may suggest that the patient might enjoy viewing a television program. The nurse may give paper and pencil to the patient with a suggestion to draw a picture. What may be drawn may be of dynamic significance. The nurse may say, "I will sit with you for a few minutes." The nurse may tell the patient that she will return at a later time, provided she is able to follow through with her promise. Such approaches have a non-threatening human element, but can transfer feelings to the patient which may lead to mental associations favoring the relationship with the nurse.

Withdrawn patients may be stimulated to relate with others when the nurse initiates or participates in some interesting group activity which the patient may be in a position to observe. Nurses who have initiated small group discussions of everyday topics with patients have observed that withdrawn patients in the social environment have often been stimulated sufficiently to move toward and listen to the group. These observations have made enough impression upon nursing personnel to cause them to refer to these onlookers as those patients who constitute a fringe group. Spectator participation is an indication that the spectators do possess inner resources for reaching out toward others.

Some writers have mentioned that it is important to make reality pleasant for the severely withdrawn patient. Because these patients are often out of contact with the environment it seems appropriate to suggest that approaches introduce elements of reality which will stimulate the special senses causing the patient to focus on reality. Bathing, feeding and dressing patients, combing their hair, introducing the smell of soap, cosmetics and flowers, and playing music within patients' hearing range are examples of the kinds of approaches that the writer would suggest. The emotional tone transmitted by the nurse to the patient during these interactions is the factor which may lead to a therapeutic nurse-patient relationship.

There are occasions when it may be therapeutic for a patient to withdraw temporarily from interaction. These are the occasions when patients feel the need to be removed from the stimulus of a highly charged, anxiety-producing environment which threatens the integrity of their self-control. Withdrawal, in such instances, is considered a self-protective device. For some persons, periodic withdrawal is also necessary to reflect upon inner experience and reorganize the resources of the personality. It is the understanding nurse who recognizes the difference between these modes of withdrawal and the more chronic, disintegrating patterns of withdrawn behavior. The independent judgment of the nurse is required in making these distinctions and determining when it is therapeutic for a patient to be permitted to withdraw.

PATTERNS OF AGGRESSION

Patterns of aggression may vary from subtle manifestations, as may be observed in passive resistance, to the more overt release of aggression through physical attack. The aggression impulse may be the motivational force underlying numerous behaviors, such as verbal threats, spreading of gossip, inciting others to aggress, and destroying property.

Some expressions of aggression are socially acceptable, for example, competitiveness in business relations. Indeed, it is believed that some degree of aggression is necessary for social adaptation. However, the socially acceptable manifestations of aggression as well as the targets at which aggression may be aimed are specified by society. Persons who do not conform to the limits set for the expression of aggression are considered maladjusted. The individual who is unable to modulate his aggressive tendencies drives others away, is often punished for his aggressive acts, and usually fails to achieve his goal. Society rewards only those who adopt the responses permitted. Buss has hypothesized the following:

When an individual is engaged in instrumental behavior that typically leads to a reinforcer and this behavior is blocked, aggression may be successful in overcoming this interference. When an individual is confronted with noxious stimuli, one way of getting rid of stimuli is to attack the responsible persons. These two classes of situations, frustration and noxious stimuli, are the antecedents of aggression.[1]

We may infer from this hypothesis that aggressive behavior may be instrumental in achieving some need. If blocking interferes with the attempt to achieve the need, the individual will experience frustration. It is said that exposure to repeated experiences of frustration influences the development of the generative power of the aggressive impulse. The more frustration experienced the stronger the impulse to aggress. We may also infer from this hypothesis that any emotionally traumatic experience may be threatening and impel aggressive behavior.

Frustration may also be an antecedent of other behavior manifestations, including withdrawal. Thus, frustration may, but does not always, lead to aggressive behavior. There are individuals who cannot express aggression owing to cultural, social inhibitions which forbid and block its release. They may develop a degree of anxiety which immobilizes them to the extent of being unable to act out their aggression. These individuals suppress or repress aggression owing to their fear of being rejected, punished, or developing guilt feelings following a release of any aggression.

Aggression may be considered an indication of improvement when it

is expressed by some mentally ill persons, particularly those having neurotic and some psychosomatic disorders. The turning point for the better
during these illnesses may occur when the patient is able to verbalize
aggression.

Aggressive behavior may be defensive or offensive. It may be aimed to
meet some need or achieve an extrinsic reward. Aggression may serve to
punish others as well as to destroy. It may be active or passive, direct or
indirect. Active aggression may be exemplified in a verbal threat or out-
right physical attack. Passive aggression may be inherent in procrastinating
behavior which often results in unnecessary delays or postponement of
some needed action. Direct aggression may be manifested in a demand
verbalized to an individual. Indirect aggression may be identified in the
behavior of an individual who incites others to aggress.

There are various types of aggression. Some investigators make reference to angry aggression. Anger is an emotional drive which may reinforce
and heighten aggressive behavior. Although it is possible to suppress an
outward show of anger, anger has mounting physiological effects and
becomes a driving motivating force. When angry aggression is released,
anger is reduced in its intensity.

Hostility may be a feeling component of some aggressive acts. Hostility is an attitude (feeling) which builds up slowly and can endure. Man has
the distinct capacity to maintain stimuli associated with former experience
and visualize it in relation to later experiences in living. Reflecting inwardly
upon rejections, humiliations, and disappointments for long periods may
increase one's reservoir of hostility which may be expressed through later
experience. Hostility may be a well-ingrained personality characteristic in
some persons. It is recognized in subtle as well as obvious patterns of
aggression. We often characterize some individuals as being more or less
habitually hostile in their responses to the social environment.

PATTERN VARIATIONS AND INTERPRETATIONS

Aggressive behavior patterns are as diversified as are their psychodynamic interpretations. Dependent upon its manner and degree of expression, aggression may be more readily detected in some variations of the
aggressive pattern than in others. Its expression in some verbal manifestations is often as distinctive as the more overt pathological acting out release
of aggression. The following interpretations made of some observations of
aggression may help the nurse to gain an appreciation for the diversity of
aggressive behavior patterns as well as the range of interpretations made in
relation to specific situations. The usefulness of the interpretations recorded

here is limited, owing to the importance of making individual interpretations of patient behavior.

In some instances, aggressive behavior has been interpreted as a response to frustration or the anticipation of frustration. On occasions, aggression has been explained as a reaction to fear, motivated by the instinct for self-preservation. In specific situations, aggression has been attributed to repressed resentment, hate, and hostility originally felt in earlier frustrating relations. The energy or tension retained from these experiences motivates an unconscious need to retaliate against and punish significant persons or substitute figures during later interactions. When society is attacked through acts of vandalism, society may unconsciously symbolize authority upon whom the aggression is displaced.

There have been instances when aggressive behavior has been explained as self-assertive behavior aimed to achieve independence and autonomy. On occasions, aggressive acting out has been interpreted as a response to frustration giving rise to feelings of helplessness, the need for being powerful and to control others. Some aggressive behaviors have been explained as compensatory actions, aimed to overcome feelings of inferiority associated with the need to raise one's self-esteem. Aggressive behavior has been viewed in some situations as an individual's manner of testing reality and the responses of significant persons. In some instances, aggression has been interpreted as behavior motivated by unconscious strivings for unmet needs of affection in relations with other persons. Aggressive rivalry and competitiveness have been explained on occasion as behavior aimed to meet needs for attention, recognition, and power.

The Freudian psychosexual interpretations of certain aggressive behaviors toward the opposite sex are of interest, but are not regarded as valid by all investigators. In specific instances the motivational source of rejecting-aggressive behavior shown towards members of the opposite sex has been traced to cultural sexual inhibitions and social taboos against incestual relations supposedly internalized during the Oedipal phase of personality development. The need to be anxiety- and guilt-free from later experiences simulating incestual longings on an unconscious level is said to produce automatically a response which wards off social relations with members of the opposite sex. These particular aggressive behaviors may be seductive or rejecting manifestations. In other instances, Freudians have identified a repressed hostility component in aggressive loving overtures made toward members of the opposite sex. These manifestations have been explained sometimes as overcompensatory behaviors unconsciously motivated by a need to be guilt-free and repress hostility originally felt in earlier relations with a significant thwarting love object, such as a parent.

Introjection (turning inward) of the aggressive impulse through self-mutilating actions and suicidal attempts has been interpreted as behavior motivated by guilt feelings giving rise to the need for self-punishment. Introjection of aggression has also been explained as behavior aimed to inflict guilt and punishment upon significant persons. It is also interpreted as a help-seeking manifestation of behavior aimed to remove some overwhelming frustrating barrier in the social adaptive path.

APPROACH TO AGGRESSIVE BEHAVIOR

Within normal limits, aggression is a requisite for successful social adaptation. When its manifestations are out of proportion to experiences in living the individual needs help in adapting to social relations. It seems pertinent to mention that aggressive behavior, considered to be out of proportion to a situation, is not always physical aggression. When the nurse is aware that other manifestations of aggression may be shown, she may be able to recognize it, speculate upon cause and effect and help to meet individual patients' needs.

It is important for the nurse to develop an awareness of her own feelings and reactions toward aggressive behavior and their influence upon the individual patient's behavior. The power of aggression heightens during early life when harsh, punitive attitudes perceived with frustrations are internalized and fused with unconscious interpretations. Thus, responses which cause the patient to feel fearful, rejected, punished, or unduly controlled may reinforce defensive aggressive behavior. More favorable attitudes which can be shown during the nurse-patient relationship may be influential in helping to change the patient's behavior.

In a psychotherapeutic setting, some approaches may be helpful in reducing aggressive behavior. Whenever possible, it is helpful to encourage the patient to discuss his behavior, thoughts, and feelings. Events which precipitate the emergence of the individual's aggression may be revealed, often providing clues to the underlying motivation for the aggression. When the patient has an opportunity to reflect upon his behavior with the nurse, cause and effect may be recognized. More appropriate ways of expressing aggression may be developed as the patient discusses his thoughts and feelings with someone. Patients have been known to ask to be excused from social activity or to be placed in seclusion when the ward environment was too stimulating an influence upon the aggressive impulse. Thus, illness may be a learning experience in which the patient is helped to recognize his potentialities for socially accepted behavior and to cope with aggressive impulses more constructively.

When aggression appears to be a self-preservation response to an environmental fear stimulus, identification and removal of the fear stimulus are indicated. All aspects of the social environment, including the patient's interactions with other individuals, should be considered in the analysis of cause and effect.

Control of verbal aggression which is out of proportion to a situation may be learned through experiences which permit some release of it. The patient may be critical or sarcastic, or use obscene language. The nurse permitting verbalization as being therapeutic must be capable of accepting its emotional impact with equanimity. Being able to absorb its effects is not always easy. If the nurse can place value upon the therapeutic effect of the release of verbal aggression she may be strengthened in accepting the patient's behavior.

Attempts made by the patient to intimidate the nurse require appropriate understanding and responses. The patient may be testing the reality of the situation, including the nurse's reaction. The patient may have a need to know whether or not the nurse will react as did earlier life authority figures who were in control of relationships. Feelings of helplessness may overwhelm the patient in the hospital setting where he is subject to certain regulations and persons who may remind him of individuals with whom he interacted formerly. The need for power and control of the situation may be reinforcing the patient's aggression. The self-control of inappropriate aggression is dependent upon the strength of an individual's internal control. There is a universal need for people to experience limitations which help to instill inner control which leads to feelings of security. Actions taken by the nurse may set limitations appropriate to the situation as well as clarify for the patient the nurse's role. When feelings of helplessness and a need for power are identified in the patient's behavior by the nurse, the nurse's response would be one which preserves the patient's self-esteem.

Tranquilizing drugs have reduced considerably the instances and intensity of overt aggressive behavior. There may be occasions, however, when attacks upon other individuals or property may appear imminent. Usually, there is some earlier indication that the patient is becoming increasingly aggressive. If the nurse is alert to and recognizes signs of mounting aggression she may be able to help the patient recognize his emotional state and redirect its potential force. The nurse may ask the patient, "Is something bothering you?" Such a query may lead the patient into a discussion of his behavior, its motivation, and a release of the feelings being experienced. A well-timed inquiry into the initial signs of aggression within the person may help to reduce or prevent its heightening and being acted out in the ward environment. In these instances, tranquilizing drugs or other sedative medications or hydrotherapy prescribed by the physician may be necessary.

There may be occasions when seclusion of the patient is indicated to

protect the aggressive individual and others in the environment from release of the patient's impulses. When the patient is placed in the seclusion
room the nurse may stand outside of the door and encourage the patient to
talk about his behavior, thoughts, and feelings. Because seclusion isolates
the individual from human contact it should never be prolonged. Observing
the secluded patient at frequent intervals, communicating with him, and
feeding and toileting him are approaches which sustain human contact and
convey the impression of providing treatment rather than punishment.

Activity therapies can be helpful in permitting the therapeutic release
of the aggressive impulse. Because frustration leads to aggressive behavior
it is important for the patient to participate in activities which can result in
accomplishment and satisfactions. Successful experience helps to reduce
the aggressive impulse. Activity therapies can also provide opportunities for
helping to meet the needs of individuals aiming for recognition and approval.

It is the sensitive nurse who recognizes when aggressive behavior is
aimed unconsciously to ward off social relations with members of the
opposite sex. The patient may experience unbearable anxiety which motivates some type of rejecting behavior, such as sarcasm, obscenity, or a
threat of attack. Dependent upon the nurse's interpretation of the particular situation, the nurse will determine whether she should remove the
stimulus of her presence. Patients having strong super egos can suffer guilt
reactions which generate anxiety following their inability to control themselves from making offending, rejecting aggressive approaches.

Allowing the patient to make some decisions is an important learning
experience for individuals who are striving for independence and autonomy. We often hear it remarked that patients should participate in their
treatment. Occasions have been observed, however, when decisions said to
be made in the patient's favor were not acceptable to or therapeutic for the
patient. Some of the so-called routines established to facilitate the management of nursing care can be frustrating to individuals striving for independence.

Passive resistance, a form of aggressive behavior, has been used successfully by some persons in their adjustment to life situations. With a
manner of graciousness these individuals can rationalize their delay or
postponement of completion of a task or the making of a decision. When
passive resistance is used habitually so that it becomes unnecessarily
thwarting for others it is considered to be inappropriate. The analysts
attribute the overlearning of this defense to a rigid habit-training period of
personality development during which the person often expressed aggression through withholding of elimination. Learning to abandon the habitual

use of passive resistance may be achieved when the patient has experiences in which a lack of persistence and force is apparent. Learning to adapt without resorting to passive resistance may also be achieved when the patient observes that some actions opposed are accomplished by others without his cooperation.

Introjection of aggressive impulses may result in physical injury to the patient or suicide, dependent upon the strength of the drive as well as the conditions in the social environment. Protective measures and observations can be helpful (see p. 294). The most effective preventive against self-injury and destruction is the establishment of a therapeutic nurse-patient relationship. The tenor of a human relationship can decrease or increase an aggressive impulse turned inward. The tone of a relationship having therapeutic potential can influence changes in the patient's feelings toward the self as well as those whom self-destruction would punish. Feelings of guilt and hostility may be tempered in proportion to the feelings experienced during interactions with others.

SUGGESTED REFERENCES

Brooks, B.: Aggression. Am. J. Nurs. 67: 2519 (Dec.), 1967.

Davies, G.: An ode to being human. Nurs. Clin. of N. Am. W. B. Saunders Co., Philadelphia, December, 1971, p. 695.

Dollard, J., Doob, et al.: Frustration and Aggression. Yale University Press, New Haven, 1961.

Evans, F.: Psychosocial Nursing. The Macmillan Co., New York, 1971, pp. 261, 293.

Lion, J., Levenberg, L., and Strange, R.: Restraining the violent patient. J. Psychiat. Nurs. 10: 9 (Mar.-Apr.), 1972.

Munro, A.: Twenty years with the problem patient. Nurs. Clin. N. Am. W. B. Saunders Co., Philadelphia, December, 1971, p. 703.

Onnembo, F.: The patient, the nurse and the "red brick mother." Nurs. Clin. N. Am. W. B. Saunders Co., Philadelphia, December, 1971, p. 715.

Tudor, G.: A sociopsychiatric nursing approach to intervention in a problem withdrawal on a mental hospital ward. Perspect. Psychiat. Care 8: 11, 1970. (Reprinted from Psychiatry: Journal for the Study of Interpersonal Processes, May, 1952.)

Ujhely, G.: Nursing intervention with the acutely ill psychiatric patient. Nurs. Forum 8: 311 (Summer), 1969.

FOOTNOTES

1. Buss, A.: The Psychology of Aggression. John Wiley & Sons, New York, 1961, p. 17.

For reviewing this chapter, grateful acknowledgment is made to Mrs. Leone Cox, R.N., Mrs. Jane Rosamilia, R.N., Miss Marilyn Schuurmans, R.N., and Miss Elizabeth Maloney, R.N.

UNIT 5

The Patient's Needs

CHAPTER 15

Meeting the Patient's Needs

Everyone has basic needs that are instinctual or have been acquired during the socialization process. Needs may be physical as well as emotional. Food, fluid, rest, sleep, warmth, and shelter are physical needs essential for survival of the individual. Emotional needs are acquired through the experiences of living and interacting with other human beings. To what degree these needs are met determines whether or not a sense of gratification is perceived by the person. Needs generate tension which causes the individual to behave in ways that direct his energy toward achievement of the goal which would meet the need. When needs are not met, tension increases; anxiety may be produced and energy transformed into physical actions and communications that may be of greater than ordinary significance.

Although most behaviors symbolize a fusion of needs and drives, a dominant need toward which the behavior is goal-directed is usually most apparent and observable. In general, behavior is aimed toward reducing tensions arising from needs which are often identified through inference. The following nurse-patient relationship interactions constitute the procedure of identifying and helping patients to meet their needs:

Observation of the patient's behavior.

Identification and interpretation of the needs inherent in the patient's actions and communications.

Establishing of nursing care goals which will help to meet the patient's needs.

Implementation of nursing actions which will help to achieve the goal needs.

179

SOME BASIC EMOTIONAL NEEDS

NEED FOR ACCEPTANCE

All persons have a need to feel accepted by other individuals in a two-way relationship, as well as by the members of a group. Acceptance does not always imply approval. At times the nurse may accept behavior which she does not approve. Accepting the patient's behavior, regardless of what it is like, will help him to realize this need. It can be therapeutic for the patient to be allowed to act out whatever he feels inclined to express, including his negative actions, within the limits of safety to himself and others.

This principle is not always as easy to apply as it is stated. Some nurses find it difficult to accept a patient's sarcasm, profanity, and obscene behavior. Inwardly the patient may be deriving satisfaction in knowing that his actions are making the nurse uncomfortable. The nurse may represent to the patient an authority figure, and perhaps the only way he could be accepted in his previous environment, prior to hospitalization, was by conforming and behaving according to the set standards therein. In the hospital, he is free to act out and release his underlying feelings of hostility without fear of punishment. While doing this, he is testing reality and the reactions of others in the environment toward him. Or a patient may make seemingly subtle or daring sexual advances. Often, when these acts are skillfully analyzed, they are discovered to be attempts by the patient to establish a relationship with another human being rather than a true desire for sexual contact. Dependent upon the particular situation, the nurse may assume a matter-of-fact attitude, or perhaps kindly remark to the patient that such behavior is not necessary in order for the patient to maintain the nurse's association. It is helpful for nursing personnel to try to develop the philosophy that, regardless of the patient's antisocial behavior, he has demonstrated a capacity to respond emotionally, which is often the first step toward recovery for some individuals. Once the patient's need to be accepted has been satisfied sufficiently, his behavior may change to socially acceptable relationships.

NEED FOR SELF-ESTEEM

People universally have a need to think well of themselves. Many persons have intense feelings of inferiority. Thus, criticism tends to undermine a patient's morale and may lead to feelings of loss of self-confidence. To raise an individual's self-esteem, the nurse may try to give honest praise in appreciable, realistic terms which will be recognized as such by others.

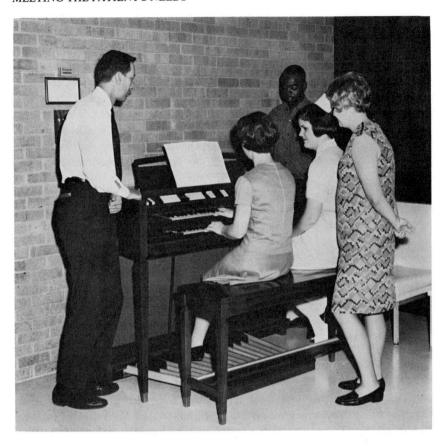

Fig. 1. Listening to the patient play the organ helps to raise the patient's self-esteem. (Courtesy of Arkansas State Hospital, Little Rock, Ark.)

When we encourage people, we stimulate their thinking and help to motivate them toward constructive and often creative behavior.

NEED FOR ATTENTION AND RECOGNITION

Attention and recognition should be given to the patient upon each contact with the nurse, although some meetings may necessarily be very brief. It sometimes happens that busy, preoccupied nurses will walk down a corridor and unintentionally ignore a patient with whom they have had a previous relationship. Hypersensitive patients interpret this action by the nurse as rejection. One should make an effort to take time to give attention and say something in passing, which indicates the nurse's recognition of the patient. Something as brief as "Good morning," or "It's nice to see you today," would be welcomed and satisfying to the patient.

Patients attempt to gain attention and recognition in various ways. For instance, we may encounter the patient who refuses to participate in activities. We may wonder why another individual deliberately refuses to dress herself, comb her hair, or feed herself. Or we may be concerned about the patient who appears to be feigning psychosomatic complaints. We may feel imposed upon by the patient desiring praise who repeatedly calls attention to some creative project she has accomplished, or we may be somewhat irritated by the person who appears to be distracting, meddlesome, and demanding.

Depending upon the particular behavior expressed, we respond to the patient's need for attention and recognition. Perhaps doing little things, like catering to the patient's physical needs, will be most effective in meeting the individual's need. Coaxing and suggestion are often successful approaches when attempting to meet this need in a patient, as are compliments given in a genuine spirit when the patient is deserving of them. Entering directly into a social activity with a patient may also help to satisfy this basic need for some patients. Anticipation of the patient's needs will supply attention and recognition before they are requested by the patient's behavior, thus reducing continuation of the patient's symptoms.

NEED FOR LOVE

The need for love is so basic to all other human needs that supplying all of the other herein-mentioned needs will automatically indicate our love for the patient. To express liking for another individual, it is essential that we avoid harsh criticism, but use instead tactful suggestion. Positive and sincere facial expressions, gestures, and the spoken word communicate to the patient that he is liked.

NEED FOR FEELINGS OF SECURITY

Maintaining consistency, giving reassurance, and setting limitations, when necessary, all help to bring about feelings of interpersonal security.

Maintaining Consistency

The patient may react acutely to an absence of consistency in viewpoints and management of his behavior by the staff, the lack of consistency produces feelings of insecurity, and the patient is unable to predict what to expect. Thus, there should not be conflict between staff members regarding the general approach to the patient.

Giving Reassurance

Reassurance may be given in several ways, dependent upon the individual situations. The nurse may remain with the patient when he appears apprehensive and frightened. She may transfer feelings of calm and confidence to the patient by remaining calm and confident herself in tension-producing situations. It is also important to explain beforehand to the patient what is going to be done, and to remember that patients want to have their questions honored regardless of how trivial some of these questions may appear to nursing personnel. Sometimes the nurse may give reassurance by simply holding the agitated person's arm as the patient, harping and whining in a talkative, hopeless mood, paces up and down the corridor. Allowing the patient to verbalize freely his feelings of guilt and unworthiness, and then later following this up with desensitizing remarks, will help to make the person feel secure. For the patient to know that a capable, interested nurse will be taking care of him strengthens his feelings of security in the hospital environment.

Setting Limitations

Sometimes it is necessary to place limitations upon a patient's activity. For instance, there are patients who may attempt to over-accomplish within a specified period and who require assistance in tempering their ambitions. There are those, also, who may try to exert control over other patients, as well as personnel, and who will require certain limitations in order to avoid the ill effects of such attempts. Limitations, such as asking to be placed in seclusion, may actually be requested by some patients who fear their inability to control their destructive and hostile impulses.

Avoidance of close bodily contact between nursing personnel and patients is another limitation requirement. In their understandably overzealous attempts to establish early rapport with patients, inexperienced psychiatric nurses sometimes place a loving arm around a patient's waist, or caress and encourage the patient to cuddle, etc. This type of relationship may be very threatening to certain patients and undermine their feelings of security. There are patients who are obsessed with the idea that they have homosexual tendencies, and fear a close relationship of any kind with the same sex. Or the patient with homosexual tendencies may actually sense an arousal of these feelings and enter into a panic state. Flirtatious, coy behavior toward the patient of the opposite sex may be interpreted by some patients as an invitation to continue in further attempts at petting; to other patients who fear their inability to control the normal sexual instincts, it may be frightening and create a defensive overactivity in the form of hostility or other types of serious behavior problems. The light touch of the hand in a friendly grasp, or an encouraging tap upon the shoulder by the nurse, may engender feelings of security within the more receptive individual patient, but more than this in a relationship may be the means of undermining the patient's feelings of security. Limitations are most skillfully set when the nurse appreciates and compares the values attached to a situation or request made by the patient with the values of the remaining patient group and hospital staff. Sometimes it is possible to be flexible and allow a patient to do as he chooses in a situation, even if the patient's desire is not in accord with the group's desire or the hospital requirements. At other times, the morale and safety of the group may be considered more important than the individual patient. Or the degree of responsibility to be assumed by the hospital staff from a legal point of view may necessarily be the determining factor.

NEED FOR UNDERSTANDING

The patient has a need to converse with others in a language he understands, and sometimes we may find it necessary to adapt our language to the patient's level of understanding. Also, we need to understand the patient's language, and this is not always an easy task; a patient's conversation may be contradictory to what he is actually thinking and feeling deeply. That is why it is important to be alert to the patient's feeling tone.

There may be times also when the patient's verbalization is filled with elements of superficially mystifying, symbolic language which does not appear to be meaningful to the observer. Listening carefully to the patient and attempting to identify key words which may serve as clues will help to bring about an understanding of what the patient is attempting to relate. Oftentimes the key words are repeated, although they may not be necessarily spoken in connected, grammatical sequence. Observing the patient's gestures and actions and hypothesizing about his past and present experiences in living may also help in understanding his communications.

To understand another, an individual must be able to empathize. This is different from the ability to sympathize which occurs when the nurse's feeling tones are like the patient's. To empathize requires that one be able to listen to the patient's expressions of his conflict, yet maintain an objective, emotionally detached viewpoint. In other words, a nurse may help the patient to feel that he is understood without becoming emotionally involved with the problem as is the patient. The nurse who develops strong emotional identification with the patient's conflict is unable to help the person rationalize his thinking but instead influences the development of a more highly charged feeling state in the patient.

When the patient's requests appear trivial, the nurse's understanding of the need behind the requests will convey positive relationship feelings to the patient. It is most important, in understanding the patient, to be able to analyze the motivation beneath the patient's behavior and the deeper or underlying meaning of his conversation.

NEED FOR COMMUNICATION

Man has a need to communicate with others for he cannot rely completely upon himself for survival. The ability to communicate has placed man above all other species and through this process he has developed and progressed.

Talking helps the patient to ventilate his feelings and thoughts, thereby relieving tension and anxiety. Some nurses are skillful in their approach when allowing the patient to verbalize freely. Listening is an art which may be acquired by those who can learn to restrain the impulse to interrupt the patient's conversation. Quite often, nurses admittedly discover themselves cutting off the patient's stream of talk by interjecting personal experiences. The patient is interested in what he has to say and has taken it for granted that the nurse will be also. Cutting off the patient's conversation may prevent him from relating his deeper anxieties.

There are occasions when the nurse deliberately attempts to change the topic of conversation because it is a subject which is painful for her to discuss. Or perhaps the patient is pressing the nurse for an answer to some inquiry, and she is unsure of her ability to reply in a vein which will be acceptable to the patient. Although the topic of conversation is apparently an emotionally charged one, nurses may employ the technique of listening, knowing that some personal feelings will have to be mastered and subjugated to the more important nursing function of helping to. meet the patient's need. Realistic replies to the patient's queries may not always be satisfying to the patient; the nurse may have to tell an inquirer, for instance, that she cannot promise to discharge him immediately from the hospital. She can, however, tell the patient that as soon as he is well, he will be given consideration to be discharged.

Since the nurse is aware that persons need reassurance, the inexperienced may attempt to "wave" away with a hand or a glib tongue the patient's expressions of fear and other feelings. Reassurance given too quickly does not allow the patient to ventilate his deeper conflicts. When the patient is allowed time to talk it out thoroughly, he becomes relaxed and may find it possible to view the situation rationally. It is interesting to note how some patients will, after venting feelings of hostility or persecution, begin to talk positively about the very persons they have been condemning. Suddenly they begin to recognize constructive elements concerning other persons in the conflict. This does not happen, however, when reassurance is communicated too quickly, because hostile feelings are not entirely released.

To encourage a patient's conversation, the nurse may use such techniques as making brief, interested comments in response to what the patient has said. She may use reflection by repeating part or all of a statement spoken by the patient, or she may simply say, "Hmm-mm, hmm-mm," or "Uh-huh." Or, if the patient has expressed some deep distress or feeling of protest concerning a situation, she might say something like, "It's not a very pleasant thought, is it?" or "It seems to bother you" or "Tell me more about it." These approaches and others of a similar nature may lead the patient to continue his conversation. Verbalization of his deeper feelings usually results.

Nonverbal communication is carried on by the nurse who simply remains with the patient so that her physical presence is a means of communicating reassurance to the patient. Holding the patient's hand or arm, also, communicates reassuring feeling tones. Doing little things such as providing literature, turning on television, or making contacts and appointments with staff members for the patient who wishes this attention are all nonverbal methods of communicating feeling tones of interest and security to the patient. (See Chap. 21 on Communication Skills.)

NEED FOR DEPENDENCE

Some people have a greater need to be dependent than others. This need may become paramount when the patient finds the problems of living too overwhelming. The longing to return to the dependency period, when little effort was required to obtain life's essentials, is not unusual; this may be expressed through passivity, inertia, demanding behavior or somatic complaints. To reactivate feelings which were satisfying during infancy, when the complete needs of the individual were met by the mothering figure, may be essential for the patient's eventual recovery. When the need to be dependent is an outstanding consideration, the nurse in her approach may, within the limits of good judgment, help the patient to meet this need by providing physical nursing care, when necessary, and helping the patient to make decisions until he is capable of doing so himself.

NEED FOR INDEPENDENCE

There are patients who have strong needs for independence. These persons are often individuals who have lived under authoritarian conditions, without choice in many matters. In order to satisfy this need, the ego begins to assert itself. The need for independence may be expressed through aggression, negativism, and refusal of nursing attentions. Meeting this need may sometimes be accomplished by the nurse's showing respect for ideas offered by the patient. Such individuals should be encouraged to make decisions and to assume responsibility for self-care within the limits of good judgment. Observations will guide the nurse in learning when these concessions are therapeutic for the patient.

NEED FOR DEPENDENCE AND INDEPENDENCE

We sometimes observe a dual need in patients who apparently foster a need for both dependence and independence. For example, the patient who has been rejected may develop an overcompensatory reaction by becoming independent of others for friendship. At the same time that the patient fears to make friends, he is inwardly desirous of companionship. These contrasting feeling tones are opposing in action. The skillful nurse will find it helpful to respect the independent behavior of the patient who rejects the nurse's association. Eventually, the nurse's repeated attempts to contact the patient in a relationship may convince the person of her sincere accepting attitude. She may later discover the patient will make the decision to accept her, thus allowing himself to become somewhat dependent upon the nurse for comradeship as a first step in establishing a social relationship. In caring for such a patient, the nurse must be prepared also to help the patient transfer dependent comradeship to others without again experiencing feelings of rejection.

Whatever mode of expression the patient uses, no matter how obscure, the nurse should keep in mind, during the interpersonal relationship, that the person's behavior is motivated by unconscious forces which he may be finding it difficult to control.

SUGGESTED REFERENCES

Aichlmayr, R.: Cultural understanding: a key to acceptance. Nurs. Outlook 17: 20 (July), 1969.

Connolly, M.: What acceptance means to patients. Am. J. Nurs. 60: 1754 (Dec.), 1963.

Ehmann, V. E.: Empathy: its origin, characteristics and process. Perspect. Psychiat. Care 9: 72 (Mar.-Apr.), 1971.

Gould, G.: Toward a philosophy of personalized care, in Maloney, E.: Interpersonal Relations. William C. Brown Co., Publishers, Dubuque, Iowa, 1966, p. 9.

Hay, S., and Anderson, H.: Are nurses meeting patients' needs? Am. J. Nurs. 63: 96 (Dec.), 1963.

Holmes, M.: The need to be recognized. Am. J. Nurs. 61: 86 (Oct.), 1961.

Holmes, M., and Werner, J.: Psychiatric Nursing in a Therapeutic Community. The Macmillan Co., New York, 1966, p. 43.

Jensen, H., and Tillotson, G.: Dependency in nurse-patient relationships. Am. J. Nurs. 61: 81 (Feb.), 1961.

Ludemann, R.: Empathy—a component of therapeutic nursing. Nurs. Forum 7: 276 (Summer), 1968.

Shea, F., and Hurley, E.: Hopelessness and helplessness. Perspect. Psychiat. Care 2: 32, 1964.

Wolfe, N.: Setting reasonable limits on behavior. Am. J. Nurs. 62: 104 (March), 1962.

Wolff, I.: The educated heart, in Maloney, E.: Interpersonal Relations. William C. Brown Co., Publishers, Dubuque, Iowa, 1966, p. 101.

For reviewing this chapter, grateful acknowledgment is made to Miss Florence E. Newell, R.N., Mrs. Selma Taxis, R.N., Mrs. Vivian S. Bryan, R.N., and Mrs. Mabel Robinson, R.N.

CHAPTER 16

The Patient's Physical Needs

The patient's physical needs include the many aspects related to hygiene, nutrition, and physical complaints which may be associated with mental illness.

HYGIENE

One of the outstanding symptoms of mental illness is the diminishing interest shown by the patient in personal appearance and hygiene. Evidences of body odor, lifeless complexion sometimes associated with acne, dull hair, unattractive nails, and foul breath may be observed. The clothing of the patient may be poorly kept, soiled, and improperly fitted, and he does not present a picture of wholesome cleanliness and grooming. There is an apparent lack of energy or ability to cope with the usual, everyday, hygienic practices of the individual. These signs are usually evident during the onset and progressive stages of many mental disorders.

The nurse will find it necessary to take over the supervision of hygiene and stimulate the patient to practice better health habits. As convalescence takes place, she gradually withdraws such supervision and permits the patient to assume this responsibility. No better description can be found of a patient's feelings regarding inability to cope with this problem than that given by Lenore McCall in her book *Between Us and the Dark:*

Little things which, in the recording of them, appear unimportant began to assume gigantic proportions because of my inability to handle them. I could not decide what to put on when I got up in the morning. I would stand in the doorway of my closet looking at the clothes hanging there and I literally could not force my brain to decide what to wear.[1]

It should never be assumed, because the patient is ambulatory, that supervision of hygiene is unnecessary. In order to give the proper amount of supervision and nursing care, the nurse must know each patient's health habits and level of ability to give self-care. Some will need complete assistance, others may respond to suggestion with partial aid, and still others may be resistive toward such procedures.

BATHING

Bathing is important and should be practiced daily whenever possible for the patient's comfort. If the patient does not bathe satisfactorily while under the shower, the nurse will have to substitute a tub bath and give necessary assistance. The closed areas of the body (axillas and genitals) should be thoroughly cleansed to reduce body odors. The nurse must also be aware of the patient with a cleanliness complex or compulsion who will repeatedly bathe herself until she is stopped. This type of patient will utilize considerable physical and psychic energy and must not be overlooked.

Acutely disturbed patients usually cannot be bathed according to schedule. The best plan is to carry out such measures at an opportune time, that is, when the patient is quiet and cooperative. It may be necessary for more than one nurse to bathe such persons in order to facilitate care in the shortest time. The protection necessary during bathing or showering consists of control of the water temperature and making certain that the tub water level is not too high. These measures will prevent accidents. Indirect, but careful observation of the patient throughout the procedure should be made.

ORAL HYGIENE

Cleanliness of the mouth and teeth is not only a preventive measure against oral-cavity disease, but definitely affects the general state of health and well-being. Patients should be encouraged to carry out good oral hygiene practices. The necessary equipment (brushes and paste) should be made available personally to patients.

The nurse must be observant of the patient who half-heartedly carries out oral hygiene. Very depressed, preoccupied, restless, or agitated patients, particularly, often need guidance and assistance. The nurse may use suggestion and persuasion in her approach to these patients.

If the very disturbed patient is offered plain water as a rinse, he may immediately swallow or expectorate it. In either event, the water coming in contact with mouth tissues will supply moisture, remove some of the bacteria and food particles, prevent drying and cracking of the membranes,

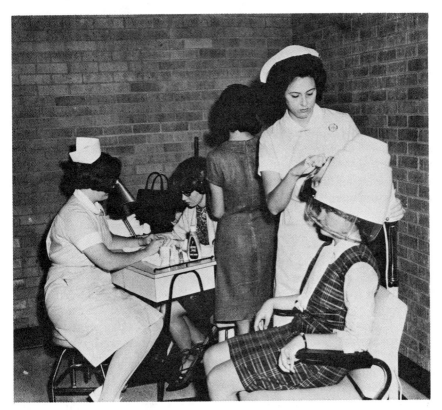

Fig. 1. Nurses help to stimulate an interest in personal appearance. (Courtesy of Arkansas State Hospital, Little Rock, Ark.)

and serve to keep them in better condition. Fruit juices, milk, and other beverages offered at intervals will supply essential vitamins and minerals necessary for dental health. A light coating of the lips, gums, and inner-cheek membranes with one part lemon juice mixed with four parts of mineral oil will help prevent cracked tissues. A slice of lemon coated with sugar may be given to disturbed patients to suck and chew when other methods of mouth care prove impractical.

HAIR AND SCALP

The threat of pediculi is ever present in large groups. Patients' hair and scalp should be observed for cleanliness regularly.

The nurse may stimulate the female patient's interest in her hair by pleasantly commenting on its appearance when it is neat and attractively arranged. Sometimes, she can be of assistance in helping the patient to arrange her hair more attractively. An occasional twist of the locks, an attempt at braiding, a hair ornament or ribbon can do much to give a person the feeling of a new look and an interest. It is never wise to urge a patient forcibly to restyle her hair. This should be brought about indirectly and born of a real desire within the patient.

Oftentimes, there are patients in the group possessing an ability for hairdressing who discover pleasure and satisfaction in helping others create new coiffures. Mental hospitals have long recognized the importance of hair grooming and have beauty salons operating on the premises to satisfy this need for patients who are well enough to take advantage of this service.

NAILS

Attention should be paid to the condition of the patient's nails during the admission procedure and whenever necessary thereafter. We think, primarily, of teaching persons to keep their nails trim and clean, but a new outlook can be given to female patients by permitting them to use gay nail polish. The variety of colors which can be applied is often a lift for some patients who have been completely disinterested in their appearance before this time. Likewise, a sense of pride in personal appearance can also be instilled in a male patient who is given a manicure.

The nurse may have to give nail care personally or the patient may be well enough to attend to this. Nail files, manicure scissors, orangewood sticks, and nail polish may be allowed at the bedside of some patients. When not allowed, they should be returned promptly to the nursing office after manicures are given. They should be used only when supervised by the nurse.

COSMETICS

Bath powder, face creams, skin lotions, and deodorants should be allowed at the patient's bedside whenever possible or given to patients to encourage good grooming. The use of these toiletries often gives patients a feeling of well-being. If the patient does not have access to these articles, he may develop feelings of lowered morale because he is denied use of personal property.

The application of cosmetics, such as powder, lipstick or rouge, is sometimes an indication of the patient's general mood. The manic patient may use an excessive amount of artificial coloring, while the depressed, apathetic patient may completely avoid the use of make-up. The under-

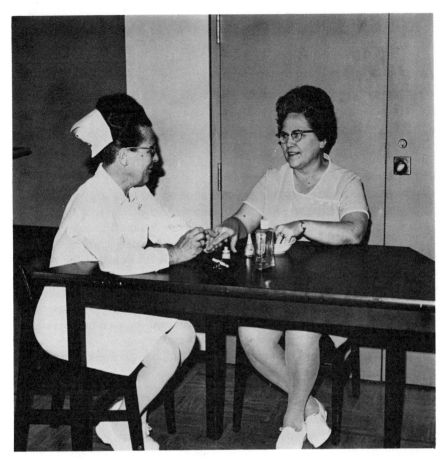

Fig. 2. The nurse helps to meet the patient's needs while giving nail care. (Courtesy of Arkansas State Hospital, Little Rock, Ark.)

standing nurse would refrain from condemning or criticizing the patient who uses cosmetics excessively since this deprives the patient of self-expression and may disrupt the nurse-patient relationship. On the other hand, the nurse can sometimes help to improve the appearance of the apathetic, disinterested person by offering to assist in applying cosmetics which simulate a healthful appearance.

SHAVING

In most hospitals a nurse, attendant, or barber always shaves the patient. A safety razor is the only type that should be used in a mental hospital. All blades must be accurately accounted for as they are used and exchanged. Some hospitals arrange to have patients shaved on specific days during the week in the central barber shop or, under the supervision of the staff on the individual wards.

CLOTHING

Clean and suitable clothing should be supplied to all mentally ill patients. Clean clothing will help to absorb body secretions more effectively, reduce body odors, and increase the person's comfort.

In small private hospitals, where laundry facilities are not always available, there is usually some arrangement for this service with a commercial concern. In some instances, relatives are required to supply clean clothing regularly. The larger institutions launder patients' clothing weekly. Having clean clothing on hand, however, is no indication that the patient will make use of it instinctively. The nurse will assume the responsibility for patients' periodic change of clothing when patients are too ill to take the initiative. Female patients sometimes launder their own underwear and hose before retiring. A drying rack can be provided for such laundering in a utility room.

The patient who is incapable of selecting a change of outer garments must be guided by the nurse's suggestions daily until he is capable of assuming this responsibility. Guidance should not be carried to an extreme. The patient should be given an opportunity to make his own choice of clothing from time to time. The interest manifested in the selection and change of clothing is often an indication of the patient's mental status, improvement, or regression. As the seasons change, the nurse should suggest to the patient's family that they bring in suitable clothing to replace garments which are out-of-season and in need of repairs and cleaning.

ELIMINATION

Proper elimination is essential to maintain an optimum state of health. A daily record of elimination should be kept for all patients.

If patients are toileted shortly after meals, it helps to prevent incontinence and to establish a time habit of elimination. It is also an opportune time for the nurse to check the elimination of patients who are incapable of assuming this responsibility.

Whenever a patient is incontinent, it is a good idea to check the elimination record as well as to make a note of it on the patient's chart. There will be no doubt about this function when cathartics are being ordered by the physician. Incontinent patients should be bathed with soap and water and kept in clean clothing to prevent chafing and sores.

If a patient becomes unduly concerned over elimination and requests daily cathartics or enemas, the nurse may seek the physician's guidance in her approach. The doctor may speak to the patient to reassure him in this respect, or he may write specific orders for the nurse to follow. This problem may be associated with the patient's symptoms, which the physician is able to appreciate and analyze most effectively.

MENSTRUATION

The menstrual cycle in female patients is sometimes disturbed during mental illness. Irregularities in the number and length of periods and the amount of menstrual flow may be observed. There also may be a temporary cessation of the menses.

The nurse may be confronted with the patient who is worried over these occurrences. She may also discover that some patients will insist that the catamenial period has failed to appear even though every evidence of its presence has been observed. The patient may be told that irregularities in menstruation are not unusual during illness. The physician frequently can be of assistance in explaining the significance of these symptoms to the patient.

It is interesting to observe behavior changes which occur and appear to be related to the menstrual cycle. These changes vary in type according to the individual patient. They are usually evident a few days prior to, during, or directly following the menstrual period. Irritability, suspicion, depression and euphoria are the most common behavior changes observed. There may also be an increase or decrease in appetite. Such changes, when noted, serve as a guide in the management of the patient's behavior. Occurrence of the menses should be noted in the nursing notes.

If the patient objects to a daily bath during this time, the nurse may assure her that a bath is not harmful, but will add instead to her comfort.

SLEEP

The nurse will learn that emotional disturbances may interfere with sleep. Therefore, efforts should be directed toward helping the patient to relax.

The day and evening treatment and social program should be well organized. Social activity during the early evening hours will help to utilize energy and bring about normal fatigue. Nourishment given just before the patient retires may help him to sleep well. Hunger can keep people awake.

The ward should then be darkened, well ventilated, and noise reduced to a minimum. When a good nurse-patient relationship exists, the patient feels secure in the presence of a nurse in whom he has confidence and who, he believes, will take good care of him.

Some patients cannot fall asleep without reading. This practice is usually a long-established habit. If reading does not grossly interfere with the comfort of others, the nurse may let the patient read. Occasionally, a patient who has not been in the habit of retiring until a much later hour may find it difficult to adjust immediately to the earlier retirement schedule. He may become irritable and insist upon sitting up until he feels sleepy. It is wise to allow him to remain out of bed rather than to insist upon conformance. Gradually, as the entire plan of organization produces its effects, the patient will adjust to the schedule and feel tired enough to go to bed when the usual time to retire approaches. If the patient requests "one last cigarette," the nurse can very often sit with him for a few minutes until he has finished smoking. Little things such as these can help to create a good nurse-patient relationship and will assist the patient tremendously in his adjustment to a schedule.

Nursing measures intended to bring about natural sleep may be employed. A glass of warm milk has a soothing effect when the patient has difficulty in falling asleep. For some patients a warm bath may be relaxing. There will also be occasions when the physician will feel that it is advisable to prescribe a hypnotic. The skillful nurse knows and implements the care which induces relaxation and natural sleep.

Various types of sleep patterns may be observed during the night. Some patients cannot fall asleep easily; others experience short, restless naps; and still others may awaken during the early-morning hours when most suicides are attempted. Close observation is required to observe sleep patterns and prevent suicidal attempts.

Sleep charts are kept in some mental hospitals. The hours when the patient is asleep and awake can be observed when the physician refers to this record. It is a guide to the status of the patient's illness and one indication for prescribing treatment.

NUTRITION

Observation of eating habits is important. A well-balanced daily diet is essential. Any irregularities should be charted as a guide to the physician.

FEEDING PROBLEMS

Feeding mental patients is frequently a problem situation. Each person presents a slightly different picture in this respect, but there are certain general problems the psychiatric nurse encounters. Some of these problems are also met on the wards of general hospitals, but the nurse will discover more of them in the psychiatric hospital owing to the degree of anxiety experienced by patients as well as disorders in thinking.

The nurse confronted with a feeding problem should aim to establish rapport with her patient. When the patient feels confidence in the nurse, the solution to the problem may be discovered. The most important step in the approach to feeding problems is to attempt to discover the reason underlying the patient's behavior toward food. Only when the reason is known can a successful approach be instituted. Sometimes, the nurse finds it necessary to try more than one remedial approach before she can cope successfully with a feeding problem.

Individual problems are best understood when the nurse has a knowledge of many known causes. From these known possibilities and observation of the patient's behavior and conversation, she can arrive at hypothetical solutions to each problem.

Other problems associated with feeding of mental patients are destructiveness, untidiness, poor table manners, throwing food about, hiding silverware and food, expectorating food, grabbing other patients' food, and tardiness.

Delusions

There are many delusions regarding food and eating which are often difficult to resolve. Patients with delusions of unworthiness and guilt may believe they have done "terrible" things in the past for which they should punish themselves by denial of food. These patients may eat if the nurse spoon-feeds them. Placement of food in their mouths by another person relieves them of a sense of guilt. Those who express the belief that they are depriving others of food may be seated with a group of patients who are eating in order to convince them that the others have not been deprived. Sometimes, if left alone with food, these persons will eat at sly intervals when they believe no one is watching.

Patients who believe they are contaminated and may contaminate others if they use eating utensils provided for a group of persons may eat if their food is served on paper plates and they are given paper eating utensils. Those who believe food is contaminated may eat if food, such as potatoes, eggs, oranges, or grapefruit, is served to them in the skin or jacket.

There is also the patient who may believe his food is poisoned. It is very necessary for the nurse to preserve this patient's confidence in every way. Sometimes, the person will eat if the nurse tastes the food first, or this difficulty may be overcome if more than one person is served at a table and the patient with the delusion that his food is poisoned is served last. It may also be possible in some psychiatric facilities to have the patient help in the kitchen in the preparation of food. When patients eat in a cafeteria, there is less possibility of their maintaining delusions of poison because they select their own food. Never suggest to the patient that you believe there is any possibility that he may not eat.

Preoccupation

It is extremely difficult to get the attention of the patient who is preoccupied with his thoughts. Preoccupation may make the eating entirely automatic, which is not desirable. If the nurse can get the patient's attention at intervals, she may be able to feed him during these moments. She may sit at the table during mealtime and engage the patient in a conversation which will hold his attention and help him to focus on the immediate situation.

Hallucinations

The patient may refuse to eat because he hears voices which command him not to eat. When a patient hears voices commanding him not to eat, the nurse may attempt to change him from that location to another section of the ward where new stimuli can be introduced. There is a possibility that a change in environment may induce him to eat. If he is engaged in conversation which requires his active response at intervals, the voices may be eliminated.

Starvation

Some patients attempt to starve themselves if they have strong suicidal drives. Fasting over long periods of time may lead to emaciation, secondary anemia, diarrhea, and lowered resistance to infection. Food served attractively, with an accompanying savory odor, will do much to stimulate the patient's desire for food so that he may overcome this idea. Any method of feeding which will establish pleasant associations in the mind of the patient is desirable. Sometimes, these patients will partake of nourishment during a social hour when the group is in a cheerful frame of mind. At this time, there may be a slight lifting of depression which accompanies suicidal tendencies. It is also a good idea to offer nourishment at regular intervals during the day.

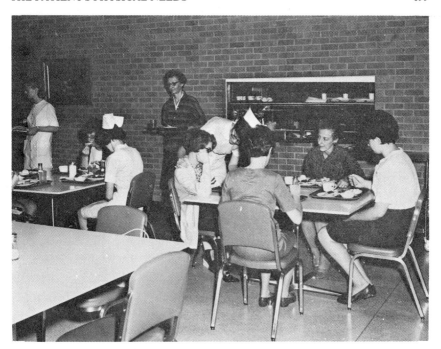

Fig. 3. Patients eat with nursing personnel in the cafeteria. (Courtesy of Arkansas State Hospital, Little Rock, Ark.)

Want of Attention

A patient who desires attention may refuse food. The following suggestions may be useful: expect the patient to eat what is placed on the table before him; do not be overattentive to his protestations of dislikes; occasionally let him miss a meal; and most important, do not focus upon his behavior.

Dental Impairment

Elderly patients who have no teeth or those who have dentures which are not properly fitted may find it painful and difficult to eat. Improperly fitted dental plates should be repaired. These patients will eat small amounts of soft, well-prepared foods, such as pureed vegetables and fruits, custards, puddings, potatoes, and ground meats. They may be given extra nourishment in the form of eggnogs in the middle of the morning or afternoon.

Physical Complaints

Nausea and vomiting may be given as reasons for not eating, and these may be organic or psychogenic in origin. Disease conditions of the gastrointestinal tract may produce these symptoms, and they are treated accordingly when detected. It is well not to show concern about these complaints or to insist that the patient eat. Consult with the doctor and seek his guidance in the approach to be used with the patient when indicated.

The patient may complain that he is suffering from a feeling of "fullness" from constipation and simply cannot "pack" more food into himself. He may complain of diarrhea which he believes is aggravated by the ingestion of food. Fear that food will produce abdominal cramps may overwhelm him. These complaints sometimes require special medical prescription. They should be reported to the physician and handled according to his suggestion.

Destructiveness

The patient who is impulsive, breaks dishes or glassware, or disrupts table decorations may be fed alone in his room where there is a minimum of stimulation. His food should be served on paper or plastic dishes.

Untidiness

The untidy patient may drop food and beverages on his clothing. Perhaps he eats too fast, or his movements may be uncoordinated. A napkin or towel used as a bib will help to keep his clothing clean. The nurse may partially spoon-feed these patients in order to regulate their rate of eating. Partial spoon-feeding also prevents fatigue if the patient's movements are uncoordinated. Such a person may be permitted to hold pieces of bread and butter, cookies and fruit in his hand and to partake of these himself. Gradually as coordination improves, he can feed himself entirely.

Poor Table Manners

Poor table manners may be in the form of the patient's not using the proper eating utensils or of eating with his fingers. Perhaps he simply gorges himself with food and completely neglects to pass food to the others at his table. He may leave his napkin in place on the table and never make use of it. The nurse may assist by handing him the proper eating utensils for each course, put his napkin in place, and wipe his lips when necessary.

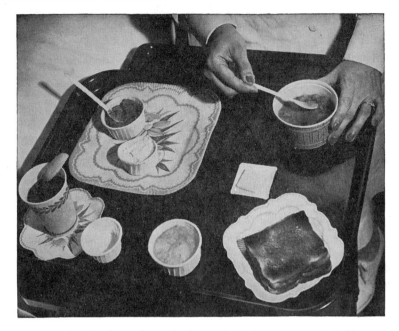

Fig. 4.   Preparation of a destructive patient's tray. Attractive paper cups and dishes are used to advantage. (Courtesy of Paper Cup and Container Institute, New York, N.Y.)

Gradually these actions will be taken over by the patient. When he is in the dining room, the nurse may stand by and softly suggest his passing food to other patients when necessary.

Throwing Food About

An impulsive patient may throw food about in the dining room. He may also resort to this action to attract attention. It is best not to focus upon the behavior observed. The patient may simply be escorted from the dining room or fed alone. Encourage him to pick up the food if he continues to carry out this action when he is alone.

Hiding Silverware and Food

Silverware and food may be desired for use at a later time. Some patients wish to save food for an in-between snack and make use of silverware to prepare personal food they may have on hand. Silverware has been known to be used in a suicidal attempt. Patients may also stuff food into their pockets and attempt to dispose of it later by flushing it down the toilet or throwing it out the window in an effort to starve themselves or deceive the nurse. The patient who stuffs food into his pockets must be observed to prevent this action. If the patient is given sufficient nourishment between meals, he may not attempt to take food from the dining room. The nurse may assure him that he will have adequate nourishment. She may also offer to prepare any personal food he may have on hand which requires the use of silverware. Many hospitals count silver before patients leave the dining room. In some hospitals, a quick silver count is taken following each course, by counting silver as soon as it is removed from the table. It is easy to do this before the silver is washed.

Expectorating Food

Patients may expectorate food if they dislike its taste. Never force the patient to eat food if he dislikes it. Those with delusions of poisoning and unworthiness must be approached as described earlier in this chapter (see p. 197). They should be fed alone, if necessary, and their clothing protected with a napkin or towel.

Tardiness

Some patients will arrive in the dining room late because they are slower in getting ready for any activity. These patients should be encouraged and assisted to prepare a little earlier than the other patients. If tardiness is persistent and appears to be deliberate, or manifested to gain attention, the nurse may ask the patient to make a greater effort to be on time. If he does not come to the dining room after a kindly, courteous request, he should be allowed to skip a meal. The nurse may find it difficult to reconcile herself to this approach, but it may be the only one which will effect a change in the patient's behavior. When this approach is not successful, the nurse should seek the guidance of the psychiatrist.

SOME FEEDING PRINCIPLES

The following principles may be helpful when feeding mental patients:

Have the dining room quiet and free from disturbances. (This eliminates external stimulation and aids in the digestion and assimilation of food.)

Have the persons who serve food appear neat and attractive. (This adds to a favorable environment which is often an incentive for the patient to eat.)

Use floral decorations and attractive dishes whenever possible. (This also increases the attractiveness of the environment.)

Do not permit the service to be rushed.

Plan dining-room seating arrangements according to the individual patient's needs. (Those persons who socialize well together make good table partners.)

Never use cracked dishes or glasses. (They are esthetically displeasing, and cracks may harbor bacteria.)

Observe patients' eating habits, manners and appetite. (These should be recorded so that remedial measures may be instituted if necessary.)

Do not focus undue attention upon the patient's appetite or eating habits. (It may be necessary to seek the guidance of the physician in the approach to such problems.)

Omit midmorning and afternoon nourishment if it decreases the patient's appetite.

Limit tea and coffee servings when patients drink excessive amounts of these beverages.

Keep food covered. (This prevents decomposition and the attraction of flies and other insects.)

TREATMENT OF PHYSICAL COMPLAINTS

In order to truly practice the philosophy of psychosomatic medicine, psychiatric nurses must ever be aware of the physical complaints their patients make to them. Physical complaints must be reported to the psychiatrist and charted as soon as possible. This is very necessary in order to give the patient the best care possible. Any immediate nursing measures or attentions which the nurse is permitted to administer to the patient without a doctor's order will often provide the patient with emotional comfort, if nothing else. When the patient can sincerely believe that someone is interested in any discomfort he may experience, he develops greater confidence in the hospital and its personnel. When this feeling is associated with physical distress, it helps to bring about relaxation and relief from tension, anxiety and worry.

The average hospitalization period for any mentally ill person is of sufficient duration to permit the development of physical symptoms. Many of the complaints encountered each day in any psychiatric hospital are very common to all of us. Patients may complain of sore throat, cold, headache, toothache, earache and backache. Nausea and vomiting may be evident. Complaints of diarrhea, constipation, menstrual cramps, localized pains, infections, injuries and dermatitis are not uncommon. Some of these symptoms may develop acutely and subside in a relatively short time, while others may recur. Whether they are emotional or organic in origin, they are still physical accompaniments of mental illness which cannot be ignored. Nurses are not adequately prepared to analyze each situation. They can, however, administer simple nursing measures permitted without a doctor's order, such as temperature taking, advising bed rest, giving fluids, a mouth rinse, an ice cap, etc., when indicated. These procedures may give some relief until the physician can investigate the complaint and prescribe the treatment which he may consider advisable. While some of these procedures are carried out for detection purposes, others may partially relieve the patient's discomfort and reduce associated feelings of anxiety. Regardless of their nature, their greatest value lies in the emotional comfort which they provide for the patient at the time. Immediate nursing measures are only temporary. The doctor will investigate each complaint and make the decision regarding the treatment and psychologic approach. If the same complaints do recur, the nurse will then know how to approach the problem.

SUGGESTED REFERENCES

Fuerst, E., and Wolff, L.: Fundamentals of Nursing. J. B. Lippincott Co., Philadelphia, 1969, pp. 178, 185.

Gragg, S., and Rees, O.: Scientific Principles in Nursing. C. V. Mosby Co., St. Louis, 1970, p. 110.

Kariel, P.: The dynamics of behavior in relation to health. Nurs. Outlook 10: 402 (June), 1962.

FOOTNOTES

1. McCall, L.: Between Us and the Dark. J. B. Lippincott Co., Philadelphia, 1947, p. 10.

CHAPTER **17**

The Patient's Spiritual Needs

That "man does not live by bread alone" but is sustained fundamentally by an everlasting, innate dependence upon his Creator for maintenance and consolation is a truism confirmed in sacred Scripture, the history of mankind, and the testimonies of eminent observers and scholars.

Many years ago William Brown, in his "Talks on Psychotherapy," said: "Sooner or later in the course of the analysis, the patient brings up the question of religion; and my impression, from the therapeutic point of view, is that religion is deep-seated in every man."[1]

In the book, "Modern Man in Search of a Soul," by the well-known late Swiss psychiatrist, C. G. Jung, we read: "During the past thirty years people from all the civilized countries of the earth have consulted me. I have treated many hundreds of patients, the larger number being Protestants, a smaller number Jews, and not more than five or six believing Catholics. Among all my patients in the second half of life—that is to say, over thirty-five—there has not been one whose problem, in the last resort, was not that of finding a religious outlook on life. It is safe to say that every one of them fell ill because he had lost that which the living religions of every age have given to their followers, and none of them has been really healed who did not regain his religious outlook."[2]

NURSING AND ITS HERITAGE

The heritage of nursing is deeply rooted in religion. "In all ages nursing has been profoundly influenced by the prevailing religious philosophies and beliefs. Though all ancient religions concerned themselves with questions of sickness and health, not all had an identical influence on nursing practice. Some rather tended to foster cruelty and intolerance, while those of an ethical type taught the duty of tenderness and compassion, and provided strong incentives to hospitality and charity."[3] Thus, we have been, from the beginning of our profession, inspired and strengthened with a reverence toward God, who dignified the individuality and worth of man. Recalling our heritage helps us to realize that the Creator provided many disciples, including nurses, with the relgous sentiments of faith, hope, and charity.

THE NURSE'S SPIRITUAL PHILOSOPHY

Holding a reverence for Almighty God automatically causes the nurses's spiritual philosophy to be reflected in all of her contacts with patients. Her spiritual strength gives rise to feelings of self-confidence and calm in the face of difficult situations. Intuitively, such a nurse views the patient as a creation of God afflicted with infirmities of mind and body which the grace of God has allowed her to escape. Thus, the nurse's spiritual philosophy may prompt her innately to console, reassure the patient and instill thoughts of reliance upon God to gain hope and confidence and face daily problems. Because concepts give rise to the development of philosophies, the patient's concept of the nurse's spiritual philosophy may foster the desire within the patient to develop a spiritual outlook.

The following words of Pope Pius XII remind us of the patient's spiritual needs:

"When it is a question of assistance to the mentally ill, there will be the added motive of generosity in giving something of your own spirit to an unhappy brother, so that he may be born again to life."[4]

Exploring this concept of transferring "something of your own spirit to an unhappy brother," we may think of the nurse's gracious manner and acceptance of others, regardless of their frailties and behavior, as an expression of her spiritual philosophy. We may consider her tone of voice and the implications contained in her verbal and nonverbal responses. And we may recognize the importance of her ability to refrain from demonstrating personal physical and emotional distress in the patient's presence. The nurse's intuitive recognition of the patient's need to experience wholesome companionship in social activities and conversation is a spiritual sensitivity to be desired. Her ability to lend therapeutic emotional support during these occasions will help to transfer something positive within her own spirit toward the recovery of the patient.

EXPRESSING RELIGIOUS SENTIMENTS

In expressing our religious sentiments of faith, hope, and charity, we accept each patient as he presents himself to us, thus reviving his declining faith in himself and others. We recognize that the individual may feel abandoned if someone does not reach out to assist him as he reaches for acceptance and security. Doing this does not mean, necessarily, that we approve at all times of that particular type of behavior on the part of the patient, but we do believe that it is only when the patient's faith in himself, in others and in God is strengthened, that such behavior may be modified or changed. Charity is extended to the patient whenever the nurse absorbs, without comment, a patient's hostile actions or words.

Sharing with a patient in social activities brings the nurse and patient into a closer relationship, and is aimed at helping to relieve the patient's feelings of tension and anxiety. The nurse's understanding and love of artistic creation in art, music, and literature, as well as her interest in current events, recreational activities, and other diversional social occasions, may be so absorbed by the patient as to provide him with feelings of genuine acceptance. This oftens leads to a restoration of faith in himself and others and in his ability to face the realities of the future.

SPIRITUAL AID TO PATIENTS AND FAMILIES

People turn to God in times of crisis, and illness is among those times when people feel the need for spiritual guidance. Nurses, therefore, are in a unique position to bring spiritual aid to their patients and to the patient's families.

The manner in which the nurse receives the family when they come to visit the patient, as well as her confidential understanding of the family relationships and their effects, may be another way of giving "something of her own spirit" to others. Families are often frightened when individual members become mentally ill. Sometimes they find it difficult to make a visit to the hospital. In addition, unfamiliar procedures such as locked doors, restrictions regarding packages, etc., may present problems in human relations. Family members may be worried that the patient will never recover because the idea is still prevalent in our society that the mentally ill may not recover. One of the most helpful things a nurse can do for members of the family is to place them at ease in her presence and give them the impression that their relative will receive loving care.

When families express the feeling that the patient will not recover and are themselves in obvious need of emotional support, the nurse may transfer to them something of her spiritual concepts of life by asking them to rely upon God for the patient's recovery. Jews, Protestants, and Catholics all appear to be in accord concerning a belief in the power of spiritual grace to cure illness. They may have different ways of expressing the state of mind of one who has found the repose which represents mental well being. It may be called "peace of mind," "serenity," or "peace of soul," but the fundamental concepts are the same.

It is important for nurses to be as sensitive to spiritual pain as to physical pain. Sometimes the nurse talks with a patient who expresses a dwindling faith in God and inability to understand why he must be afflicted with illness and other adverse situations. The nurse with a spiritual outlook may express recognition of the patient's sentiments, stating that it is not unusual for one to feel this way when experiencing unfortunate circumstances. At the same time, however, she might well comment that there are many things in life which happen to everyone which cannot be understood, but that through God's grace they can work for some good purpose.

There are some patients who believe genuinely in their religions, utilizing many acts of reverence and faith to ensure the feeling of emotional support which religion alone affords. Others waver in confidence, will question the existence of a Supreme Being, and may even confess a lack of religious feeling or of a religious creed. Quite often these persons are striving unconsciously to resolve uncomfortable religious conflicts. The nurse who can allow the patient to verbalize all of these feelings, without attempting to give advice or to steer the patient into any particular path of religion, may be the ultimate means of assisting the individual to arrive at a rational decision in regard to the conflict. The person must sincerely want a religion; it must never be forced upon him. That is why the nurse may only inquire of the patient, at the proper time, if he or she would care to talk to one of the religious chaplains about the matter. The choice is then left to the patient, who will probably not make an immediate response but who may, at a later date, decide to talk it out with one of the members of the clergy.

RELIGION

Religion is a guiding influence within man. It is a strong anchor for many patients during emotional crises. When God holds the position of supreme importance for an individual, he has reason to live and, therefore, appreciates the meaning of earthly life and of his own ultimate destiny. When such knowledge is genuinely accepted by the patient and based upon deep conviction, it is of immense value in maintaining mental health. The patient then views himself as part and parcel of God's plan. Therefore, it is wise to encourage patients to be faithful to their religious tenets and to attend, if possible, the services of their respective faiths.

RELIGIOUS SERVICES

Participation in religious services strengthens and helps people to relieve their anxieties through the attainment of Divine help. One's morale is lifted from the ordinary existence of every-day life. Religious holidays and sermons serve to reinforce a love of God, and are known to be powerful forces in maintaining family unity.

If possible, nurses of the same faith as the patients should accompany them to their respective church services. The nurse's participation in religious ceremonies with patients is always spiritually pleasing and comforting to the sick. If a nurse of a different faith must escort patients to certain religious services, she is not obliged to participate in the services.

Patients who attend religious services should be encouraged, and assisted individually, if necessary, to bathe and dress appropriately for these occasions. Attendance by the individual at these ceremonies implies respect for God; thus, the patient should be properly dressed and groomed. Appropriateness and cleanliness of one's attire are indications of self-respect which, in turn, reflect reverence for God.

CONVERSION

As for actual conversion to another religion, this is such a serious step that the patient should not be encouraged to consider the move while he seems emotionally incapable of realizing its full significance. In such instances, the doctor and the chaplain of the religion he contemplates embracing should be consulted by the nurse, as they are the people who would be best qualified to advise the patient in this matter. Chaplains consulted on such occasions will often provide the patient with literature concerning the particular faith. It is also customary for a chaplain to advise the patient to wait until he is discharged and then discuss the matter with the clergy in his home community. To engage in efforts to influence the patient's opinion or actions in this respect might only serve to confuse him further, thus creating a situation where inner conflict is heightened instead of resolved.

PRAYER

Prayer is one of the most helpful forms of sublimation. All religions rely upon the power of prayer to obtain comfort in trial, and favors which are sought from a higher being. Mankind has always recognized the need for reliance upon something greater than himself. Not only does the practice of prayer serve to divert the patient's mind from distressing thoughts, but it actually strengthens his resistance to fear.

There are occasions when a patient may feel extremely anxious and tense and ask the nurse to say a prayer or to pray with him. The writer recalls one occasion when a Catholic patient requested a Protestant aide to say the rosary with him, explaining that he could not seem to get the prayer words to flow from memory. The aide, unable to assist the patient, asked a Catholic nurse to do so, thus providing the necessary spiritual aid which the patient so desperately needed. If the patient does not request a particular prayer, any charitable nurse may recite with the patient the Lord's Prayer. Praying with the patient is often spiritually strengthening. If the patient should ask the nurse to read a prayer of his faith or a passage from the Scripture, regardless of the nurse's religion, the charitable response would be to read for the patient.

ARTICLES AND EMBLEMS OF FAITH

Certain articles and emblems may have sacred significance to patients who possess them. They should be allowed to keep these on their persons. Among such articles, the wedding ring is the most precious symbol to a married woman or man, the circular shape of the wedding band being symbolic of a continuous union. Aside from its intrinsic value, which may be great, the sentiment attached to the wedding ring is indeed a spiritual one. For this reason, married persons should be allowed the privilege of wearing the wedding band, unless, of course, they have destructive tendencies toward it. Some patients deliberately attempt to hide or discard the wedding band owing to marital conflicts. Families are sometimes willing to assume the responsibility for possible loss when the patient appears too disturbed to take proper care of the wedding ring. Patients who wear their marriage bands are being sustained thereby with the assurance that the marriage vows bind them securely to their families, and thus they may be strengthened and encouraged in the desire to recover.

A much valued religious article, especially for Catholics and which the patient should be allowed to keep, is the string of prayer beads known as the Rosary.

Another custom which is sometimes misunderstood is the habit of wearing religious medals. To the genuinely devout person, medals are not regarded as "good luck charms." Instead, the one wearing such an emblem, is, by that action, availing himself of the blessing attached to medals.

Rosary beads and devotional medals may be obtained for Catholic patients who are in need of them from a Catholic priest. Likewise, other religious emblems and devotional articles may be obtained from the clergy of a patient's particular faith.

The history of many American hospitals commenced with some disaster or emergency which prompted church elders to convert church basements into infirmaries. The early hospitals usually displayed, in the vestibule, a picture of Christ. Later generations removed these pictures. Only lately are the founders' descendants learning that the spirit which motivated the construction of our early hospitals was not, primarily, the spirit of science.

Some persons have a misunderstanding concerning the significance of religious pictures and statues. Persons who pray before statues, for instance, are not worshiping the statue which, they realize, is an inanimate object. Instead, the statue serves only as a reminder of whatever saint the individual desires to address in prayer. Statues and pictures brought into the hospital are, therefore, worthy of respect. If an American shows respect for the picture or statue of some great former President, it is certainly not idolatry for an individual to hold an attitude of veneration toward an artistic representation of someone whom he considers to be great in the eyes of the Lord. Statues and religious pictures are now being made of unbreakable plastic materials and do not present problems in protection of the patient.

RELIGIOUS LITERATURE

If the patient desires a Bible, the nurse can usually procure one from the chaplain representing the patient's particular faith. Family members will often be pleased to bring or mail a Bible to the hospital for the patient if the request is made verbally or through correspondence. Patients will find modern versions of the Bible the easiest to understand.

Religious leaflets circulated by groups visiting the hospital should be distributed only with knowledge and approval of the hospital's administrative and religious representatives. To understand the reason for this, one has merely to read Reverend Granger Westberg's account of the very ill patient who awakened from a sound sleep to discover a religious leaflet upon his bed with the following caption, "Are You Ready to Die?"[5] Psychiatric nurses will readily realize that patients often misinterpret what they read or may see only that which will strengthen their delusions or reinforce their repressions. Distribution of religious pamphlets, therefore, should be permitted only after they have been approved by the hospital authorities in view of the adverse effects such reading may have upon certain patients.

Many books which may aid patients in need of spiritual assistance have been published. These, too, may have a more beneficial effect when they are carefully selected with the particular person in mind.

FASTING

Abstinence (or refraining from the eating of flesh meat, though not of fish) is a custom observed on specific holy days of obligation by Catholics and members of some other faiths.

Catholic patients who intend to receive Holy Communion are obliged to fast from solid food for one hour before receiving Communion. They must refrain from drinking any alcoholic beverages for at least three hours. Nonalcoholic beverages may be taken until the time of communion. Fasting is not required when Holy Communion is administered to the patient who is seriously ill.

Jewish patients abstain from food from morning until evening on certain days of religious observance during the year. They also fast from sundown the evening prior to, and until sundown of, Yom Kippur. Orthodox Hebrews observe "the traditional Jewish dietary regulations which permit the eating of the flesh of only those animals that are ruminants and have divided hooves (cows, sheep, goats, etc.) and, among the fowl, primarily those that are not birds of prey (chickens, ducks, etc.). Animals or fowl must be slaughtered, dressed, and prepared in a prescribed manner to be considered "kosher," that is, permissible. Dairy products, fats, oils, and shortenings are kosher if they are derived from the animals mentioned or from plants and vegetables. Fish that have both scales and fins (carp, salmon, whitefish, etc.) are kosher, and they do not have to be slaughtered or dressed in any prescribed manner."[6]

The various religions usually excuse the sick from having to observe fasting and abstinence regulations, but there are many patients who would be most uncomfortable if they could not adhere to such rules decreed by their faiths. Whenever possible, the nurses should assist the patient in carrying out his fasting and dietary rules. At the end of the period of fast, the patient should be given some nourishing food, even if this is only bread and butter, fruit, or some other staple food which might be available at the time.

HOLY COMMUNION

Patients should be encouraged to receive Communion as often as possible in their respective faiths. Most mentally ill patients are able to attend religious services at which Holy Communion is given to them. However, when the patient is too ill and confined to the ward, the priest or minister will usually bring Communion to the patient. The patient should be left quietly alone for a brief time prior to and after receiving Communion.

To assist the Protestant chaplain it is necessary for the nurse to place at the foot of the patient's bed a stand or table which is covered with a clean white cloth. If possible, flowers may be placed upon it, as a small service is conducted by the minister in which both he and the patient participate. A spoon is required to serve the grape juice or wine, whichever is used.

The nurse may assist the Catholic priest by covering a stand or table in the patient's room with a clean, white cover. Upon this she should place a glass of water and a spoon. To these she may add a crucifix, if one is available, and a candle, to be lighted by the priest, if the patient's condition will permit the safe use of a candle. The priest carries the Host, a wafer which has already been consecrated, in a pyx (a small gold container) and distributes it to the patient.

Nurses may indirectly encourage patients to attend religious services and partake of Communion by themselves engaging in the services and taking Holy Communion.

BAPTISM

Occasionally, a mentally ill woman confined to a psychiatric hospital is pregnant. Most institutions arrange for the transfer of the patient to a general hospital in sufficient time for the birth of the child. However, there may be a rare occasion when, through unforeseen circumstances, the child will be born in a mental hospital. A Catholic infant must always be baptized. Not all religious faiths practice infant baptism; therefore, the nurse should be guided by her knowledge of both the patient and the patient's family with regard to their religious preference in determining what to do.

For the Catholic child, "If the nurse feels that the priest will not arrive before an infant dies, she should administer the sacrament herself, or get a Catholic who is present to do so. A sufficient quantity of water must be used to insure flowing, and it should be poured on the head of the person to be baptized, preferably on the forehead, to be sure that the water touches the skin. At the same time, the person pouring must pronounce the form of Baptism: 'I baptize thee in the name of the Father, and of the Son, and of the Holy Ghost.' The person administering baptism must also have the intention of doing what Christ intended when he instituted the sacrament."[6]

For members of Protestant denominations, "if there is danger that the clergyman may not arrive in time, baptize any unbaptized person, adult or child, in the following manner: pour water on the patient's head, making sure that it touches the skin, while saying, '(Name), I baptize thee in the name of the Father, and of the Son, and of the Holy Ghost. Amen.' "[6]

Whenever possible, baptisms should be witnessed by one or two members of the nursing or medical staff. These persons should enter a note of the Baptism into the official records and sign a statement indicating when and where it took place. This statement may be given to the family or the parish pastor by the hospital administrator. The parents of the infant and members of the previously unbaptized patient's family will be consoled to learn that the baptismal rite was performed.

ANOINTING OF THE SICK

The anointing of the various parts of the patient's body with oils by the priest, is often referred to as the Last Rites of the Catholic Church. This sacrament is administered once during any critical illness of a Catholic patient. Therefore, the nurse should consider it most important to ascertain the patient's religion so that if he is a Catholic and becomes critically ill, a priest may be called to administer the Last Rites. The priest should be left alone with the patient.

Although it is not an ordinary occurrence, there are times when death comes suddenly to a Catholic patient. In such instances a priest should be called immediately, because Church law permits the administration of this sacrament as long as the body of the deceased has not yet begun to decompose.

According to Reverend Granger Westberg, a few Protestant churches are placing increasing emphasis upon anointing in times of illness.[5] Therefore, the nurse should consult with the patient's family and have them determine whether or not they wish to have the patient anointed by the minister. The presence of the clergyman at such times is always consoling to the patient and his family.

CALLING THE CLERGY

Nurses and members of the clergy can work together with a more beneficial effect upon the patient if the nurse understands the importance of knowing when to summon the clergy of the patient's particular religious faith. Sometimes patients are emotionally distressed about entering a psychiatric hospital or receiving treatment as recommended by the attending psychiatrist. When all approaches have failed to gain the patient's cooperation, the minister, priest, or rabbi may be found to be the only individual in whom the patient will express sufficient confidence to accept hospitalization and treatment. Members of the clergy have often been most helpful in encouraging the patient to discuss underlying reasons for antisocial behavior which may have created feelings of prejudice in others instead of an understanding of the motivational forces involved. There are other times when the nurse should ask the clergy to visit. These are as follows:

When a patient asks to see the minister, priest, or rabbi. Such a request should never be denied.

When a patient has few or no relatives or visitors and appears to be lonely.

When a patient receives news of a sudden and unexpected death of a relative, or some tragic incident in the family of the patient.

When the patient appears to feel hopeless and to have lost faith in his religion.

When the patient is to be discharged and returned to the community.

When the patient is critically ill.

When the patient has expired and relatives are emotionally distressed.

Since the clergy are extremely busy people, nurses can be most helpful in assisting them by providing privacy for their visits and by not keeping them waiting after they arrive in the hospital.

THE INCURABLE PATIENT

Sometimes a mentally ill patient will be afflicted with an incurable and painful disease, such as cancer. Relatives may bemoan the patient's suffering and question the wisdom of giving strengthening treatments and medications which prolong the patient's life. The nurses should recognize that these situations are distressing to families and should never condemn them for expression of feelings which would probably not be demonstrated in times other than stress. At the same time, the nurse has only to remember that life is the Lord's most precious gift, "He giveth and He taketh away." It is not for human beings to decide when life should be over. What seems incurable today may be curable tomorrow. In addition, doctors and nurses are committed to support the Hippocratic and Nightingale oaths. As healing instruments of the Almighty, they are compelled to do whatever the doctor feels is essential. Nurses may also dwell inwardly upon these thoughts, thus strengthening their own convictions concerning their part in treatment.

THE DYING PATIENT

Patients and relatives sometimes ask if the patient is going to die. The nurse may feel uncomfortable when queried about such an emotionally distressing situation, but it is better to face reality and realize that attempts to evade the question will only heighten the patient's and family's fears. Since none of us know when the last hour will come to anyone, the nurse might say something such as, "There doesn't seem to be much hope but only God alone knows." She might add that on occasions people who are very ill often recover and that we must never give up hope for recovery. She can encourage the patient and family to be hopeful and dependent upon God's grace and remind them to pray and accept the will of God, whatever it may be.

SPIRITUAL AID IN THE COMMUNITY

Rabbis, priests and ministers play a large preventive role in the community. Many times persons who are emotionally distressed will visit the clergy to seek counsel and assistance. The amazing number of problems in human relations discussed with members of the clergy is an indication that such discussions often lead to relief of anxiety and the resolution of mental conflicts. By no means, therefore, should the role of the clergy in the prevention of emotional illness be underestimated. A nurse working in a community agency, such as the visiting nurse association, or industry may well remember this. Nurses may refer patients to their pastors when it is apparent that the patient will not seek mental health assistance anywhere else. Sometimes it is only a member of the clergy who is able to convey to the patient that he should see a psychiatrist or be admitted to a mental hospital.

SUGGESTED REFERENCES

Drummond, E.: Communication and comfort for the dying patient. Nurs. Clin. N. Am. 5: 55 (March), W. B. Saunders Co., Philadelphia, 1970.

Essentials of a Hospital Chaplaincy Program (Editorial). American Hospital Association, Chicago, Ill.

Fulton, R., and Laugton, P.: Attitudes toward death: an emerging mental health problem. Nurs. Forum 3: 104, 1964.

Phillips, C.: Meeting your patients' religious needs. R.N. 29: 61 (April), 1966.

Piepgras, R.: The other dimension: spiritual help. Am. J. Nurs. 68: 2610 (Dec.), 1968.

Quinlan, J.: The psychiatric nurse's responsibility to the chaplaincy program. J. Psychiat. Nurs. 1: 392 (Sept.), 1963.

Spitzer, S., and Folta, J.: Death in the hospital. Nurs. Forum 3: 85, 1964.

Ward, A., and Jones, G.: Ministering to Families of the Mentally Ill. National Assoc. for Mental Health, Inc., New York.

FOOTNOTES

1. Brown, W.: Talks on Psychotherapy. University of London Press, London, 1923.
2. Jung, C.: Modern Man in Search of a Soul. Harcourt, Brace & Co., New York, 1936, p. 264.
3. Dock, L., and Stewart, I.: A Short History of Nursing. G. P. Putnam's Sons, New York, 1938, p. 8.
4. Pope Pius XII: The True and Sacred Ministry. The Pope Speaks, October 2, 1953.
5. Westberg, G.: Nurse, Pastor and Patient. Augustana Press, Rock Island, Ill., 1955, pp. 43, 95.
6. Schorr, H., Nagle, R., and Priest, B.: The patient's spiritual needs. Am. J. Nurs. 50: 64 (Feb.), 1950.

For reviewing this chapter, grateful acknowledgment is made to Reverend Clarence Bruninga, Reverend Father Raymond G. Stewart, Reverend Herbert M. Randall, Th.D., Very Reverend Father Raymond J. Wahl, J.D.C., Mrs. Manolia Schult, R.N., Sister Marian Catherine, S.C., Miss Florence E. Newell, R.N., Mrs. Vivian S. Bryan, R.N., and Mrs. Mabel Robinson, R.N.

UNIT 6

Nursing Approaches and Responsibilities

CHAPTER 18

Integrating Basic Psychiatric Concepts in Nursing

A concept is a mental image of interwoven philosophies, beliefs, ideas, principles, attitudes, and ideals. The concepts discussed in this chapter may be relevant to nursing situations and actions wherever nursing is practiced. Certain knowledge, basic to their formulation, is derived from the biological, social, and physical sciences.

LEARNING AND IMPLEMENTATION OF CONCEPTS

A concept is learned through experiences having meaningful associations with the integral or interwoven aspects of the concept. Personal involvement in nursing situations provides the most realistic learning experience for the nurse. Reading literature related to specific concepts may also heighten one's understanding. Examples of the implementation of these concepts may be helpful in demonstrating their relevancy to a function or functions associated with the nursing role. For that reason, a number of examples have been included.

The learning and implementation of a concept are dependent upon the nurse's ability to discriminate and intellectually visualize the relationship between a concept and the nursing approach. Concepts learned influence the nurse's personality development to the extent that their integral aspects are naturally woven into the functions associated with the nursing role.

THERE IS AN INTERRELATION BETWEEN MIND AND BODY

Pre-Christian philosophers and physicians were aware of the inseparability of the body and mind. The human organism is a complete entity in its construction and functioning. Physical and mental health states influence each other's balance. Anxiety is an emotionally distressing feeling reaction to anything which threatens the self-security of the person and stimulates a fear response. The kinds of threats which produce anxiety vary widely with different people. They may be physical illness states as well as various types of conflictual life situations. The intensity and duration of anxiety reactions are in proportion to the particular threat as it is perceived by the individual, to the ability of the afflicted person to cope with anxiety-producing conditions and situations, and in proportion to the alleviating responses which may be made by individuals who give help through supportive relationships (see Chap. 10, Psychodynamics of Personality Development). The objective of medical and nursing care is to effect in the patient equilibrium or stabilization of the body's physical and mental processes.[1] Nurses, in supportive relationships, provide care which meets the physical as well as the emotional needs of patients. The interrelation concept may be inherent in the actions of the nurse who permits a patient to ask questions and to talk about illness and its treatment. This nursing approach allows the patient to release anxiety feelings and need cues. It is a therapeutic response aimed to identify and help meet the patient's needs. Simply explaining to the patient what is going to be done is a circumscribed approach having obvious limitations which exclude the patient's participation in treatment.

EVERY INDIVIDUAL HAS INTRINSIC WORTH AND DIGNITY

The aims and objectives of medical and nursing care stem from the high value placed upon the creations of God. Human beings are one of the most complex and valuable of divine creations. In dignifying man, we dignify God who created him and ministered to his needs. Nurses who believe in this concept harbor a value and respect for human beings as they minister to their needs during health and illness. Helping the underprivileged person without injuring his pride, showing attention to the less attractive and less talented individual, preventing unnecessary exposure of the patient's body, permitting a patient to select wearing apparel, sharing the satisfaction of a person's achievement, refraining from probing into the intimate details of an individual's life, avoiding punitive approaches, and relieving a person in an embarrassing situation are some of the many examples of how this concept may be woven into nursing care.

EVERY LIVING ORGANISM POSSESSES A DYNAMIC LIFE-GIVING FORCE

Human beings need the feelings of emotional support which can be transferred to them during relationships with significant persons. Observations have been made of infants separated from their mothers who, following separation, suffered marked loss of body weight, developed lassitude, and manifested feelings of mistrust, insecurity and fear.[2] Whenever it was possible to restore the warmth and love of the supporting, mothering, nurturing relationship, the symptomatic effects of the former loss disappeared.[3] The nurse is a significant person to the patient who is ill. The nursing role may be a mothering relationship. This concept may be implemented when the nurse relates to patients with attitudes of acceptance, understanding, and support. During interactions the nurse releases an inherent dynamic, life-giving force which is perceived by and influences patients' recovery. Acceptance, understanding and support may be shown by the nurse through various nursing approaches which are determined by the individual situation. The nurse may accept the patient's behavior through such actions as listening to what is said, refraining from penalizing actions, or simply tolerating behavior until the patient feels secure enough to relinquish inappropriate responses. It is well to remember that acceptance of behavior does not always imply the condition of approval. Food, medicine, and specific therapy are important in the treatment of sick persons, but their effects are complemented by supportive emotional relationships with significant persons.

HUMAN BEINGS HAVE COMMON PHYSICAL AND EMOTIONAL NEEDS

Shelter, warmth, food, clothing, sanitation, and environmental conditions are known to influence the health status of individuals. Whether or not the person experiences satisfaction in meeting his spiritual, social, and emotional needs also influences his health state. This concept is relevant to the nursing function of identifying and meeting patients' needs. Nurses may be able to identify patients' needs during the nurse-patient relationship. The identification and meeting of patients' needs are sometimes dependent upon knowledge shared and gained in association with interdisciplinarian health team members. Helping patients to meet their needs may also be a function which is carried out in cooperation with personnel of other community agencies. The identification of needs sometimes requires observation and interpretation of behaviors which actually mask their underlying motivation; for instance, a patient who does not make requests of the nurse may have fearful feelings of rejection which immobilize his capacity to make help-seeking overtures. In this situation the concept may be implemented if the nurse assumes the initiative in offering a relationship and ministrations which meet the patient's need for acceptance and nursing care.

COMMUNICATION IS THE BASIS OF SOCIAL EXCHANGE

When two or more persons interact, their communications constitute the basis of social exchange. What each one says and does makes up the content of the interpersonal situation. Conversations, voice tone, facial expressions and gestures exchanged between the interacting persons influence the tenor of their relationship, the feelings experienced, and the interpretations made by them of each other's behavior. Nurse-patient relationship communications are social exchanges. The nurse's awareness of the effect of her own as well as the patient's verbal and nonverbal communications can be helpful in guiding nursing behavior during exchanges. (See Chap. 21, Communication Skills.)

PERCEPTIONS OF REALITY ARE INDIVIDUALISTIC

Perceptions are gained through the special senses. What is seen, heard and felt in a situation is influenced by what is happening to the person at the time as well as what has happened in the past. If the immediate event stimulates the recall of former experience, the emotional responses associated with the past may be reactivated. The nurse may view her role as that of the kind, supporting, mothering relationship. The patient, having been reared by an authoritarian mother, may perceive the nurse as an authoritarian figure and respond accordingly.

Unmet personal needs for acceptance, security, recognition, attention, and the like, dependent upon the situation, may narrow the sphere of an individual's perception. Owing to the anxiety generated and to meet personal needs the individual may become consciously or unconsciously selective about what is seen, heard, and felt. The nurse may perceive a treatment as therapeutic and interpret it as such to the anxious patient. The patient may perceive it as painful or punishing and communicate only his selective perception as he seeks support for his protests.

When anxiety feelings are aroused, they may obscure the reality aspects of a situation experienced or cause its denial. Some persons become emotionally uncomfortable when another individual assumes an attitude of indifference or maintains social distance. When confronted with a show of lack of warmth or support, the uncomfortable rejected person may withhold the expression of anxiety feelings by seeming to ignore the reality aspects of the situation or by rationalizing an interpretation of its perception to other individuals.

What the nurse does in response to a patient's perception of reality will depend upon her ability to recognize and validate the motivational aspects of a situation. In some instances, patients may be helped to widen their perceptive spheres as they live through realistic experiences which permit them to test, without fear, nursing actions as well as aspects of the treatment regimen. A specific role or the tenor of a role assumed by the nurse may influence changes in the patient's perception. Attitudes shown, such as the acceptance and overlooking of a patient's hostile projections, may alter the individual's perception. Gentle persuasion, coaxing, giving attention, refraining from force, or extending time to test a situation may be approaches which enlarge the person's perceptive capacity. Any nursing action which meets the person's need is the choice approach.

SELF-AWARENESS INFLUENCES ONE'S UNDERSTANDING OF OTHER PERSONS

When an individual is aware of why he behaves as he does it helps him to understand the behavior of persons with whom he relates. In this concept there are implications for the nurse to develop an awareness of her own feelings and her behavior and its motivation in the nurse-patient relationship. A nurse who is aware that she is fatigued may recognize the importance of not permitting her feelings to influence her reactions to patients' comments, queries, and requests.

The self-awareness concept may also be exemplified in the actions of the nurse who has learned to conform for the sake of receiving approval and recognizes what motivates her mode of behavior. She may feel uncomfortable when others do not conform because their actions arouse in her feelings of insecurity and fear of disapproval from authority figures. If she has developed an awareness of why she feels uncomfortable when patients do not conform to regulations she may be able to handle the anxiety felt by her in these situations. Otherwise her need to conform and have others conform so that she may feel secure may cause her to practice inflexible approaches which motivate and reinforce nonconforming behavior.

SELF-CONCEPTS ARE INFLUENCED BY SOCIAL INTERCHANGES

A person's self-concept is the mental image which the individual has of himself as a person, a citizen, and a member of a family, sex, or occupational group and various social groups. How the person thinks and feels about himself in relation to these aspects of the self-concept is influenced by the interaction which takes place between him and significant persons from infancy until the end of life.

Sick people develop images of themselves as patients during interaction with significant medical and nursing personnel and family members. Because what goes on in the nurse-patient relationship may strengthen or weaken some aspect of the patient's self-concept to the extent of influencing subsequent behavior, these phenomena are relevant to nursing.

The patient's image of himself as a sick, dependent person for whom others feel compassion and a desire to help may be conceptualized as dependency needs are recognized, accepted and gratified through nursing actions. These approaches can be therapeutic for patients whose dependency needs were not met in the mother-child relationship or primary group.

If the nurse perceives the dependent-acting patient as a neurotic or malingerer she may unwittingly communicate this image to other personnel. Such infectious communications influence the staff's interactions with the patient. Through verbal and nonverbal communications the patient perceives the image which staff members have of him. To get personnel to relate to him as a sick person having needs the patient may consciously or unconsciously resort to some type of regressed behavior, such as mutism, vomiting, fainting, self-injury, or mutilation.

It has been recognized that there are individuals who cannot permit a sick person to conceive of himself as being ill or to act out his sick role. This behavior may be observed on occasions in relationships with patients' relatives. The dynamics of these situations are related to what illness means to the censoring persons and its influential relationship to the stimulation of fear and anxiety reactions. Illness may mean weakness to some individuals who cannot tolerate its expression owing to their personal feelings of insecurity. For other persons, illness may pose the threat of the loss of a loving, supporting relationship. Some individuals may conceive of illness as a condition which incurs unwanted or feared responsibilities. Mental illness may mean a threat to the integrity or social status of a patient's relatives. Thus, it is not unusual to observe relatives trying to hasten a sick person's recovery, telling the patient to "snap out of it," or instituting actions to remove the patient from his sick environment and social group which reinforce his concept of himself as a patient.

IDEATION, FEELINGS, MOODS, AND ACTIONS CONSTITUTE BEHAVIOR

Behavior is complex in its totality, being constituted of a person's ideas, feelings, moods, and physical actions. Its identification is dependent upon the nurse's sensitivity to these integral aspects of reaction to human experience. This concept is relevant to the nursing function of observation.

Ideas may be directly verbalized or simply inferred in the content of communications. They may also be communicated indirectly to the nurse through persons who have interacted with the patient during the nurse's absence. Inferred, as well as indirect, reports of ideation should always be

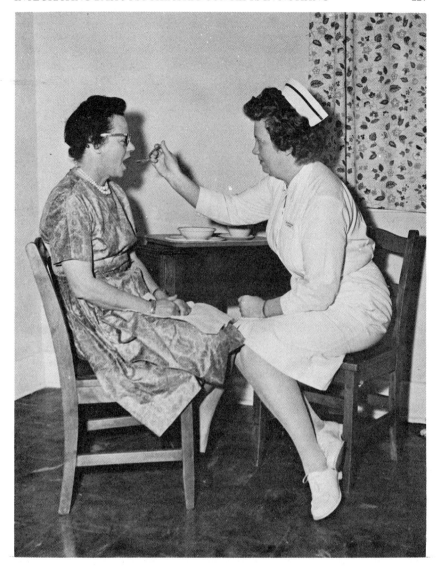

Fig. 1. The patient's image of herself as a sick person may be conceptualized as dependency needs are met by the nurse. (Courtesy of New Jersey State Hospital, Greystone Park, N.J.)

validated through the process of exploration. To explore, the nurse may make use of selective communication techniques which encourage individuals to talk and validate ideas. Quite often it is the less obvious, inferred ideation which is difficult for the person to verbalize freely owing to the immobilizing force of its associated anxiety feelings.

Feeling responses to human experience may intensify or stimulate the formulation of additional ideas. Feelings may be identified in the language an individual uses to verbalize, in voice tones, facial expressions, gestures, mood manifestations, and body actions. When feelings can be verbalized, without fear of censor or rejection, their release often strengthens the person's ability to think rationally, make judgments and decisions, change attitudes, and initiate action considered appropriate to specific situations.

The duration of a mood state may serve as an index for making distinctions between appropriate and inappropriate behavior reactions to life situations. For instance, feelings of grief and depressed mood are appropriate reactions to bereavement. With the passing of time, release of feelings through talking, weeping, and the investment of energy in the demands of living, we anticipate that grief and depression will subside. Persistence of grief and depression beyond a reasonable time period is an indication that the person is in need of competent medical assistance.

ALL BEHAVIOR IS MEANINGFUL

There is a meaningful explanation for everything a person says and does. This concept is relevant to the desirable nursing attribute of understanding people and the function of helping patients to meet their underlying needs. Meeting needs is dependent upon the ability of the nurse to interpret the meaning of individual patient's behavior. It has been said that people spend a considerable portion of their lives attempting to avoid or alleviate anxiety. Any behavior which reduces or relieves anxiety is rewarding. Owing to the law of effect, rewards favor the learning or "conditioning" of defensive behaviors which alleviate anxiety.[4] Defensive behaviors may be conscious or unconscious reactions to anxiety perceived. For instance, the person who talks freely about an emotionally distressing situation relieves anxiety through communication releases. Need cues may be identified in key words or specific references verbalized. An individual who anticipates that an anxiety-producing topic of discussion may be brought into a nurse-patient relationship may avoid introduction of the topic by talking continuously about another subject or subjects. Another defense may be an attempt by the patient to maneuver the conversation into an interview of the nurse. The nurse's interpretation of the dynamics underlying defensive behaviors may be utilized as a guide for a dynamic nursing response. The nurse may recognize the merit of selecting a listening response, avoiding attempts to change the conversation topic, or simply removing her presence until the patient appears to be relatively anxiety free. When the patient is uncommunicative the nurse may decide to remain with the patient—an approach which conveys understanding and emotional support.

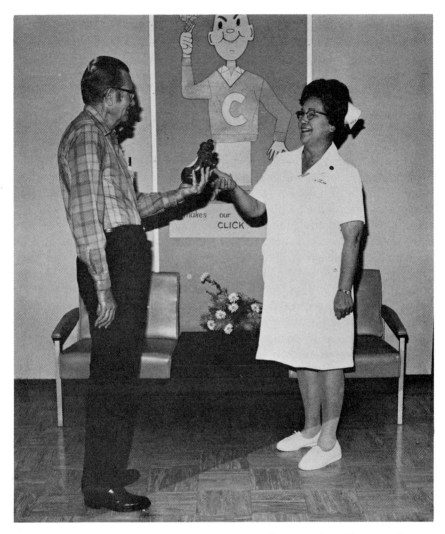

Fig. 2. The person seeking a warmer relationship may offer some token object as a gift to the nurse. (Courtesy of Arkansas State Hospital, Little Rock, Ark.)

Symbolic behaviors mask their hidden motivation and meaning. Their interpretation requires astute observation and interpretation. The patient who becomes anxious when medication is overdue may aim to be tactful and avoid the nurse's rejection by asking, "What time is it?" The question may actually be a reminder to the nurse. The person seeking a warmer relationship may offer some token object as a gift to the nurse. Deep-seated hostility feelings, the release of which are feared as anxiety- and rejection-producing, may be held in check by the individual who is warmly receptive and complimentary toward another person. The examples cited are just a few of the many nursing situations which may provide an understanding of the concept that all behavior is meaningful even though the dynamics may or may not be obvious in surface behavior.

BEHAVIOR IS NEVER STATIC

Behavior is never at a standstill owing to the changes which take place in time and space causing individuals to react to them. Anxiety is often associated with responses to change. During illness the patient's behavior changes as he reacts to his environment, treatment, and interpersonal relations. Recognition of this concept helps the nurse to be alert to as well as to anticipate patients' behavior response to what is happening and its influential relationship to the production of anxiety and the recovery process. Some changes may not be difficult for patients to accept. Others, especially treatment ones, require the giving of nursing support through listening, explanations, reassurance, and the conveying of feelings of trust to the patient.

Some reactions to change are unpredictable owing to the immediacy of the causative stimulus. Changes which can be anticipated offer the possibility of predicting the patient's response as well as planning nursing approaches. Planned approaches are helpful in reducing or eliminating physical and emotional discomfort for the patient. A person who is going to be transferred to another ward environment can be prepared for the change so that its reason and advantages for the patient are understood and accepted. Changes in nursing personnel often create anxiety and insecurity feelings in patients because of one's inability to predict the tenor and trust of unknown relationships. It is helpful for nurses to be aware of feeling responses to changes in human relations and to appreciate the importance of establishing rapport in the nurse-patient relationship. Rapport strengthens security feelings, alleviates anxiety, and favors the patient's recovery.

EMOTIONAL EQUILIBRIUM (HOMEOSTATIS) MAY ALTER WITH INTERNAL AND EXTERNAL CHANGES AND DEMANDS

Any internal or external change which requires the human organism to adapt to new conditions or situations may alter a relatively stable emotional state of existence. There are implications in this concept for the nurse to develop a sensitivity to the emotional status of the patient's behavior. Emotional responses indicate the presence of change, the patient's capacity to adapt, and the need for medical and nursing investigative approaches. These observations are prerequisites for therapeutic interventions which may effect equilibrium or stabilization of the body's physical and mental processes.

STRESS AND STRAIN MAY BE PRODUCED BY BOTH INTERNAL AND EXTERNAL CHANGES AND DEMANDS

Whenever the human organism is exposed to anxiety-producing conditions of stress and strain, its physical and psychic defenses are mobilized to protect against as well as to attract attention to the presence of threat. Stress and strain may be produced by both internal and external changes and demands for adaptation. This concept is relevant to the nursing functions of observation and investigation and also to therapeutic interventions which may relieve anxiety by strenghthening or supplementing the patient's capacity to adapt. Clues relative to the origin of stress and strain may be identified in observable somatic symptoms, examination reports, patients' communications, unique behaviors, analysis of the interpersonal situation, and immediate and remote happenings.

Remote happenings, those situations removed by distance or time from current behaviors observed, are sometimes overlooked when immediate manifestations are being investigated. Anxiety responses to remote happenings may gain momentum if the influencing situation remains unresolved. For instance, a hospitalized patient discovered weeping was reacting to a change which had occurred in her home environment. Another example is that of a patient who became severely agitated and thrust her head against the wall with such force that she required medical treatment. Investigation of the behavior revealed that for several days the patient had been talking about "feeling terrible." Her communication, which was actually a plea for help, had not been explored. Literally speaking, the patient had to bang her head against the wall to create a situation which would attract attention to her distress and need for therapeutic intervention.

COPING WITH STRESS AND STRAIN IS AN INDIVIDUALISTIC ABILITY

Being able to cope with stress and strain and relieve the anxiety which they produce in a person is an individualistic quality of behavior. The appropriateness and strength of a person's natural and acquired defenses determine success or failure in overcoming threats to unified, integrated body-and-personality functioning. This concept is relevant to nursing attitudes of understanding and acceptance of patients' behavior, considered a prime requisite for quality nursing.

Some individuals have developed natural immunities to specific illnesses. To resist the same illnesses, other persons must acquire immunity through the ministrations of medical personnel. When illness develops in the absence of natural or acquired immunity, the afflicted person requires supportive, alleviating treatment. Likewise, some persons have developed psychic defenses sufficiently strong to resolve mental conflicts which produce anxiety, and thus are able to maintain emotional stability. Other individuals, unable to cope successfully with the stress and strain of psychic conflict, resort consciously or unconsciously to inappropriate defensive behaviors which release anxiety, but do not resolve mental conflict. Thus, the symptoms observed during periods of emotional and mental disturbance are inappropriate defensive behaviors. Their intensity and duration varies, dependent upon the severity of the conflictual situation, the availability and effectiveness of tension-relieving emotional support given by significant persons, and the ability of the patient to reorganize and unify his personality functioning.

Inappropriate defensive behaviors are not always overtly pathological. Some defensive behaviors are relinquished by patients within a relatively short period of time when remedial, supportive care is promptly administered and effective. This belief has been aptly demonstrated in the psychiatric services of general hospitals and mental health clinics. Nurses are in a unique position to provide the care and emotional support which help to reduce patients' anxiety, tensions, and need for defensive reactions. Each situation, however, requires nursing judgments relative to actions to be taken which are based upon observations and interpretations of the individual patient's behavior and the underlying needs communicated.[5]

ILLNESS CAN BE A LEARNING EXPERIENCE

The emphasis placed upon health teaching and learning has contributed to the impression that teaching and learning in the sick environment are focused upon physical aspects of illness and health. Actually, learning experiences during illness may be those which are related to the learning of new attitudes and behaviors which reduce the incidence of anxiety-producing situations. This concept is relevant to the nurse-patient relationship. Recovery from illness is essentially a growth process. Personality growth is fostered through satisfying learning experiences with significant persons. Emotionally disturbed people often do not trust or have confidence in themselves or other individuals—feelings which are basic to the development of successful human relations. Trust and confidence are learned behavior attitudes acquired in relationships with others. The manner in which the nurse speaks to patients, accepts them, and permits them to express feelings, without retaliating, as well as to participate in treatment may actually be learning experiences which foster trusting relationships leading to personality growth.

INTERESTS AND APTITUDES REPRESENT
GROWTH POTENTIALITIES

A person's natural interests and aptitudes (abilities) are considered to be potentialities for his personality growth. Because illness can be a learning experience this concept has implications for the nursing functions of observation and helping to plan patients' treatment. Interests and aptitudes may be identified in the observations made during interaction of a patient's preference for conversation subjects and activities. When identified, interests and aptitudes constitute a readiness and foundation for learning leading to personal growth. To provide growth-inducing learning experiences the nurse may require the counsel and assistance of other health workers. When learning experiences contribute to the patient's acquisition of social, diversional, or vocational skills they produce satisfaction feelings which influence favorably the patient's rehabilitation and recovery.

HUMAN GROWTH AND PERSONALITY DEVELOPMENT
REPRESENT THE RESULT OF A COMPLEX PROCESS

Everything an individual is exposed to during his life experience, including his culture, environment, health conditions, and interpersonal relations, influences his growth and personality development. The health state and personality characteristics, traits and defenses observed in the nurse-patient relationship are the result of this lifelong complex process. The forces which have impinged upon the patient's growth and development affect his reactions during illness, treatment, and interactions with other individuals. These factors constitute what is often referred to as the psychodynamics of personality development and behavior. Thus, it should be obvious that a dynamic nursing approach must be based upon an understanding of the individual patient's past and present life experiences, including the immediate experiences associated with medical and nursing care. There are no available clear-cut, stereotyped nursing interpretations or responses to observations made of patterns of behavior or symptoms manifested by sick persons. When the nurse is imbued with an understanding of this concept, she is prepared to make objective instead of subjective interpretations of behavior in attempting to meeting individual patient's needs.

KNOWLEDGE OF PERSONALITY DEVELOPMENT STRUCTURE PROVIDES A FRAMEWORK FOR STUDYING BEHAVIOR

Frames of reference are helpful in making comparisons between what is being studied currently and what is already known in relation to the subject of study. From the comparisons made, conclusions are drawn concerning the current object of study. A framework for the study of personality development has been structured by investigators who have made observations of human growth and development as it proceeds from birth to old age. Certain manifestations of physical and emotional growth have been identified as normal sequential life-stage developments. Physical growth usually proceeds without interruption so that the physique of the infant develops into that of the adult. Emotional growth may proceed in unison with physical growth or it may be arrested at a specific stage of personality development, dependent upon the person's inborn capacities as well as the life experiences to which the individual is exposed in his culture, environment, and relationships with other persons. Thus, the behavior of the physically mature individual may be emotionally immature to the extent of being equated with an identifiable earlier stage of emotional growth. The comment that a person is behaving like a child is testimony to the comparison being made between the individual's behavior and a personality development frame of reference. What is important, however, is to discover what happened during the earlier period of life which stymied the person's emotional growth sufficiently to subsequently influence adult behavior.

Through education, nurses learn the frame of reference associated with personality development. Its use as a basis for comparison in evaluating and attempting to understand behavior is dependent upon the nurse's obtaining pertinent information concerning the individual patient. To learn about the patient's unique life experiences and present illness situation the nurse may utilize professional sources of information as well as skillful communication techniques during interactions with patients and their relatives.

INDIVIDUAL CONCEPTS OF SPECIFIC ILLNESSES MAY BE OF CULTURAL, SOCIAL, OR FAMILIAL ORIGIN

The ideas and beliefs an individual associates with illness in general or a specific illness may stem from the person's culture, or community, society, or family group. Because individual concepts of illness may influence a person's reactions to illness, treatment, and recovery, it is helpful for the nurse to discover how the patient thinks and feels about his particular illness. This knowledge may be related to the patient's present and possible future health state.

McCabe described patients receiving care in a modern general hospital who conceived of their illness as the "miseries" associated with human existence, a concept most likely having its roots in the patients' ancestral primitive culture. These patients endured their discomforts as if they were to be expected and rarely requested nursing attention.[6] Some persons consider cancer incurable and manifest fear, anxiety, and hopeless feelings. Mental illness is regarded by some individuals as a heredity affliction. They fear its familial transmission.

Nurses may harbor concepts of specific illnesses which influence their care of patients as well as patients' responses. If a nurse has fearful or hopeless ideas, beliefs and feelings about an illness she may reinforce already existing fearful or hopeless concepts in a patient. Thus, it is helpful for nurses to be aware of their personal concepts of illness and to recognize the possibilities of their influence on patients' responses to and recovery from illness.

CHANGES WHICH ALTER OR THREATEN THE CAPACITY FUNCTIONING OF THE HUMAN BODY EVOKE PHYSICAL AND EMOTIONAL REACTIONS

Illness may alter a person's capacity to function or make it necessary to rely upon substitute or supportive devices for functioning. Such changes may evoke feelings and thinking which may be threatening to the person's image of the self. Feelings of fear, anxiety, inadequacy, and loss of confidence may be manifested by the patient. Concern may be expressed about future relationships, acceptance by others, and the ability to be self-reliant and financially independent. For instance, a patient having an open colostomy may be required to wear a receptacle for elimination purposes. An individual having a leg fracture may use crutches for walking. Anxiety may interfere with a person's ability to concentrate or perform other functions requiring certain intellectual activities. Nurses can help to provide the care and emotional support which alleviate negative feeling reactions and alterations in the person's image of the self. A professional understanding of specific illnesses, their possible accompaniments, and degrees of incapacity enable the nurse to recognize and appreciate threatening-feeling influences of illness. Nursing approaches may be aimed to help the patient overcome defects in functioning, accept limitations, or learn new ways of functioning.

These approaches are anxiety-reducing and alleviating. Adaptations and adjustments are achieved with a minimum of distress when the nurse is capable of transferring feelings of acceptance, hope, and confidence to the patient through nursing actions.

ATTITUDES INFLUENCE BEHAVIOR

Attitudes are expressions of a person's feelings and thinking concerning people, events, places, or abstract ideas. They predispose an individual to be motivated to behave in specific ways. Attitudes may be acquired as responses to life experiences or learned through association with other individuals. A person may adopt an attitude shown by another individual or may express one which reflects the emotional impact of a specific happening or relationship. This concept is relevant to the nursing investigative approach. When it is accepted it may cause the nurse to speculate upon or query into the relationship between the patient's attitude behavior and his past or present experiences. Speculation and queries may include a focus upon the attitudes shown by the nurse during interaction with the patient. The nurse's attitude may influence her own behavior as well as that of the patient.

ATTITUDES CAN BE CHANGED

It is sometimes beneficial for patients to be helped by nurses to change attitudes which negate favorable responses during illness. It is well to remember that attitudes which do not favor recovery are often the result of experiences which have caused the patient to feel pushed, rejected, threatened, or abandoned. Consequently, the individual develops anxiety and a need to protect and preserve his individuality, independence, and personal identification in a group. Direct verbal appeals to the patient's reason and logic are ineffective approaches toward changing attitudes because they lack the elements of realistic experiences which are conducive to effecting desirable changes in thinking and feeling. Attitudes are more likely to change through nursing approaches having inherent attitudes which motivate changes in the person's thinking and feeling. For instance, a patient who manifests an attitude of disinterest in a social activity may become interested when he is invited instead of told to participate because the activity is part of treatment. A patient who demonstrates a critical attitude toward personnel may develop an approving attitude when shown that the staff does not avoid or penalize him owing to his attitude.

REHABILITATION IS A VITAL PART OF THERAPY

Rehabilitation is an important phase of treatment aimed to restore the patient to an optimum level of physical and mental functioning. It is an individual approach based upon a study of each patient's impairments, potentialities for achievement, aptitudes, interests, and needs. The objective is to help the patient become self-reliant and self-sustaining in the community. Learning activities are selected to restore normal aspects of body functioning as well as to foster the learning of social, recreational, and vocational skills. To implement this concept, special therapists plan and teach physical, vocational, and rehabilitative technics. In the treatment environment, nurses assist the health team by planning for and participating with patients in selected physical, social and recreational activities. They may provide opportunities for patients to study and practice vocational skills. A patient who is capable of making a fuller contribution to society while meeting his own personal sustenance needs is strengthened in his capacity to avoid and resist anxiety-producing life situations.

REHABILITATION IS INFLUENCED BY SELF-PARTICIPATION

Successful rehabilitation depends upon the patient's acceptance of the treatment program as well as the degree of interest and participation placed in rehabilitative learning experiences. This concept is relevant to nursing practice because the nurse in her relationships with patients is in a unique position to influence their participation. Nursing approaches may be aimed to encourage the patient to make therapeutic use of his intellect and reasoning and to willingly participate in accepting and adapting to a rehabilitation program designed to raise his self-sustaining level. The degree to which the person is able to function independently in the management of his daily occupational and social needs influences his feelings of confidence, security, satisfaction, self-esteem, and dignity.

REHABILITATION IS INFLUENCED BY
FAMILY PARTICIPATION

When members of the patient's family participate in rehabilitation conferences and activities conducted by the medical and allied treatment staff, it helps them to achieve a better understanding of illness and the patient's responses. Participation offers opportunities for them to ask questions and seek advice. What is learned often helps to dispel misconceptions and fears, and fosters the acceptance of illness. Relatives may learn what to anticipate in the patient's behavior and how to respond to help meet the patient's needs. Family participation may be a source of emotional support which stimulates, strengthens and reinforces favorable responses in the patient. Nurses may participate in rehabilitation programs designed to teach and assist family members. They also have occasion to meet and talk with relatives who visit patients in the hospital or whom they may meet in patients' homes. Nurses who accept this concept may utilize communication and teaching approach opportunities to encourage interest and participation of the patients' relatives in rehabilitation programs.

SOCIAL INSTITUTIONS ARISE TO MEET SOCIETY'S NEEDS

Each era of human existence has its values, philosophies, emphases, scientific discoveries, and advancement in knowledge. These cultural developments give impetus to the establishment of social institutions designed to meet society's needs. We live in a humanitarian period. In keeping with the times, society places high value upon the health, comfort, happiness and betterment of the individual. The emphasis upon prevention and early treatment of illness and rehabilitation has led to the creation of many new health institutions. Various types of mental health clinics and treatment centers have been established to prevent long-term illness and to assist in the rehabilitation of mentally ill patients. The hospital, formerly considered the headquarters for treating illness, has become one of a network of related community health agencies. This advance has caused the practice of nursing to expand into the community. Nurses become acquainted with, and nurse in cooperation with, community health and allied agencies to assist in the prevention of illness and in meeting patients' health needs.

COMMUNITY EDUCATION INFLUENCES SOCIETY'S REACTIONS

Historical accounts reveal the influence of education upon the rise and fall of social regimens. Education is recognized as a system for conveying information and motivating social change, opinion, and action. Realizing that the health of a nation is vital to its preservation, health specialists have introduced community education. This concept is relevant to the teaching role of nurses. Professional nurses participate in plans and organizations designed to educate community residents concerning illness, its treatment and prevention, and the availability of special services in local health facilities. Examples of community education programs in which nurses participate are those provided by heart associations, mental health societies, and the like. Through community education programs, participants may be motivated to adopt health practices learned and to assist the organizations in their aims and achievement of objectives.

SOCIETY IS IMPROVED THROUGH
JOINT EFFORTS

Groups of people having mutual interests may institute social reforms and controls or give support to a cause which benefits their society. Nurses have professional, personal, and citizen obligations. As members of citizen groups, nurses have opportunities to participate in activities which foster social improvement. The nurse may attend citizen meetings, interpret health needs, support appropriate legislative action, and vote upon matters related to social and health improvement. For instance, the nurse may support citizen action favoring the establishment of a mental health clinic; she may interpret the need for a community youth recreation center, school lunch program, rehabilitation facility for physically handicapped persons, or a day social center for aged residents.

TREATMENT AND CARE OF THE MENTALLY ILL ARE NOW
CONSIDERED MORAL, SOCIAL, AND
COMMUNITY RESPONSIBILITIES

When interpreting mental illness and the needs of the mentally ill to succeeding generations of professional nurses and citizen groups it is important for nurses to perpetuate the ideal. The latter half of the twentieth century will be recorded historically as a period during which treatment and care of the mentally ill are considered moral, social, and community responsibilities. Individual citizens, social groups, and community governments have advanced in their thinking, contributions, and organized activities to meet the needs of the mentally ill. For more than 2,000 years previous to this century, attitudes toward the mentally ill, their treatment, and their care have fluctuated in accordance with prevailing philosophies, interests, and resources. Humane periods of attitudes and treatment have never been charted in a straight line of ascent. Contemporary philosophies, interests, and resources greatly favor the continuance of moral viewpoints and treatment. Whether or not there is a break with the record of the past depends greatly upon the nursing profession. Never before have the resources and sentiment for improvement of the treatment and care of the mentally ill been more favorable or more challenging.

It is hoped that the nurse who has read this chapter has gained an appreciation for the concepts discussed herein and their relationship to the nursing process.

SUGGESTED REFERENCES

Bier, R.: Rehabilitation on a shoestring. Am. J. Nurs. 61: 98 (Aug.), 1961.

Blanton, S.: Love or Perish. Simon & Schuster, Inc., New York, 1955, p. 52.

Bressler, B.: The psychotherapeutic nurse. Am. J. Nurs. 62: 87 (May), 1962.

Brownberger, C.: Emotional stress connected with surgery. Nurs. Forum 4: 46, 1965.

Carlson, C.: Behavioral Concepts and Nursing Intervention. J. B. Lippincott Co., Philadelphia, 1970.

Committee on Therapeutic Care, Group for the Advancement of Psychiatry: Toward Therapeutic Care. Springer Publishing Company, New York, 1970.

Fleming, R., and Grayson, D.: An aftercare program for patients discharged from mental hospitals. Nurs. Outlook 9: 544 (Sept.), 1961.

Gorton, J.: Behavioral Components of Patient Care. The MacMillan Company, Collier-MacMillan Limited, London, 1970.

Hays, J.: The psychiatric nurse as sociotherapist. Am. J. Nurs. 62: 64 (June), 1962.

Ingles, T.: Understanding the nurse-patient relationship. Nurs. Outlook 9: 698 (Nov.), 1961.

Jackson, J.: The role of the patient's family in illness. Nurs. Forum 1: 1187, 1962.

King, S.: Beliefs and attitudes about mental illness, in Perceptions of Illness in Medical Practice. Russell Sage Foundation, New York, 1962, p. 134.

Lewis, J.: Reflections on self. Am. J. Nurs. 60: 828 (June), 1960.

Madden, B., and Affeldt, J.: To prevent helplessness and deformities. Am. J. Nurs. 63: 59 (Dec.), 1962.

Mahaffy, P.: Nurse-parent relationships in living-in situations. Nurs. Forum 3: 52, 1964.

Maloney, E.: Does the psychiatric nurse have independent functions? Am. J. Nurs. 62: 61 (June), 1962.

Martin, H., and Prange, A.: The stages of illness—psychosocial approach. Nurs. Outlook 10: 168 (March), 1962.

McCabe, G.: Cultural influences on patient behavior. Am. J. Nurs. 60:1101 (Aug.), 1960.

Mercita, Sr. M.: Rehabilitation—bridge to a useful and happy life. Nurs. Outlook 10: 581 (Sept.), 1962.

Monterio, L.: The patient had difficulty communicating. Am. J. Nurs. 62: 78 (Jan.), 1962.

Neylan, M.: Anxiety. Am. J. Nurs. 62: 110 (May), 1962.

Otto, H.: The human potentialities of nurses and patients. Nurs. Outlook 13: 32 (Aug.), 1965.

Peplau, H.: Interpersonal techniques. The crux of psychiatric nursing. Am. J. Nurs. 62: 50 (June), 1962.

Roslyn, E., and Diers, D.: The patient comes to the hospital. Nurs. Forum 2: 89, 1963.

Ross, E.: On Death and Dying. The MacMillan Company, New York, 1969.

Schmahl, J.: Ritualism in nursing practice. Nurs. Forum 3: 74, 1964.

Smith, S.: The psychology of illness. Nurs. Forum 3: 35, 1964.

Stillar, E.: Continuity of care. Nurs. Outlook 10: 584 (Sept.), 1962.

Tarnower, W.: Psychological needs of the hospitalized patient. Nurs. Outlook 13: 28 (July), 1965.

Trail, I., and Monke, V.: Psyche sequelae of surgical change in body structure. Nurs. Forum 3: 13, 1963.

Tryon, P., and Leonard, R.: The effect of the patient's participation on the outcome of a nursing procedure. Nurs. Forum 3: 79, 1964.

Ullman, M.: Disorders of body image after stroke. Am. J. Nurs. 64: 89 (Oct.), 1964.

Wolfe, N.: Setting reasonable limits on behavior. Am. J. Nurs. 62: 104 (March), 1962.

FOOTNOTES

1. Johnson, D.: The significance of nursing care. Am. J. Nurs. 61: 63 (Nov.), 1961.
2. Blanton, S.: Love or Perish. Simon & Schuster, Inc., New York, 1955, p. 52.
3. Film: Grief—A Peril in Infancy. New York University Film Library, Washington Square, New York City.
4. May, R.: The Meaning of Anxiety. The Ronald Press, New York, 1950, p. 103.
5. Maloney, E.: Does the psychiatric nurse have independent functions? Am. J. Nurs. 62: 61 (June), 1962.
6. McCabe, G.: Cultural influences on patient behavior. Am. J. Nurs. 60: 1101 (Aug.), 1960.

CHAPTER 19

Effect of the Environment upon Behavior

The importance of the effect of the environment upon the patient's behavior should not be underestimated. This includes the physical aspects of the environment, as well as the interpersonal ones (see Chaps. 20, 21, and 23). The society in which a person lives, whether it be a hospital, a hotel, or a home, is one of the major determinants of his behavior. Patients and relatives coming into a hospital must discover how people are going to perceive the patient in his sick role. They must know how people are going to help the patient and especially under what conditions. The very architecture of the institution is going to influence patients' and relatives' concepts.

Creating a therapeutic environment in our present mental hospitals challenges the integrity, ingenuity, resourcefulness and intellect of the entire staff. We live in an age in which there is striving between old and new concepts of patient care. Some of the problems we face in attempting to create a therapeutic environment may appear to be insurmountable to some individuals. There is, however, every indication that new treatments and concepts of rehabilitation will eventually reduce sufficiently or eliminate some of our major obstacles. Community mental health centers, psychiatric wards in general hospitals, mental hygiene clinics, day and night treatment centers, halfway houses, and integrated plans for community facilities and care are increasing. Special hospitals for alcoholics and the aged, recreational day centers for elderly persons, vocational rehabilitation agencies, and foster homes are also increasing in numbers. More patients are being cared for in their homes. In addition, the emphasis upon prevention of mental illness, early treatment, and enlightenment of the general public concerning psychiatric disorders will undoubtedly manifest their assistance effects in the creation of a therapeutic environment in the mental health facilities of the future. Authorities view the outcome of these developments in terms of reduced number of patient admissions and population in our larger psychiatric hospitals. Integrated plans for community facilities and care have already resulted in the commencement of construction of smaller community mental health centers to replace the present state type of structures. Sociologists have recommended that our remaining larger hospitals be divided into two or more separate institutions to be administered by individual superintendents.

OLD AND NEW CONCEPTS

Some personnel are still governed by the momentum of past thinking, and have not attempted to make use of the great wealth of modern knowledge available to us concerning the management of human behavior.

Some of our public hospitals are still large, overcrowded, unattractive and isolated from the community with its normal aspects of living. While we may be imbued with a desire to help those who need help and to develop in them the desire and ability to help themselves, the environment has, in many instances, forced us into the position of being our brother's keeper instead of his helper. Change is difficult, especially for those staff members who have achieved feelings of security in caring for patients who are domiciled behind locked doors and subjected to certain limitations and restrictions. There is often the tendency to impose and perpetuate the same restrictions in living upon all patients regardless of their individual capacities and needs.

The open hospital which has developed considerably in both England and Canada appears to be inevitable in the United States. Some of our institutions have opened many of their doors. Others are moving cautiously and slowly toward this change. There are certain security and legal complications to overcome in some areas before the open-door policy becomes an absolute reality.

Our cultural heritage has endowed us with a democracy which respects the dignity and personal freedom of man. Thus, the restrictions upon human behavior which still exist in many of our hospitals will undoubtedly be removed some day in the future. New discoveries and methods of treatment will, most likely, assist in making this revolutionary change which is already upon the psychiatric scene. The real key, however, to the creation of a therapeutic environment lies in the ability of all personnel to relate beneficially with patients in a warm, comfortable, homelike atmosphere, and to allow them the attainment of individual needs and the privilege of self-activity. To do this requires preparation of all personnel to function effectively as social therapists in group and team relationships. Outmoded custodial approaches of vigilant watchfulness must yield to skillful interpersonal contacts with patients which inspire faith and confidence leading to a desire for recovery and a return to the larger community.

Fortunately, we lean toward change at a time when new concepts regarding patient care and treatment developments have proved, to a considerable degree, effective in providing an optimistic outlook toward the recovery of the mentally ill. Problematical behavior has been reduced to the extent that it has become possible to replace much of the formerly absent normal accessories of everyday living in many of our hospital environments. More and more we are reaching out into the community from which we were formerly largely isolated. As we increase our contacts and inspire the assistance of citizens we will eventually have the means to acquire a therapeutic environment. Therefore, nursing personnel must possess the know-how to revise and create.

ARCHITECTURE

Many of our older psychiatric institutions date back to colonial times. Architecturally these structures are frozen in an antique ideology which is out of harmony with our present concepts of adequate space, freedom, privacy, and remotivation. This fact, however, should not deter personnel from attempting to introduce change whenever possible in the present hospitals. In the details of some environments lie potentialities for improvement of patients' living. It is important for all staff members to be acquainted with desirable aspects of a social setting in order to assist with plans for renovation of some of our older structures and the construction of new psychiatric facilities.

RECEPTION LOUNGE

First impressions are lasting. The general hospital has recognized for some time the need for an attractive, warm environment in a reception lounge. Unfortunately, a number of psychiatric hospital reception foyers are cold, austere, and too business-like in appearance. Consideration for this area is necessary because it produces feeling reactions in visitors which may cause them to respond negatively to the entire hospital environment.

A spacious, comfortable entrance can do much to make visitors feel welcome, at ease, and necessary to the patient's recovery. As changes are made and new hospitals constructed it is hoped that this important part of the psychiatric institution will receive the attention it deserves. Colorful walls, floors, drapes, pictures, flowers, plants and other furnishings help to enhance the reception foyer. Toilet facilities should be easily accessible to visitors.

Reception personnel should be carefully selected individuals who like people and have a deep appreciation for the frailties of human beings and their need to be understood and accepted. The manner in which relatives are received and assisted is of utmost importance. It should be recognized that some personnel are just naturally adept at meeting strangers and making them feel welcome and comfortable in the hospital environment.

VISITING ROOMS

One of the most striking inconveniences for relatives and patients is the lack of suitable visiting rooms in many mental hospitals. In some institutions there is absolutely no place for relatives to visit privately with patients. This problem is more obvious in open wards and dormitories where several patients live together. Living rooms may be used by some persons, but owing to overcrowded conditions it has been necessary to use some of these areas for other purposes. If there is a dining room on the ward, patients could be allowed to visit there with relatives and friends. Some personnel have found it possible to convert one sleeping room into a visiting area even though this change required that one or two beds be moved into a dormitory. Making such a provision requires that the staff weigh the value to patients and visitors of this area with other values, such as health conditions and fire prevention in the larger dormitory. Experience in some hospitals has proved a change of this type to be entirely safe and emotionally beneficial.

WARD ENVIRONMENT

It is much easier for the person to accept hospitalization and adapt to the environment when security measures are reduced to a minimum. Deviations from a normal environment creat feelings of fear, insecurity, anxiety, and doubts about one's mental capacity. Stripping the ward of normal living accommodations and furnishings, conveniences, eating utensils, toilet articles, and restricting patients' movements reduce their feelings of self-esteem, confidence, and faith in the hospital. Symbolically, such practices convey to the patient: We cannot trust you. We expect the worst of you.

It has been demonstrated that overactive behavior is at a minimum when disturbed patients live in an attractive, comfortable furnished environment. Appealing color tones, comfortable chairs, tables, lamps, and window curtains and/or drapes constitute an important aspect of the general ward environment. A piano, sheet music, current magazines, books

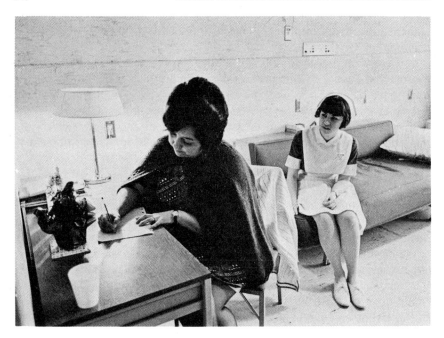

Fig. 1. An attractively furnished and pleasant bedroom. (Courtesy of Sweedish-American Hospital, Rockford, Ill.)

and televisions are excellent diversional provisions. Natural or artificial flowers, plants and pictures are esthetically pleasing to human beings. A calendar and ward clock are of much value to patients because people have a need to be in contact with the date and time and feel anxious when these articles are absent. Proper ventilation and light are essential health provisions. Nursing personnel should be sensitive to the ward temperature. Assistance may be obtained from the maintenance department, when necessary, to make adjustments on individual wards.

BEDROOMS AND DORMITORIES

Single bedrooms furnished attractively in hotel style with a bed, bedside table, writing desk, dresser, lamps, mirrors, chairs, and window curtains and/or drapes are desirable. Toilet, bathing facilities, and clothes closets are essential. Some patients need and desire this privacy. Others crave companionship and prefer to live in a double room or small dormitory. Many hospitals are not constructed to offer patients a choice in living arrangements. Whenever possible the individual's needs for living alone or in company with others should be taken into consideration. Some of the present, larger, open wards could be converted easily into cubicle arrangements which allow privacy as well as group association.

An obvious lack in the older institutions is clothes closets. To meet patients' needs for clothing storage, some wards are equipped with large, general clothes rooms which are usually kept locked. Patients are frequently unable to choose their own wearing apparel and access to clothing may be had only if some member of the nursing staff is available to unlock the door of the clothes room. Therefore, it becomes difficult and often impossible to rehabilitate patients in a normal environment in which one is able to exercise initiative, make decisions, and engage in self-activity. Perhaps this practice exists in many instances because we have simply adhered to past practice and failed to investigate the possibilities of desirable change. It may be entirely possible to remove clothing restrictions for many patients. Individual metal clothes lockers which require little additional space at the bedside might be substituted in a number of areas. Single lockers are preferable to section arrangements, especially when patients are confused and tend to misplace their clothing in another person's compartment. While developing self-reliance in clothing selection and dress, patients would automatically relieve the nursing staff of unnecessary attentions. General clothes rooms usually require the space allocated for two bedside units or single rooms. A ten-ward hospital, for instance, may actually be reducing its number of available beds by twenty when such a clothing plan exists.

BATHING AND TOILET FACILITIES

Group bathing and toilet facilities still exist in many of our older hospitals. It has been recognized that the number of plumbing fixtures is inadequate when compared with the patient census. Open toilet and shower facilities are a common observation and, no doubt, were originally provided for protection purposes. This arrangement, however, is not in keeping with our concepts of striving to meet patients' needs. Inspection committees have viewed some of these areas and are to be commended for their recommendations to increase toilet and bathing facilities. Most important, however, is the need to separate individual fixtures with partitions so that necessary privacy is provided.

The system of locking water valves and designating certain days of the week and hours to bathe should be recognized as outmoded and unnecessary for many patients. Encouraging individuals to develop desirable hygienic practices depends a great deal upon the availability of resources. Many persons who are accustomed to and enjoy a daily bath or shower are often unable to use bathing facilities. Sensitive people resent these limitations because they indicate that the patient is unreliable and unable to make simple decisions. A well-prepared nurse is able to recognize immediately patients who fail to attend to their daily hygiene and are in need of some suggestion and supervision. Restrictions upon bathing in all wards is unnecessary and fails to provide patients with feelings of personal comfort, trust and the incentive to recover. Instead, such limitations simply increase nursing duties.

PERSONAL PROPERTY

Combs, hair brushes, toothpaste, toothbrushes, deodorants, and cosmetics are often locked away from patients' bedside units. For years it has been assumed that these articles are implements of self-destruction and they should be allowed only under supervision at stated times, usually upon arising in the morning and prior to retiring in the evening. Nursing personnel are often so busy that they find it impossible to unlock these articles and supervise their use. Patients are frequently unable to attend to personal grooming to effect a presentable appearance. Such limitations leave much to be desired if the patients' efforts toward self-improvement are hampered by this method. Whenever possible, modern nursing personnel should attempt to change these practices. Quite often administrators are not aware that some limitations exist, and it may be possible to remove some of these restrictions. When requested, relatives will usually be happy to purchase cosmetics in unbreakable containers.

Some institutions have realized the value to women patients of having available on the ward a shampoo sink and hair dryer. When these facilities must be located in a general beauty parlor, it does seem as if a plan could be devised to make them accessible to patients who are able to make personal use of them as they desire. Often patients are skillful in the art of hair styling and enjoy assisting less capable patients with their coiffures.

Some institutions do not allow patients to carry money upon their person. All purchases must be made with money certificates or charge accounts. Both systems create tremendous paper work for hospital personnel while denying all patients a small human privilege, trust, and an opportunity to exercise responsibility. A small number of patients may be too confused and bewildered to assume this responsibility and for them a substitute method is desirable. To be able to purchase such items as cigarettes, newspapers, candies, soft drinks, and the like on a money exchange basis would do much to heighten some patients' morale.

LAUNDRY FACILITIES

Making light laundry facilities accessible to patients is most helpful in encouraging them to attend to their personal appearance. Experiments have demonstrated that mentally ill women patients enjoy the privilege of washing and ironing certain articles of clothing and frocks which are difficult to handle with care in the large, central laundry. When it is not possible to equip the individual ward with these facilities, patients may be allowed to launder and iron some of their clothing if a special room can be provided for this purpose in another area of the hospital.

LIVING AND GAME ROOMS

Quite often patients using the living room desire to relax in a restful environment where they may read, sew, knit, crochet, write letters, listen to music programs, or just meditate. For this reason some of the modern institutions have added a game room or general recreation room to the ward environment. The game room is equipped with tables, chairs, and cabinets containing playing cards, various games, and puzzles. A ping pong table also may be included. Additional recreation space makes it possible for patients to express their individual social needs with less concern for patients who sometimes feel distressed in the presence of some competition and hilarity.

DINING ROOMS AND KITCHENS

Anything which will increase the attractiveness of dining rooms is helpful in creating a therapeutic environment. Flowers, plants, and other seasonal decorations have a very appealing effect when they are placed on tables and buffets. Colorful walls and window drapes afford pleasing surroundings at meal time. Some of the newer institutions have decorated these areas with painted murals of interesting design. Small group table service for four persons is desirable for a friendly dining atmosphere. Whenever possible, patients should be allowed the use of customary eating utensils, including knives, forks, and spoons.

Having a ward kitchen equipped with facilities for the storage of staple food items is advantageous. In some of our older hospitals, many of the wards do not have kitchens because food service is provided in large, congregate dining rooms. There are times, however, when it is socially advantageous to have heating equipment to warm foods and beverages. A refrigerator is necessary to preserve foods which decompose readily at normal room temperature. Patients enjoy planning small parties on the

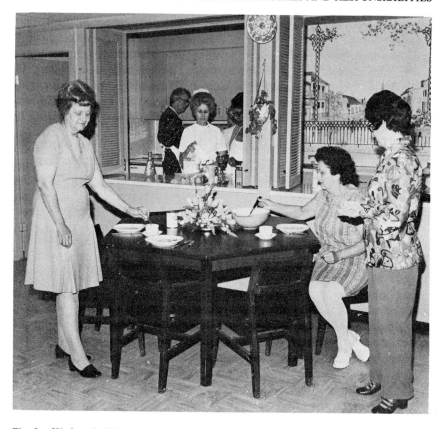

Fig. 2. Kitchen facilities make it possible for patients to plan a small party in the ward. (Courtesy of Arkansas State Hospital, Little Rock, Ark.)

ward, and kitchen facilities make this pleasant, intimate type of family association possible. Nursing personnel will discover that usually patients who are allowed this privilege gladly assume the responsibility for maintaining the appearance and health conditions of a small kitchen. As the hospital takes over the care of the patient in his sick role it must endeavor to provide more of the functions provided formerly by the family.

OFFICE, CONFERENCE AND TREATMENT ROOMS

Remaining in a closed office which obstructs the nurse's observation of patients and their activities contributes to difficulties in ward management. Newer types of offices make it possible for personnel to carry on record functions while being able to view at a glance the ward activities and

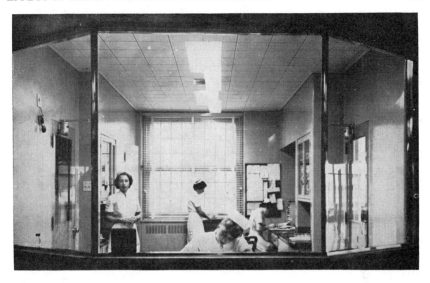

Fig. 3.   Modern nursing office with excellent view--Allan Memorial Institute of Psychiatry. (Courtesy of Royal Victoria Hospital, Montreal, Canada.)

patients. This arrangement also offers to patients a certain amount of security in knowing the location of staff members whom they may wish to approach for various reasons.

Conference rooms are valuable, particularly for conducting group therapy and team meetings in a quiet environment. These rooms can also be used for individual patient interviews and psychological testing.

A ward treatment room eliminates the necessity of removing patients to another area of the hospital when it becomes necessary to administer some treatment in the care of the patient. It is also helpful for conducting physical examinations.

THE OPEN HOSPITAL

The open hospital concept attracted world-wide attention. American doctors visited the British institutions during the summer of 1957 and were enthusiastic about many of their observations.[1] The open hospital is the most outstanding symbol of the new philosophy in the treatment of the mentally ill. Until the 1950s administrative and legal considerations overshadowed the possibility of change in philosophy and treatment. This was because none of the treatments as we know them today were available.

Discussions concerning the open-door policy evoked both positive and negative reactions in some administrators, but we began to move gradually toward this change. Some investigators estimated that between 80 and 90 per cent of the mentally ill could be treated in open hospitals. Certain problems are still being solved in connection with the establishment of the open door concept in some psychiatric institutions and facilities. Depending upon the individual psychiatric hospital and the philosophy which predominates, nurses may assist in moving rapidly or slowly toward the conversion into an open institution. In some instances it is necessary to temper one's enthusiasm and move in accordance with administrative direction. It will be helpful for personnel to have some knowledge concerning the aspects of conversion from a closed to an open hospital so that they may assist effectively with its development.

Investigators who favor open wards say that locked doors, railings, and fences do much to destroy relationships between the staff of a mental hospital, patients, and society, perpetuating the insecurities and anxieties felt towards one another. Patients feel hostile and resentful and tend to become isolated and completely dependent. Experiments have demonstrated that living in a normal environment raises the individual's self-esteem and the morale of the entire ward.[2]

Authorities point out that personnel involved in converting to the open hospital should recognize their own tendencies to develop anxiety, insecurity, and fear during the conversion process. Such a venture will require confidence and integrity on the part of all staff members. Perhaps we may take courage by reviewing the past, especially the example of Doctor Philippe Pinel who released the mentally ill from their chains.

Contemplating such a change presents the possibility that in the years to come medical personnel will look back upon our present security methods as inhuman. Undoubtedly, the future will present more and better treatment discoveries which will eliminate our present problems, making it possible to treat the mentally ill exclusively in open hospitals. Time and changes will eliminate our present difficulties and reduce future generations' sympathy and appreciation of our current problems. Our viewpoints will vanish into oblivion. Thus, some day we may very well be thought of and spoken of as the keepers of the mentally ill.

According to the literature, the average hospital can be opened in about ten months' time if a well thought out plan is prepared in advance. Three steps are considered important when making such a change. First, the patients who are security risks are transferred to a special institution. When such facilities are not available immediately, it may be assumed that the individual institution would have to rely upon placing these persons in special security wards. The second step is to segregate patients according to their behavior tendencies and abilities.* A third and very important step is to develop a well-organized daily schedule of social activities which patients may help to plan and initiate on the wards.[2]

Ward doors are kept open during the day, but locked at night. Patients are allowed to come and go as they please and have access to porches, lawns, gardens, and their personal property. They assume the responsibility for their personal needs and are encouraged to help less able patients to dress, move out of doors, and socialize.

Many advantages of the open hospital are cited in various reports. Contact between patients and staff is improved; mutual trust and sharing develop. Voluntary admissions to the hospital increase. Newly admitted patients are less fearful. Hostile, impulsive, disturbed, and regressed behavior are reduced. Escape and suicide attempts are decreased. Opportunities to improve social interaction and rehabilitation are made possible. Patients live a more normal existence and can move about freely, and the community reacts more favorably toward mental illness and the mentally ill. Routine security nursing functions are eliminated, thereby reducing the number of personnel required. This makes it possible to place more staff on the infirm wards where they can concentrate on making patients ambulatory, active, useful, and occupied socially. Eventually, nursing functions are reduced on the infirm wards when groups of patients become partly or completely ambulatory. Reduction of bed rest, sedation, and physical treatment results.

PRESENT NEED

There is still a need in some psychiatric hospitals to review current ward practices, especially those which pertain to restrictions. Outdated, abnormal procedures should be eliminated whenever possible. Recognizing the importance of normality in the environment and making it possible for the patient to express independence and to make decisions to a reasonable degree are necessary if we hope to truly rehabilitate patients. When this is done, it will be possible to measure accurately the required ratio of nursing personnel to patients. The present figures are not realistic and simply make the nursing shortage problem appear to be more acute. Some staff members are still spending much of their time performing purely perfunctory duties. This also affects greatly the cost of nursing service.

Creating a therapeutic environment in our mental hospitals is depen-

---

*I believe that failure to segregate patients, especially security-risk individuals, when converting to the open hospital, is the cause of hazards and lack of success with the change. Well-trained nurses and aides who are familiar with their patients can give invaluable assistance to professional personnel charged with the responsibility of segregating patients.

dent upon our philosophy, abilities, and, above all, our willingness and courage to remain flexible and open-minded toward change.

SUGGESTED REFERENCES

Briggs, D., and Wardell, M.: A locked ward was opened. Am. J. Nurs. 61: 102 (Sept.), 1961.

Cole, L.: Institutionalitis. Ment. Hosp. 6: 16 (Feb.), 1955.

Cumming, J., and Cumming, E.: Ego and Millieu. Atherton Press, New York, 1962, p. 89.

Hoch, P., Hunt, R., Snow, H., et al.: Observations on the British "open" hospitals. Ment. Hosp. 8: 5 (Sept.), 1957.

Holmes, M., and Werner, J.: Psychiatric Nursing in a Therapeutic Community. The Mac-Millan Company, New York, 1966.

Maloney, E.: Interpersonal Relations. William C. Brown Co. Publishers, Dubuque, Iowa, 1966, p. 84.

Mandelbrote, B.: An experiment in the rapid conversion of a closed mental hospital into an open-door hospital. Ment. Hyg. 42: 3 (Jan.), 1958.

McKeighen, R.: Communication patterns and leadership roles in a psychiatric setting. Perspect. Psychiat. Care 6: 80 (Mar.-Apr.), 1968.

Stainbrook, E.: Hospital atmosphere is a definite treatment measure. Ment. Hosp. 8: 8 (Feb.), 1957.

Sushinsky, L.: An illustration of a behavioral therapy intervention with nursing staff in a therapeutic role. J. Psychiat. Nurs. 8: 24 (Sept.-Oct.), 1970.

FOOTNOTES

1. Hoch, P., Hunt, R., Snow, H., et al.: Observations on the British "open" hospitals. Ment. Hosp. Bull. 8: 5 (Sept.) 1957.
2. Mandelbrote, B.: An experiment in the rapid conversion of a closed mental hospital into an open-door hospital. Ment. Hyg. 42: 3 (Jan.), 1958.

For reviewing this chapter, grateful acknowledgment is made to Mrs. Lorne Cameron, Sister Mary Renee, R.S.M., and Mrs. Vivian S. Bryan, R.N.

CHAPTER 20

Relating with Patients

The dynamic nature of interactions between people as well as the variations in individual reactions to a situation complicates the task of describing the kinds of relationships that are beneficial to sick persons. It is equally difficult to identify those specific nursing actions or behaviors that promote therapeutic relationships. Many individuals regard the ability of the nurse to communicate skillfully with patients as the essence of good nursing care (see Chap. 21, Communication Skills).

Each interaction that takes place between the nurse and patient is just one of a series of steps that lead to the establishment of a nurse-patient relationship. Some interactions may be helpful to patients, others may not. In what is considered to be a therapeutic nurse-patient relationship, the needs of the patient are met unconditionally. Everything the nurse says and does for and with patients constitutes the process through which the purpose of nursing is accomplished. This includes the interaction that takes place while the nurse is feeding and bathing the patient, giving medication, dancing, playing games, listening to, and talking with the person.

Evaluation of the effectiveness of the nurse-patient relationship is a measurement of the extent to which individuals and families have been helped to face and resolve the inevitable problems and sufferings associated with illness.

PARTICIPATING, OBSERVING, INTERPRETING
DURING INTERACTIONS

Relating with patients is a two-way process in which both the patient and nurse interact as participants and observers, each assuming an active part in the particular situation and observing the reactions of the other.

Sometimes the relationship is widened to include other patients and personnel so that there is interaction within a group. What goes on between persons during interactions may become therapeutic for the patient if the nurse is skilled in recognizing and understanding why the patient feels, thinks, and acts as he does and why the nurse reacts toward the patient as she does. It is important for the nurse to analyze feelings, including her own, because these reactions do influence an individual's thinking and behavior. This essential attribute of nursing is known professionally as the operation of self-awareness. It is the ability to connect one's immediate feelings and responses during interactions with people to past experiences in living. For example, if a person begins to talk about divorce, an individual who has had an emotionally distressing experience with divorce in the family may develop anxiety. Unconsciously, that person may try to change the topic of conversation because it is emotionally painful. Specific types of situations and discussion topics may reactivate from the unconscious mind repressed experiences and feelings that are emotionally unbearable at the conscious level of behavior.

INTERPERSONAL SKILLS

Although some persons appear to have natural interpersonal skills, there is no magic formula for learning how to conduct satisfying human relationships. Each nurse, patient, and situation is individualistic. We can never predetermine exactly how others and ourselves are going to feel and behave or the circumstances which will surround each and every developmental nurse-patient relationship. We may, from past experiences, observe similarities in situations and the reactions of others. What we learn through our observations of behavior and approaches during these times may serve as very useful guides in later, similar situations. However, we must always be prepared for new elements in thinking, feeling, and acting which may enter into the particular relationship as it develops.

In striving to create therapeutic relationships, it is helpful for nurses to be aware of some basic principles. First, it is commonly agreed that all persons have certain basic emotional needs which are expressed through individual behavior. These needs are not unusual, but are required by all human beings. In attempting to assist others emotionally, it is necessary to develop the ability to observe well and identify the needs inherent in patients' behavior (see Chap. 15, Meeting the Patient's Needs).

THE INITIAL NURSING APPROACH

Actually, no one can tell another person exactly what it is best to say or do or what attitude one should assume in each interpersonal relationship. These aspects of the nurse's response cannot be turned on and off at will. Therefore, only some general principles and ideas are expressed herein for the nurse to be aware of and to add to her general knowledge of approach techniques.

One may think of the initial approach to the patient as primarily the nurse's function. There are extroverted persons who will take the initiative on occasions, and this is to be expected. If the nurse considers the initial approach as her function, however, the patient who is frightened of others, timid, or lacking in courage will not be forgotten or neglected. There are patients who want relationships with others very badly but who have been so hurt by rejection or failure in previous relationships that they fear making contact with other persons. Withdrawing from association is the patient's method of protecting himself from psychic trauma. Knowledge of the dynamics of this response might be recalled when the nurse discovers that establishing a relationship with a patient is extremely challenging. It will also serve to preserve the nurse's morale if she is aware that all persons do not establish relationships easily and quickly, and that, insofar as her nursing ability is concerned, she should not consider this a personal failure.

Failure to establish contact that is enduring should not deter the nurse from making additional attempts. In fact, it may take several or more approaches to gain the patient's acceptance. At times, nurses find it necessary just to sit in a patient's room, commenting now and then, perhaps, on something in the environment. Although the patient may not respond verbally, there is an awareness of the nurse's presence which can be emotionally gratifying to the sick person. It is as if the nurse were, by her actions, demonstrating to the patient that she is interested in him as a person and understands the individual's reluctance or inability to communicate. Eventually, the repetitive, visiting approach may lead to a nurse-patient relationship which may be therapeutic for the patient.

MEETING THE PATIENT'S MOOD

Being prepared to meet the patient's mood of the moment is important. A downcast patient may be made to feel irritated and frustrated when the nurse approaches in a highly optimistic, overly vibrant manner. Conversely, the gay-hearted patient may feel antagonistic toward the indifference of the nurse who does not possess at least a small sense of humor. We think of these types of nurse-patient interactions as requiring common elements of mood if they are to develop into successful relationships.

On the other hand, there are occasions when the nurse will observe a patient to be excited, loud voiced, and sometimes threatening. To respond in a like manner will only increase the patient's inner feelings of fear and being threatened and thus intensify his behavior. Just listening to the patient in a calm manner, allowing him to ventilate his feelings, will help to allay his underlying tension and anxiety. We may remember that patients who feel threatened often project this feeling onto others in the environment in order to gain feelings of comfort. In this type of relationship, the nurse's mood is not in common with the patient's, but instead she remains passively alert and skillful in her aim to modify and change the patient's mood.

STRUCTURED, SUSTAINED, THERAPEUTIC NURSE-PATIENT RELATIONSHIPS

The general aim of nursing actions is to establish rapport, to provide comfort, and to promote feelings of confidence, trust, and security in the patient to the degree that the patient's needs are met and recovery from illness favored.

In the psychiatric field, there has developed the belief that professional nurses should become skilled in the art of initiating and developing interactions which lead to a more structured, sustained, nurse-patient relationship that is therapeutic. This belief is based on the concept that illness can be a learning experience. The objective is to help the patient gain insight into his illness and his behavior and to learn more satisfying ways of adapting to stressful life situations.

Working under the guidance and supervision of a psychiatrist, the nurse relates with a selected patient whom she visits by appointment. While interacting, she makes use of approaches gained from a theoretical frame of reference. Her objective is to establish a relationship which will ultimately be therapeutic for the patient. In working with a patient, a nurse should always seek clues concerning traumatic events in the patient's past which may prevent him from relating satisfactorily with others. After gaining the patient's confidence and trust, the nurse encourages the patient to verbalize about himself. From this data she identifies those emotionally traumatic and conflictual life situations which the patient has experienced to an overwhelming, anxiety-producing degree. Patient and nurse explore these experiences for the purpose of identifying and clarifying those experiences and their feeling reactions which resulted in mental conflict for the patient. Through counseling approaches the nurse may help the patient to learn new ways of behaving in a specific situation which the patient may test and which may help to resolve conflict. During this experience the patient may cast the nurse into roles, such as mother, father, or sibling and relate to the nurse as the patient related to these significant persons in the past.

The trend toward developing therapeutic nurse-patient relationships is based on the widely held belief that mental illness is fundamentally a disturbance in an individual's relationships with other human beings. Satisfactory relationships are considered essential for the maintenance of mental health. Attentions to nutrition, rest, and medication are necessary and helpful nursing actions to be performed for any sick person, including the mentally ill. These approaches help to stabilize physiological body processes which, in turn, do have an influential effect upon the person's general state of health. However, the manifestations of mental disturbances which symbolize an underlying mental conflict and produce anxiety are often relieved when social, psychological, and communications techniques are skillfully used during nurse-patient interactions.

The nurse-patient relationship is also a learning experience for the nurse who is expected to analyze her own behavior during interactions with patients. It is essential for the nurse to identify those actions of hers which influenced the patient's behavior, their motivation, and whether or not her actions were helpful to the patient with whom she is relating. During this part of the experience, the nurse may experience some anxiety. Talking over the details of the interactions which have been anxiety producing for her and reviewing the printed record of the experience with an experienced advisor may be very helpful.

The same concepts, framework of theoretical reference, and approaches used in the one-to-one, nurse-patient relationship with a mentally ill patient may be used by the nurse in any health facility and nursing situation. Hopefully, learning derived by the nurse in the structured, sustained nurse-patient relationship will become an integral part of all of her nursing actions and enable her to give understanding and comprehensive care to patients.

PHASES OF A THERAPEUTIC RELATIONSHIP

Four interlocking phases have been identified in the nurse-patient relationship that is therapeutic. These may be observed as one reviews the detail in the printed record kept by the nurse who is interacting with a patient. When the nurse relates by appointment with a selected patient, she is expected to inform the patient in advance about the plan she has for visiting on a regular basis for a specified period of time. An agreement is reached by them concerning the days and hours when the nurse will visit. The patient is informed that the time is to be used in his interest and that the nurse may be able to give greater assistance in helping the patient to get well.

The orientation phase is a period in which the nurse and patient get acquainted. It is a time when both observe each other, hypothesize privately about the meaning of actions, and generally move with caution toward the second phase of the relationship. The patient will usually test the nurse in various ways as he seeks trust in the relationship. Both the nurse and patient may experience anxiety as they exchange information which is of an impersonal nature. How the patient's time has been occupied on a daily basis during his hospitalization is often the point of reference for conversation. The fundamental aim is to establish contact, maintain rapport, gain the patient's acceptance and gradually work into the second phase of the relationship.

If the relationship endures and the second phase is reached, there is a lowering of anxiety owing to the feelings of trust perceived by the patient. Some persons view this phase as one of emerging identities. Generally speaking, the nurse and patient get to know each other well enough to anticipate the possibility of specific feeling reactions during situations which may develop. It is not unusual for some patients to continue to test the nurse's trust. For instance, the nurse may visit one day and discover that the patient is busily occupied with some activity which delays or postpones the nurse's visit. It is important for the nurse to recognize the meaning of such behavior and to accept it. During phase two, the nurse encourages the patient to verbalize, clarify, and extend his discussions and gives emotional support needed by the patient to continue verbalizing. These meetings may be helpful to the extent that the patient looks forward to the nurse's visit as a time for unburdening himself emotionally. On occasions a patient who verbalizes with ease may develop a fear of having talked too much. He may be rejecting and hostile toward the nurse when she next visits. The nurse's understanding of this development, her show of acceptance, and ability to keep confidences is important for continuing the relationship and moving into the next phase.

During phase three, the patient may become more vocal and active as he relates with the nurse in the role into which he has cast her as a significant person. It is a period when the patient may vacillate between being dependent upon the nurse and trying to become independent. This is a stage which can be difficult for the patient and nurse and in which the nurse will need to make use of all her communication and other interpersonal skills. The patient is allowed to act out his feelings and discuss situations freely. The nurse may identify unhealthy pressures the patient has experienced that have stymied his mature emotional development. She may also recognize distortions and exaggerations of events that may have caused the patient to be rejected and feel threatened when he behaved in a similar manner during his past relationships. Understanding shown by the nurse toward the patient helps to deepen the patient's trust. Learning may take place owing to the reduction of anxiety which occurs when interpersonal trust is perceived. The nurse and patient continue to discuss his problems and behavior, and he is encouraged to try new ways of resolving them.

The fourth phase is that of termination. Actually, the patient should have been prepared for the final stage in the beginning of the relationship during the orientation phase. In the earlier period the nurse tells the patient how long she expects to be able to visit with him on a regular basis. Throughout the relationship she refers, at intervals, to the date of termination in order to prepare the patient with realistic expectations of what is to develop and to keep him reminded about it. If the nurse is unable, for any reason, to continue regular visits while the patient is still dependent upon her, arrangements are made to have another nurse work with the patient. During this period, the nurse gradually reduces her visits and encourages the patient to relate and socialize with other individuals and groups. Sometimes the termination of a relationship is a spontaneous development. The patient may have benefited by the experience to the extent that his behavior indicates that he no longer needs the nurse's support or he may be discharged from the hospital.

SUGGESTED REFERENCES

Albiez, A.: Reflecting on the development of a relationship. J. Psychiat. Nurs. 8: 25 (Nov.-Dec.), 1970.

Holsclaw, P.: Nursing in high emotional risk areas. Nurs. Forum 4: 36, 1965.

King, J.: The initial interview: assessment of the patient and his difficulties. Perspec. Psychiat. Care 5: 256, (Nov.-Dec.), 1967.

Maloney, E.: "One to one"—who needs it? Perspect. Psychiat. Care 7: 9 (Jan.-Feb.), 1969.

Melat, S.: The development of trust. Perspect. Psychiat. Care 3: 28, 1965.

Mertz, H.: How the nurse helps the patient in his experience with psychiatric care. Perspect. Psychiat. Care 6: 260 (Nov.-Dec.), 1968.

Nehren, J., and Gilliam, N.: Separation anxiety. Am. J. Nurs. 65: 109 (Jan.), 1965.

Peplau, H.: Psychiatric nursing skills and the general hospital patient. Nurs. Forum 3: 28, 1964.

Rouslin, S.: Interpersonal stabilization of an intrapersonal problem. Nurs. Forum 3: 69, 1964.

Sene, B.: Termination in the student-patient relationship. Perspect. Psychiat. Care 7: 39 (Jan.-Feb.), 1969.

Siegel, N.: The impact of patient interaction on behavior. Ment. Hosp. 16: 19 (Sept.), 1965.

Stastry, J.: Helping a patient to learn to trust. Perspect. Psychiat. Care 3: 16, 1965.

Stockwell, M. and Nishikawa, H.: The third hand: a theory of support. J. Psychiat. Nurs. 8: 7 (May-June), 1970.

Stringer, M.: Therapeutic nursing intervention following derogation of the nurse by the patient. Perspect. Psychiat. Care 3: 37, 1965.

Thomas, M., Baker, J., and Estes, N.: Anger: a tool for developing self-awareness. Am. J. Nurs. 70: 2587 (Dec.), 1970.

Travelbee, J.: Interpersonal Aspects of Nursing. F.A. Davis Co., Philadelphia, 1966.

Younkin, B.: Empathy. Am. J. Nurs. 71: 104 (Jan.), 1971.

For reviewing this chapter, grateful acknowledgment is made to Mrs. Gloria Matulis, R.N., Mrs. Jane Rosamilia, R.N., and Mrs. Rosemary Wynn, R.N.

CHAPTER 21

Communication Skills

PROCESS OF COMMUNICATION

Communication is an important, integral aspect of human relations, including the nurse-patient relationship. Nurses, having a basic understanding of communication skills and the ability to utilize them in their relationships with patients, may be able to identify and help patients meet their needs.

Facts, feelings, and meanings may be transmitted during interaction through words, gestures, facial expressions, or other means. Communication must carry with it the transmission of feeling if it is to be meaningful in nurse-patient relationships. Thus, there is a relationship between the communication process and the nursing aim to communicate therapeutic attitudes of understanding, acceptance, interest, and a sense of trust to one's patients.

Communication involves all the modes of behavior that an individual employs consciously or unconsciously to affect another. This includes the spoken or written word, gestures, body movements, somatic signals, and symbolism in the arts.

LEARNING COMMUNICATION

Learning modes of communication commences during infancy and is progressive. Three types of language are learned sequentially during the maturation process: somatic, action, and verbal.

SOMATIC—The infant communicates distress through increased respiration rate and flushed skin reactions.

ACTION—He walks or crawls toward a wanted object.

VERBAL—He makes use of words which may supplement earlier learned modes.

Ideally, an adult should be able to use well all three modes of communication appropriately. The early acknowledgment received by the child during the developmental stages of communication levels will influence his mastery and choice of a communication mode. Communication exchanges with parental figures, especially the mothering figure who spends considerable time with the child, are important during the learning process. If action language is acknowledged more favorably or to a greater degree than verbal language the individual will tend to make use of action communication because the acknowledgment received achieves gratification for the child. Thus, the learning of higher-level verbal communication may be retarded if the child's efforts to verbalize new statements when learning a language are not acknowledged to a gratifying degree. Progressive participation in communications which are inhibited results in impairment of the communicative ability. Communication failures lead to frustration. If frustration is extended or becomes intense, the individual's thinking, feeling, and reaction become progressively disorganized and inappropriate. Prolonged frustration reduces the person's ability to establish satisfying social relations. Therefore, it is important for nurses to recognize communication modes, understand their development, and acknowledge patients' use of them. Acknowledgment conveys understanding which is gratifying to patients.

When patients' communications are disturbed, the fundamental aim should be to help the patient experience satisfaction and success during communications. When satisfaction is achieved through communication, the individual is encouraged to engage in and seek human relations.

TYPES OF COMMUNICATION

Generally speaking, there are two classical types of communication: verbal and nonverbal.

VERBAL COMMUNICATION

Attitudes, thoughts, and feelings may be communicated through the spoken or written word. They may be inherent in informal conversation, planned speeches, letters, and printed forms of communication addressed to specific readers.

NONVERBAL COMMUNICATION

Nonverbal aspects of communication may be deliberate or unintentional ways of communicating thoughts, attitudes, and feelings. They may be detected in a person's tone of voice, volume of speech, gestures, posture, body movements, facial expression, and the like. Nonverbal communication is considered to be a more reliable expression of true feelings than verbal because the person has less conscious control over his nonverbal behavior. A variety of emotions may be expressed, dependent upon who is communicating with whom, when the individual is communicating, and the communication content.

CHARACTERISTICS OF SUCCESSFUL
COMMUNICATION

Communication is successful when the person has a feeling of being understood. This feeling is the result of and is dependent upon the presence of four characteristics of communication. The absence or malfunction of one or more of these characteristics leads to disturbed communication and, usually, disturbed relations with others.

Feedback

The return response. There is opportunity for the listener to make a response which indicates the effect made upon the listener by the communication received. It may serve to clarify, extend, or alter the original idea contained in the communication.

Appropriateness

The reply is fitting and relevant to the communication received. There is neither too much or too little stimulation (what is said, feelings expressed, etc.) in the response made.

Efficiency

The language used by the communicators is understood. There is enough time between verbal responses for the listener to perceive and evaluate them.

Flexibility

There is an absence of overcontrol or undercontrol. Overcontrol occurs when there is checking and counterchecking of communications exchanged and deliberate prescribing of one's responses. Undercontrol exists when the participants do and say as they wish to the extent of disregarding the influential effects of feedback, appropriateness, and efficiency.

INTERPRETING COMMUNICATIONS

Valid interpretations of communications are dependent upon the nurse's ability to listen and observe well all that goes on during interaction with other persons—that is, listening to what is said, observing movements and actions, and being sensitive to feeling expressions. They are also dependent upon the nurse's ability to make appropriate responses which aid in extending, exploring, and validating interpretations of what has been heard, seen, and felt.

The nurse-patient relationship is a two-way communication process. The patient also perceives and evaluates the nurse's communications. What the nurse says and does influences the patient's interpretation of the meaning of the nurse's communication. The skillful nurse is as aware of the effect or the possible effect of her communications as she is of the patient's communications. The nurse's language, voice tone, gestures, facial expressions, posture, and body movements are noticed by the patient who interprets their meaning.

The nurse's degree of self-awareness may influence her communications as well as her ability to interpret communications. Self-awareness of the nurse is developed through the process of reflecting upon what went on during interaction and attempting to visualize a connection between the nurse's communication and some former life experience which may have stimulated the nurse to respond as she did during the interaction being analyzed. This process can be helpful in guiding the nurse's future responses, but it can also cause the nurse to feel uncomfortable, particularly if distressing elements of former experience are recalled. Sometimes the nurse can learn to recognize and handle her feelings through talking about a situation with an experienced person who has not been involved in the interaction being discussed, can view it objectively, and can offer helpful suggestions.

The immediate interpretation of another individual's communication may not be correct. Clarification and validation may be achieved by extending and exploring the communication. The following is a brief example of an early misinterpretation of a patient's communication.

Patient: "I don't like my room." (Nurse's interpretation—doesn't like rooming with another patient.)

Nurse: "You'd rather be in a room by yourself?"

Patient: "It's not that. It's other things."

Nurse: "Could you tell me what these other things are?"

Patient: "Well, like during the night, especially."

Nurse: "And things are different during the day?"

Patient: "Well, during the day people talking don't bother me."

Nurse: "You can hear people talking?"

Patient: "Well, I don't like to say it, but I can hear the nurses talking."

Sometimes a person means exactly what is verbalized, such as, "That medicine makes me feel sleepy all the time."

On other occasions what the person is thinking and feeling may be the opposite of what is verbalized. What is spoken may be a "cover up" for thoughts and feelings being experienced which are difficult to verbalize directly, such as, "It would be better if you didn't tell the doctor what I said." The patient may actually be seeking a communication channel through which information could reach the doctor. Making interpretations of such communications depends upon the nurse's sensitivity to feeling expressions as well as underlying needs and the various ways in which needs are communicated.

On occasions the individual initiates conversation through an indirect approach aimed to stimulate a discussion which would meet the person's need for information, clarification of a situation, and perhaps reassurance, such as, "They say that if you're in this ward you're not as sick as the other patients in the hospital."

Sometimes the individual's conversation symbolizes a need as that indicated by a child, needing attention and affection, who says, "The other nurse reads us a story when she puts us to bed."

Language which sounds unintelligible and disorganized in content may sometimes be interpreted if the nurse focuses her listening on clue words and actions. Emphatic pronouncements, words repeated, rambling connections between thoughts expressed, and associated gestures and movements should be observed.

Feelings may be interpreted through observation of voice tones and speech volume; for instance, the excited person may speak loudly, sometimes rapidly. Anxiety is obvious, but the nursing approach would be aimed to explore and determine the underlying motivation of the feeling shown—listening to what is said and making appropriate responses which help to identify causative factors.

A person feeling insecure may talk a great deal. The general content of the individual's conversation may provide clues for understanding the

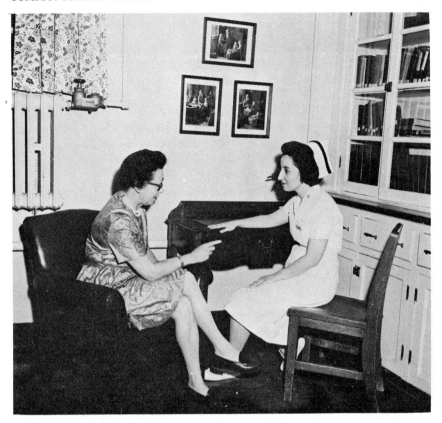

Fig. 1. Attentive listening includes observing conversation as well as actions, gestures, movements, and feelings. (Courtesy of New Jersey State Hospital, Greystone Park, N. J.)

motivational aspects of the communication. Clues may sometimes be detected in key words spoken or repeated.

Gestures made by a person may indicate an attitude felt, a reaction being expressed to a communication received, or a request for action by the person to whom the communication is directed. A shoulder shrug may communicate a reaction felt. A come-hither or go-away gesture is an obvious communication. Glancing at one's wrist watch or looking up at the clock may be a request for the other person to depart and terminate an interaction.

Body movements may be feeling communications as well as need communications. Coughing and twitching during an interaction may be communications of anxiety being experienced.

Positions assumed may be obvious or not so obvious communications. A mute patient who positions himself close to and in view of the nurse who is standing behind a serving table while pouring and passing beverage may be communicating a request for nourishment. The nurse may acknowledge the patient's language by handing a container filled with beverage to the patient. She may make a brief comment to the patient as she responds to his communication.

A restless person who is walking up and down the corridor may be communicating some personal discomfort. The nurse may acknowledge the patient's language by making her observation known and following it with an inquiry: "Miss _____, I notice you've been walking up and down the hall. Is something bothering you?"

Posture, such as lying curled in the fetal position, is thought by some analysts to indicate dependency longings and needs. The position is supposedly symbolic of the embryonic phase of human development when needs were met without having to struggle for existence. Implementing the mothering nursing role through bathing, dressing and feeding procedures establishes a communication channel which may help to meet such an individual's needs.

Facial expressions may communicate feelings of pleasure or displeasure, reactions of doubt, agreement or disagreement, and so on. The appropriateness of the nurse's response requires an evaluation of the language observed and its possible meaning in the individual situation.

INTERPRETING WRITTEN COMMUNICATIONS

Written communications are more difficult to interpret, owing to the absence of personal contact between senders and receivers of messages. When reading communications it is advantageous to seek out the less obvious as well as the very obvious meanings conveyed in the individual written communication. Much can be communicated in the choice of words used, the inherent implications of the words, and the general tone of the message. It is also helpful for the reader to know the roles occupied by the senders and receivers so that relationships may be visualized between the communication content and the participants' roles and their possible reactions to a message.

Sometimes the writer of a communication will pose a question or quote something said or written by another individual in order to convey indirectly an idea or an attitude felt, to stimulate a reaction in the reader, or, possibly, to instill some thought. Thus, written communications may contain hidden thoughts, attitudes, feelings, motivations and meanings which may be identified through careful observations. Examples of such observations may be those interpretations offered by newspaper analysts who study and report upon correspondence exchanged between interna-

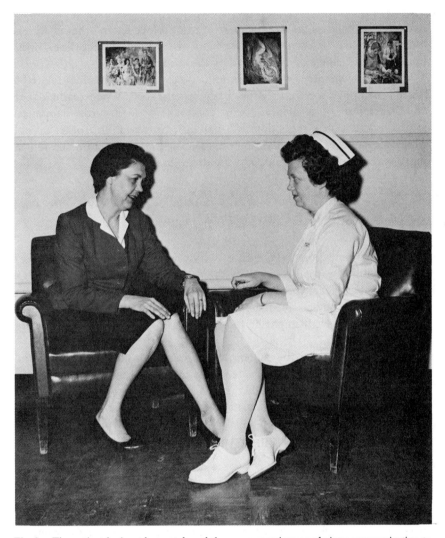

Fig. 2.   The patient looks at her watch and the nurse perceives an obvious communication to depart from interaction. (Courtesy of New Jersey State Hospital, Greystone Park, N. J.)

tional diplomats. During the Cuban crisis of October, 1962, the communications exchanged between American and Russian chiefs of states were carefully studied by news analysts who aimed to evaluate the feeling tone of the international situation as well as to make predictions concerning its outcome.

I recall with some amusement the advice offered several years ago by an unknown author who stated that we ought to learn to read communications as efficiently as the average person reads a love letter—that is, to read them as a love letter is read, over and over, between the lines, while examining the choice of words used by the sender.

Patients sometimes write communications which reveal clues related to hidden meanings, needs, or stress being experienced. When reading these communications it is helpful to be observant of key words, capitalized symbols, underlines, repetitions of thoughts expressed, and other aspects which may convey more than the obvious superficial content. The following communication was handed by a patient to a nurse.

Honey Beautiful lady Lovely one of mine I love you. How I love onlee you an no other. Why do I have to think for you.

In this communication the choice of words, repetition of the word "love," and the symbols capitalized convey the patient's feelings and thoughts. On the surface it appears to be an affection-seeking communication as well as a query of the nurse's feelings. If one knew the circumstances and the sender and receiver, it might be interpreted as having elements of frustration and hostility.

The letters written by patients may reveal considerable information concerning the patients' feelings, response to hospitalization and treatment received, relationships with other individuals, progress made toward recovery, regressive manifestations, or actions contemplated.

INTERPRETING THE ARTS

Creative productions convey the feelings, especially, of their creators as well as their thoughts. Dancing and music may convey communications of these aspects and also may stimulate the responses of observers to the extent of influencing their behavior. Dancing and music are sometimes used in the treatment of the mentally ill to create or change a mood and to stimulate other responses. Patients may communicate through their personal creations or observations of these arts.

Communications may also be inherent in patients' arts-and-craft creations, such as drawings and paintings. The subject of the art creation, figures sketched, and colors selected may be expressions of feelings, thoughts, attitudes, and conflictual situations being experienced. Interpretations of the arts are usually made well by specifically skilled therapists with whom the nurse may discuss their interpretations.

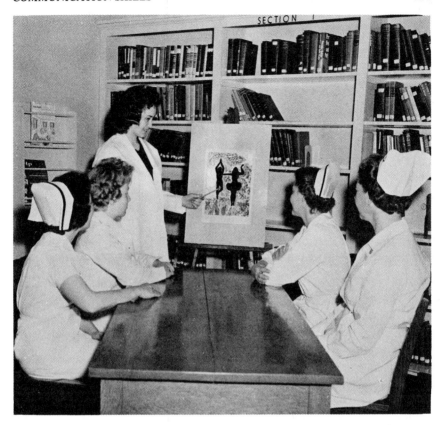

Fig. 3. Discussing the communications (feelings, conflictual elements) inherent in a patient's painting. (Courtesy of New Jersey State Hospital, Greystone Park, N. J.)

TALKING WITH PATIENTS

There are no specific verbal responses available for the nurse to use in her day-to-day interactions with patients because of the individuality of situations and communications. Often the naturalness and sincerity of the nurse's reply is the therapeutic element of the communication exchange. When in doubt about what to say or do, the nurse may be guided by the knowledge that good intentions and respect for people's feelings are favorable responses to convey in a relationship; that is, responses which offend, challenge, reject, or inflict emotional wounds should be avoided.

COMMUNICATION TECHNIQUES

There are some techniques which may be useful to the nurse who desires to improve her communication ability. Their use, when indicated, is aimed to encourage the patient to take the communication lead and to extend and clarify communications so that information which helps the nurse to identify and meet the patient's need may be obtained. Techniques may also be useful in helping patients to focus upon initial communications. There may be times when patients can focus upon the communication topic, take the lead, and verbalize without being prompted or encouraged. On other occasions the patient may have a need for silence which may be preferred to the nurse's use of a technique which has a prompting quality. Thus, the use of selective communication techniques by the nurse is dependent upon the ability of the nurse to evaluate the need for using a technique as well as to determine its potential value as a therapeutic approach. Generally speaking, the nurse may select the technique with which she feels most comfortable, but caution must be maintained to avoid its overuse to the extent of causing unfavorable reactions in the patient.

LISTENING

Listening provides the opportunity for the patient to take the communication lead. Ventilating by the person aids in releasing and alleviating uncomfortable feelings. The nurse acts as a sounding board for projected thoughts and feelings. The power of controlling emotions may be reduced to a degree which helps the patient to relax and reflect more objectively upon a distressing situation. The nurse may receive information which helps her to evaluate communications and understand better the person with whom she is relating. Quality listening requires attentiveness of the nurse who is seeking clues which may be inherent in verbalizations. The nurse observes all modes of language used as she listens. The willingness of the nurse to listen as well as a show of attentiveness conveys to the patient the feeling of being accepted and understood which is important in the conduct of successful communications.

FLASHBACK

This technique is sometimes referred to as "reflection." A flashback may be the return of the content verbalized by the individual in whole or in part. For instance, the person may say, "I relied on the wrong people." The flashback may be, "You relied on the wrong people," "The wrong people," or "Wrong people." A flashback may also be used to reflect feelings, such as, "You seem to be upset about something." This may lead to communication which is effectively therapeutic. This technique has a prompting and encouraging effect and aids in helping the person to focus upon the communication topic. However, its repeated use in the same communication setting can cause the tone of the nurse's responses to become monotonous and irritating to the patient.

SILENCE

The person's silence may be an attempt to think through a situation, recall information, or evaluate the effect of the communication upon the listener. The counterpause of the nurse may indicate acceptance and understanding of the patient's immediate need. It may also convey the impression that the nurse is interested to hear more and serve as a cue for the individual to continue the conversation. Sometimes the silence of a pause in communication stimulates talking because some persons feel uncomfortable when a degree of anxiety is reached, which may happen when silence is maintained.

COMMENT

Interjecting a timely, appropriate comment now and then indicates attentiveness and interest of the listener. The comment has an encouraging effect which helps the person to continue the conversation; for instance, the nurse might remark, "That interests me," "Go on," or "Tell me more."

OPEN-END STATEMENTS

This technique may be useful in referring to a topic from which the person has shifted momentarily or mentioned previously and about which the listener would like to hear more. Sometimes communications following the change in topic may cause the listener to visualize a relationship to the former topic which could be of interest. The open-end statement has a prompting quality, such as "You were saying something about _____." The topic may or may not be mentioned at the end of the statement dependent upon whether the technique is an immediate or delayed feedback. This technique provides an opening for the patient to take the lead and continue the discussion.

QUESTION

Questions should be used carefully. Deep probing should be avoided. Trying to force out information places the patient on the defense. "Why" and "How" questions ask for information, reasons or causes which a patient may not be able to or want to give; for instance, a compulsive-behaving patient may not be able to tell why he touches a door knob three times. If he is asked why he does it and he says, "I just know I have to," and the nurse asks, "How do you know?", he may give some equally uninformative reply, such as, "I don't know." The answers to some "why" and "how" questions require analytical ability and information which the patient does not have. "Why" can sometimes reactivate feelings of being disapproved of or reprimanded, especially in an individual who has had unfavorable, earlier experiences with authority figures. For instance, if the patient says, "I didn't want to go to O.T. today," and the nurse asks, "Why?", or "Why didn't you go?", this can sound like a challenge to explain actions or the forerunner of disciplinary action by the nurse. In some situations, therefore, "why" and "how" do not have a reaching effect because there is nothing to connect with on a conscious level or the question provokes the hostility barrier to communication.

Some questions may be appropriate. If a patient keeps making reference to third persons, such as "They," "They did that," or "They said," the nurse may ask, "Who do you mean by 'they'?", or "You said 'they.' To whom does 'they' refer?" Patients may use the question to interview the nurse about her personal life. In such instances the nurse may give a brief, factual reply which is appropriate. The nurse may say, "No, I am not married," if that is the factual reply. If the patient continues to pursue informations such as, "Why?", or "Do you have a boy friend?", the nurse may reverse the direction of the interview by responding, "Is there some purpose for which you need this information?" This type of response requires the person to whom it is directed to focus upon the purpose and may result in abandonment of the attempt to elicit personal information from the nurse. To stimulate, as well as increase the volume of communication, and to get more information, it is essential to avoid asking questions which may be answered with one word, such as, "Did you have a good weekend at home?" More information would be obtained by saying, "Tell me about your weekend at home." The use of specific lead words in questions, such as who, when, where, and what are helpful when clarification and specific additional information are needed.

TO IMPROVE COMMUNICATION

Acknowledge the patient's mode of communication (somatic, action, or verbal) with appropriate responses which convey interest, acceptance, and understanding. Listening and observing are important, but communication is not established unless the nurse responds through some talking or action approach.

Appreciate that nurse-patient communications may help to reduce or alleviate anxiety and other controlling feelings.

Use language that is appropriate to the person's level of understanding.

Minimize verbal participation so that the opportunity for the patient to take the lead in verbalizing is made available.

Employ suggestion when its use appears to be indicated, such as, "Perhaps we can talk about that."

Allow individuals to express their negative feelings, the release of which may be therapeutic for the patient.

Accept periods of silence as preferable to trying to force patients to talk through the use of techniques which may be helpful at times but which are not always appropriate to the situation.

The nurse should appreciate that her mere presence can communicate support to a patient who is unable to verbalize well. Some nurses are more skillful in the use of nonverbal approaches than are others. They seem to know intuitively when the patient needs them.

Refrain from offering reassurance too quickly, changing the patient's conversation topic, or defending individuals whom the patient may criticize, including family as well as staff members. Such responses to communications convey anxiety in the nurse and tend to "cut off" the patient's verbalizations of deeper underlying thoughts and feelings. They may cause the patient to feel ashamed, guilty, fearful, and increasingly anxious.

To be avoided is the sharing of personal life experiences which may cause the patient to lose respect for, and doubt the integrity of, the nurse as well as destroy the confidential nature of the nurse-patient relationship.

Select topics which may be of interest to the patient when attempting to introduce a subject of conversation, but refrain from the choice of topics which could be emotionally distressing for the patient.

Help the person to strengthen his personal identification in relation to other individuals by speaking of "I" and "You" when the use of these pronouns is appropriate. Talking about "we" is appropriate only when the pronoun refers to actual associations in action or thoughts; for instance, the nurse would not say, "We will now take a bath," but would say instead, "You may take your bath now."

Making interpretations or offering explanations of behavior or communications observed should be avoided. These are more than is required of the nurse.

It should be recognized that communications and their interpretations are important in all human relations as well as the nurse-patient relationship.

SUGGESTED REFERENCES

Alexander, K.: Nonverbal communication. RN 29: 59, 1966.

Arteberry, J.: The disturbed communication of a schizophrenic patient. Perspect. Psychiat. Care 3: 24, 1965.

Barbara, D.: The Art of Listening. Charles C Thomas Publishers, Springfield, Ill., 1966.

Cook, J.: Interpreting and decoding autistic communication. Perspect. Psychiat. Care 9: 24 (Jan.-Feb.), 1971.

Cuthbert, B.: Switch off, tune in, turn on. Am J Nurs. 69: 1206 (June), 1969.

Faust, J.: Body language. M. Evans & Co., New York, 1970.

Freund, H.: Listening with any ear. Am. J. Nurs. 69: 1650 (Aug.), 1969.

Goldin, P., and Russell, B.: Therapeutic communication. Am. J. Nurs. 69: 1928 (Sept.), 1969.

Jones, E.: The use of speech as a security operation. Perspect. Psychiat. Care 3: 18, 1965.

Kron, T.: Communication in nursing. W. B. Saunders Co., Philadelphia, 1972.

Lewis, G.: Nurse-Patient Communication. William C. Brown Co. Publishers, Dubuque, Iowa, 1969.

Lewis, G.: Communication: a factor in meeting emotional crises. Nurs. Outlook 15: 36 (Aug.), 1965.

Nagai, M.: Communication is the key. J. Psychiat. Nurs. 2: 47 (Jan.), 1964.

Linehan, D.: What does the patient want to know? Am. J. Nurs. 66: 1066 (May), 1966.

McKeighen, R.; Communication patterns. Perspect. Psychiat. Care 6: 80 (Mar.-Apr.), 1968.

Muecke, M.: Overcoming the language barrier. Nurs. Outlook 18: 53 (April), 1970.

Phillips, L.: Language in disguise: nonverbal communication with patients. Perspect. Psychiat. Care 4: 18 (July-Aug.), 1966.

Roehler, S.: The therapeutic milieu of the art department at the Allan Memorial Institute. J. Psychiat. Nurs. 5: 545 (Nov.-Dec.), 1967.

Smith, V.: I can't believe I said that! Nurs. Outlook 18: 50 (May), 1970.

Stoneberg, C.: Communication through art on a psychiatric ward. Perspect. Psychiat. Care 2: 12, 1964.

Travelbee, J.: Interpersonal Aspects of Nursing, ed. 2. F. A. Davis Co., Philadelphia, 1971.

For reviewing this chapter, grateful acknowledgement is made to Mrs. Leone Cox, R.N., Miss Laura Davidson, R.N., Mrs Ura Ann Lazaroff, R.N., Miss Elizabeth Maloney, R. N., and Mr. William A. Nace. R.N.

CHAPTER 22

Group Nursing and Activities

Investigators who studied the social structure of mental hospitals during the 1950s concluded that we had been treating patients in crowds instead of groups for too long. We are now in an era of change that has its impetus in the challenge to determine how we can best structure a group society.[1] Some authorities believe that the apathy manifested by schizophrenic patients results from a crowd type of structure which provides little opportunity for individualized attention and group association. Social scientists have implied in some of their writings that catatonic schizophrenic mutism exists only in hospitals in which the atmosphere is one of neglect.[2]

To structure a group society involves first a consideration of the hospital administration's philosophy, particularly its willingness to accept change, and the inevitable problems which arise and necessitate giving emotional support to personnel who are assisting with social reconstruction. Studies have demonstrated that whenever social reconstruction is attempted in the mental hospital environment, personnel manifest a tendency to feel anxious, insecure and threatened. Certain changes, especially those which involve more freedom in patient movement, may be difficult to make unless the ward personnel feel confident that they will be supported by the hospital administration. Other considerations involved in social reconstruction include the physical plan of the ward, available equipment, patient census, personality structures of both patients and personnel, number of ward personnel, number of nursing personnel, method of assigning staff to patients, interest and ability of personnel to relate with individual patients and conduct group techniques, leadership ability, assistance available from members of other departments, and the level at which social activities are structured for the group.

A preferable group structure consists of 6 to 10 patients. If the group must be larger, owing to the ratio of available personnel to patients, it is recommended that the number of patients not exceed 20.

Nursing personnel in charge of the ward must possess leadership ability as well as the willingness and capability to delegate successfully certain functions to assistants. Routine written records, requisitions and other perfunctory duties should be assigned to ward clerks and house-keeping and maintenance personnel who do not have responsibility for patient care. Nurse leaders and aides should be free to initiate and partici-pate in ward activities and interpersonal contacts. The skills of psychiatric nursing personnel should not be wasted on clerical and housekeeping duties.

It is highly recommended that all nursing staff members be prepared and able to carry on various types of social activities. Separate functioning of personnel as aides, nurses, and occupational, recreational and social therapists places limitations on the development of individual staff mem-bers' skills. In addition, such a plan limits opportunities for interpersonal contacts and the range of activities which may be utilized.

Authorities believe that it is best to assign nursing personnel to small groups of patients instead of having the entire staff responsible for the care of all patients on the ward. Patients should be grouped according to their personality structures; recognizing their individual potentialities and abili-ties to socialize in certain groups is an important consideration. The per-sonality structure of staff members and their ability to socialize and relate successfully with certain types of patients is also important. Some person-nel are understanding and skilled in the management of various types of patient behavior. Intuitively they appear to be able to establish rapport in certain groups and bring about social relationships.

A written plan of social activities is a helpful guide for both personnel and patients. These programs are developed best through group planning. Some hospitals employ a supervising social therapist who coordinates the activities being conducted by the various departments and wards. A master program of social activities is structured at the hospital level by the super-vising therapist and departmental directors, including occupational, recre-ational and social therapists and volunteer services.

Individual wards structure a basic schedule of social activities which patients sometimes help to plan in team meetings. Activities are selected, when suitable, from the published master program and integrated into the ward activity schedule. When social activities are structured at the ward level they tend to be helpful in meeting individual patients' needs. The supervising social therapist may, by request, meet with ward teams on occasion to suggest activity choices or to offer suggestions concerning the

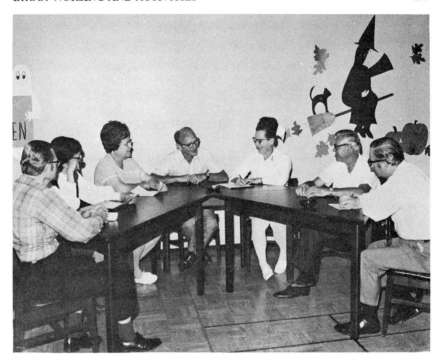

Fig. 1.   A group meeting with the nurse to plan recreational activities. (Courtesy of Arkansas State Hospital, Little Rock, Ark.)

procurement of assistance from any of the special departments in order to facilitate a ward plan. I have observed a successful experiment which functioned through the joint efforts of ward and special department personnel. It was possible to conduct an active program without adding extra personnel to the regular ward staff. When the ratio of ward personnel to patients is low, it may be very helpful to consult the supervising social therapist and work out a joint plan with other departments.

One of the important functions of a nurse supervisor in a group setting is to assume the responsibility for observing social activity programs in action to make certain that implementation occurs according to schedule. Supervisors should observe when patients fail to participate because the plan may not assist in meeting the individual's needs. This is just as important as the supervisor's function of personally visiting patients who are physically ill and require attention from a professional nurse. The late C. C. Burlingame, who served as Psychiatrist-in-Chief of The Institute of Living (formerly known as the Hartford Retreat), where he organized an excellent group society of patients, often remarked, "Five per cent is having ideas. Ninety-five per cent is putting ideas into action."

GROUP THERAPIES

Planned group psychotherapy sessions are conducted by well-trained personnel. Psychiatrists, psychologists, social scientists, members of the clergy, and sometimes nurses guide these group discussions.

NURSE-PATIENT DISCUSSION GROUPS

These ward group meetings which are scheduled and conducted, usually weekly, by nursing personnel may include topics related to current events, literature, music, sports, art, sciences, hobbies, or just conversation which ultimately develops into something of general interest to the patients. Controversial subjects, such as religion and politics, are avoided. This is a simple, practical type of group discussion which requires no special preparation and can be initiated by the average member of the nursing staff. The leader assembles a small group of patients and makes an everyday, ordinary statement, such as, "I've been thinking about making a dress. Has anyone had such an experience?" or "I planted a small garden the other day. Do we have any gardeners among us?" It is surprising how such simple leading statements can produce learning as well as enjoyment in the group and stimulate discussion.

THE TECHNIQUE OF REMOTIVATION

Remotivation is essentially a technique of simple group interaction between a member of the nursing staff and a group of patients. Most remotivation sessions are conducted by psychiatric aides who have had special instruction in the technique. The primary aim of the technique is to stimulate patients into thinking about and discussing topics associated with the real world. Discussion methods are used to motivate the group's interest and participation. A meeting is held with a group of 10 to 12 patients once a week for about an hour, each meeting being focused on a specific topic chosen for discussion. Advance preparation for the discussion is made by the remotivator. A remotivation series consists of one meeting each week for 12 weeks. After a short interim a new series may be started. Interaction develops between the remotivator and the group members as the following steps of the procedure are carried out:

1. *The climate of acceptance* is developed when the meeting opens. The remotivator makes personal introductions and warm friendly comments and demonstrates a pleasant attitude as he circulates in the group. The objective is to establish rapport between the remotivator and patients and among the participants.

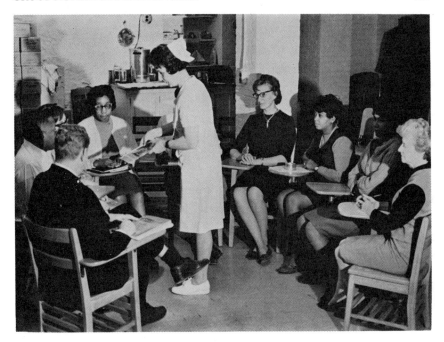

Fig. 2.   A remotivation meeting. Remotivator starts to show the visual aid for the purpose of motivating communication responses from participants. (Courtesy of Essex County Overbrook Hospital, Cedar Grove, N. J.)

2. In the second step, *a bridge to reality*, the remotivator aims to start the group thinking about a selected topic of the real world. The remotivator may ask a thought-provoking question and exhibit a visual aid for the purpose of motivating responses from individual members. A poem related to the topic may also be introduced and each patient may be asked to read a part of the poem.

3. In the third step, *sharing the world we live in*, the remotivator uses questions and visual aids related to the topic which are prepared in advance of the meeting in order to enlarge and enhance the discussion.

4. *Appreciation of the work of the world*, the fourth step, is carried out in a fashion similar to step 3, but the discussion is geared toward occupations related to the main topic. An attempt is made to get the members to think about and discuss work in relation to themselves.

5. The completion of the discussion and meeting is carried out in step 5, *the climate of appreciation*. The remotivator briefly summarizes the highlights of the meeting. He thanks individuals who have made special contributions as well as the entire group before announcing the time and date of the next meeting. There are no recess periods between steps; the

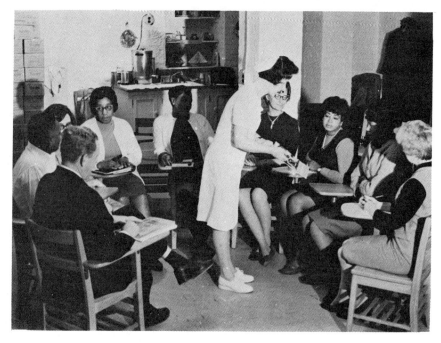

Fig. 3.   Remotivator moves around the circle continuing to show the visual aid to the other participants. (Courtesy of Essex County Overbrook Hospital, Cedar Grove, N.J.)

meeting flows as one continuous structured discussion. The basic technique can be broadened to include some activities, such as garden projects, picnics, and trips to the community. A more inclusive reference on this group technique is Gibson's *The Remotivator's Guide Book*.[3]

PATIENT GOVERNMENT

Government by patients exists in some hospitals, particularly smaller institutions. Each ward selects a representative to the general council of governing patients which meets regularly. The organization has guiding principles and keeps written minutes of the meetings which are sent to the chief administrative officer. Patients may discuss and request certain changes in already established policies and practices, or they may ask for some special social equipment. Some governing groups assume the responsibility for recommending a patient's discharge from the hospital. According to published reports, patient government has improved morale and strengthened confidence and cooperation between patients and administration. Other institutions, especially larger ones, find it difficult for a group to function successfully. When the council's suggestions and requests cannot be met, owing to administrative policies over which the individual hospital may not have control, patient government attempts may result in frustrating experiences. The success of this type of group function depends very much upon the attitudes, interest, and philosophy of administrative officers and personnel as well as any higher, centralized authority which may have control over the hospital's functions.

WARD PATIENT-STAFF MEETINGS

A more recent development in group activities has made it possible for patients living in wards of large mental hospitals to participate in a group organization. These sessions, attended by the patients and all ward staff members, are held for one hour twice a week on each ward. Meetings are chaired by a patient whom the group elects. Minutes are kept by a recording secretary.

The purposes of the meetings are to provide an opportunity for patients to talk and learn about their situation in the hospital, the functions of the staff, the patients' relationships with staff members, and the operation of special departments, and to propose suggestions for improvement in ward living. The meetings are guided by a psychiatrist, psychologist, or nurse, dependent upon the staff available. Once a week the staff members meet for about an hour to discuss the meetings attended, the recommendations made by the patient group, and what may be done about them. This type of organization differs from patient government meetings which are composed of representatives sent from each ward who present matters on behalf of the patients in all wards whom they represent. The effects of patient government meetings are more far-reaching owing to the number of wards participating through representatives.

Patient-staff meetings may include discussions of such matters as problems experienced by newly admitted patients and the functions of staff members and other department personnel. Individuals may wish to know about privileges given to patients and how to get them. Some persons may be interested to know how a discharge from the hospital is obtained. Functions of the institution's Social Security representative may be of interest to those patients who wish to inquire about benefits during illness. A variety of matters may be of particular interest and concern within a group.

A ward meeting is not a favorable occasion for patients to discuss their individual problems. Patients may inquire which staff member they should confer with about special types of problems during a meeting. The standing committee responsible for arranging appointments may be authorized to contact the staff member who ordinarily provides the type of assistance needed. Some ward groups are composed of members who are capable of and interested in organizing a more formal group structure. A constitution may be written by a special committee and then presented to the patient group for approval. The purposes and functions of the group are included as well as the duties of officers and standing committees. Copies of the constitution are distributed to all patients and staff participants. Terms of office are usually for a three-month period. The chairman is authorized to appoint people to vacancies created when a patient resigns or is discharged from the hospital.

Standing committees provide excellent opportunity for patients to function actively in the interest of the group. Participation helps them to engage in social relations, assume responsibility, develop abilities, such as creativity and initiative, and to strengthen self-esteem.

The program committee may assume responsibility for orienting new patients and plan for talks by special department personnel. Community citizens who are specialists in discussing specific topics of interest to the group may be invited to a meeting. The proposal committee recommends changes desired in the physical environment of the ward, involving the procurement of equipment, furniture, and other items that would, in their view, improve living conditions. The housekeeping committee sets expectations for patients in the care of their individual living units. Daily assignments may be given to individual patients and followed up by the housekeeping committee. The recreation committee plans the social program and may be especially helpful in planning for ward activities, such as table games and community singing, during the hours when therapists are not available.

Patients are given printed notice well in advance when the organization of a ward group is being contemplated. Each one is made acquainted with the purposes, functions, and limitations of the organization. The decision to organize is made by the patients. Guidance is given when a group wishes to write a constitution.

Generally speaking, ward meetings are one of the most effective means of resocializing and revitalizing patients and the ward environment through a group process that can by dynamic.

SOCIAL, RECREATIONAL GROUPS

Social groups may engage in table and circle games, singing, dancing, various types of handicrafts, and informal social gatherings on the ward,

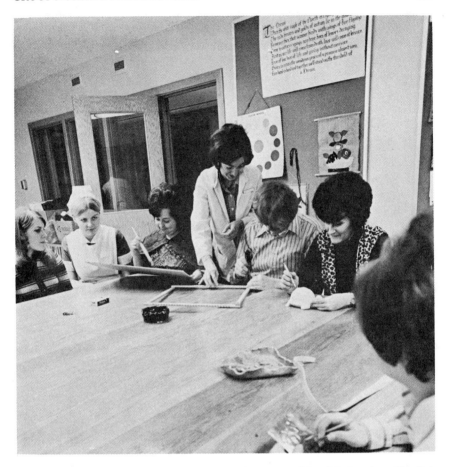

Fig. 4. Enjoying handicrafts, ceramics, and art. (Courtesy of Swedish-American Hospital, Rockford, Ill.)

such as coffee snacks and afternoon tea. Mixed groups of men and women patients are part of normal living and should be encouraged. Invitations to social gatherings on wards may be extended to members of the opposite sex.

Special projects, such as designing holiday decorations for the ward, presenting a short skit, planning a social, or planting a small garden, may be undertaken by group members.

Extending the social activity program beyond the ward environment is recommended because this plan provides a change in atmosphere and

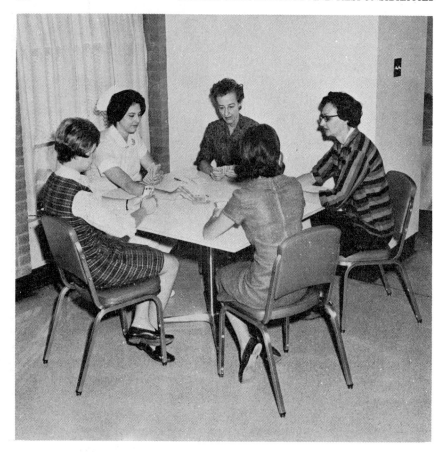

Fig. 5. Group participants in a card game. (Courtesy of Arkansas State Hospital, Little Rock, Ark.)

socialization in mixed groups. Patients may attend some of the activities scheduled in the published master program when these functions are considered suitable for members of individual groups. Motion pictures, pageants, and competitive sports, such as football and baseball games, are enjoyable spectator events. Some hospitals plan weekly dances for larger groups of patients. Picnics may also be scheduled in warm weather for one or more groups. Groups of patients may be allowed to socialize in the main recreation room of the hospital on selected evenings of the week. Games, juke box music, dancing, general conversation and other informal activities may be enjoyed there.

Morale is often built by what one is able to do for other people. Patients can help each other in various ways and should be encouraged to do so. The physically able can assist the less capable individuals with dressing, toileting, walking around the ward, and similar activities. Patients who possess special abilities in the arts and crafts can help others to improve their talents. Assignments may be given in connection with ward management, such as the maintenance by patients of the appearance of certain areas of the ward, including such sections as the game room and snack kitchen.

Some hospitals have managed to evoke the interest of community volunteers to visit lonely patients who do not have visitors. Volunteers have been known to escort groups of patients to community functions and to invite them into their homes for a social hour.

STAFF RELATIONSHIPS

Staff relationships affect the ward atmosphere. Patients are sensitive to the emotional climate of the environment and react to feeling tones expressed by personnel. The development of a serene atmosphere, free of tensions and anxiety among staff members, requires mature, socially conscious, understanding, inspirational leadership.

Ward team meetings and incidental discussions between personnel help to increase one's understanding of the main treatment objectives of meeting patients' needs and rehabilitation. When the staff can be assisted to realize that every relationship between staff and patients, whether positive, negative, passive, or aggressive, is a treatment relationship, each individual on the team conceives of his role as important in the rehabilitation process. A constant exchange of information related to patients' problems and progress is important for the development and maintenance of a common, consistent treatment approach. Personnel also need to be familiar with each other's duties, problems and goals. Frank discussions may reveal difficulties between staff members, but when these are brought out into the open during a team meeting they are often solved effectively. Tensions are reduced when information and problems are shared.

An optimistic attitude among the staff concerning recovery is important. The team leader can do much to stimulate desirable attitudes and optimism. Professional growth occurs when the group is encouraged to review current literature and discuss experimental reports which stimulate new ideas and effect harmonious staff relationships.

COMMUNICATION

Communication affects the staff and patients' perception of situations and feeling reactions. Irrational communication flows much more rapidly

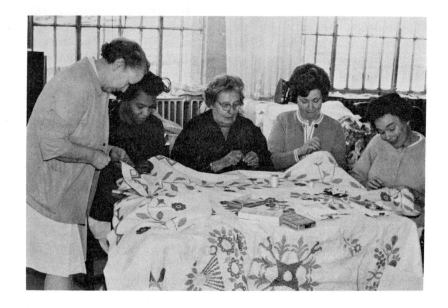

Fig. 6.   Therapist conducts a group embroidery project. (Courtesy of Essex County Over-brook Hospital, Cedar Grove, N. J.)

through an organization than does rational communication. When people are concerned about changes and situations, rumors spread rapidly. Rumors are attempts of people to find answers to questions or create a new situation which may relieve anxiety. Established channels of communication which keep personnel well-informed are effective in dispelling rumors. Staff members need to develop the ability to recognize distortions in communication which may be corrected before negative reactions and situations develop.

Therapeutic results depend upon communication skills of the personnel. Allowing patients to verbalize is effective in relieving their tensions and anxiety. It is important to recognize when the maintenance of silence by a staff member may benefit the patient. Reflecting upon and repeating a statement made by the patient may encourage some individuals to verbalize further. Knowing when the patient's verbal communication is contradictory to his deeper feelings may be very helpful in determining immediate and subsequent approaches by personnel. Recognizing the meaning of nonverbal communication gestures increases the nurse's sensitivity to the needs of individual patients as well as the ability to approach behavior successfully.

MANAGEMENT OF BEHAVIOR

Skill in the management of patient behavior depends very much upon the ability of personnel to recognize behavior changes as they begin to emerge. Mood swings, impulsiveness, paranoid trends and suicidal drives gain momentum when they are allowed to progress for days and weeks. Serious disturbances in behavior are usually later expressions of some deeper, underlying need which was previously unrecognized. The immediate causes of acute behavior are much less significant than the remote causes. Therefore, it is necessary for all personnel to possess an understanding of the meaning of behavior and especially what it means to the patient. When early behavior changes are recognized and analyzed, appropriate responses may be made by the staff to assist the patient in meeting his needs.

Serious disturbances of behavior are poorly managed when the only solution available is to restrain or seclude the patient. Restraint and seclusion are interpreted by the patient as punitive measures. Authorities point out that this type of management fails to relieve the patient and represents failure on the staff's part to understand and treat the person effectively. Medical personnel respond immediately to the development of acute physical symptoms and regard them as emergencies which must be treated promptly. Psychiatric personnel should consider emerging, deviate behavior trends as emergencies which should be placed under control to prevent the development of acute disturbances.

For additional information on group activities see Chapter 26, Social, Recreational, Art and Music Therapies.

SUGGESTED REFERENCES

Bell, R.: Activity as a tool in group therapy. Perspect. Psychiat. Care 8: 84 (Mar.-Apr.), 1970.

Eddy, F., O'Neill, E., and Astrachan, B.: Group work on a long term psychiatric service. Perspect. Psychiat. Care 6: 9 (Jan.-Feb.), 1968.

Gauron, E., Proctor, S., and Schroder, P.: Group therapy training: a multidisciplinary approach. Perspect. Psychiat. Care 8: 262 (Nov.-Dec.), 1970.

Geller, J. J., et al.: Staff tensions increase during therapeutic interventions. Ment. Hosp. 16: 40 (May), 1965.

Gibson, A.: The Remotivators's Guide Book. F. A. Davis Co., Philadelphia 1967.

Gough, J.: How a group reacts. Am. J. Nurs. 69: 2396 (Nov.), 1969.

Holmes, M., and Werner, J.: Psychiatric Nursing in a Therapeutic Community. Macmillan Co., New York, 1966, p. 3.

Hubbard, J.: The hospital ward: an exciting therapeutic setting. Perspect. Psychiat. Care 3: 8, 1965.

Hutton, G.: It all began with talk. Am. J. Nurs. 63: 107 (Dec.), 1963.

Marshall, R.: A guide toward establishing patient government. Ment. Hyg. 49: 230 (April), 1965.

Racy, J.: How does a group grow? Am. J. Nurs. 69: 2396, (Nov.), 1969.

Robitaille, N.: The organization of a patient council. Perspect. Psychiat. Care 3: 23, 1965.

Schaefer, A.: Participants—not patients. Am. J. Nurs. 65: 94 (Feb.), 1965.

Stevens, L.: Nurse-patient discussion groups. Am. J. Nurs. 63: 67 (Dec.), 1963.

FOOTNOTES

1. Stainbrook, E.: Hospital atmosphere is a definite treatment measure. Ment. Hosp. 8: 8 (Feb.), 1957.
2. Greenblatt, M., York, R., and Brown, E.: From Custodial to Therapeutic Patient Care in Mental Hospitals. Russell Sage Foundation, New York, 1955.
3. Gibson, A.: The Remotivator's Guide Book. F. A. Davis Co., Philadelphia, 1967.

CHAPTER 23

Nursing Care of Suicidal Patients

Suicide is one of the leading causes of death as well as a major public health problem. For these reasons and because of the reported increase in suicidal threats and deaths, medical and nursing personnel cannot afford to underestimate the scope of the problem.

It is impossible to compile accurate statistics of the number of deaths resulting from suicidal acts. Authorities believe that some deaths listed as accidental may actually have been suicides. Accidental deaths reported as a result of taking a lethal dose of a sedative, self-inflicted gunshot wounds, falling from high places, and being struck by a moving vehicle are examples of the circumstances which often cause doubtful reactions in persons studying mortality reports.

UNDERLYING DYNAMICS

Dynamically, a suicidal attempt is a communication, a "cry for help." The person who attempts self-destruction is involved in an intensely emotional, psychological struggle concerning an overwhelmingly frustrating life situation with which the individual cannot cope. The suicidal act is the most desperate, final attempt to resolve the problem when all other defenses have failed. Some suicidal attempts have been recognized as mere gestures made by a distressed person to attract attention to the need for help, instead of behaviors motivated by deep self-destructive impulses. However, these actions may get for the individual the assistance and emotional support he needs from relatives and friends because they arouse feelings of anxiety, guilt, and fear of what may happen to the patient. They may bring about changes in the life situation which help to resolve the patient's overwhelming problem.

CULTURAL CONCEPTS

Cultural viewpoints and attitudes may influence and reinforce an individual's selective use of defense mechanisms. In the American and most western cultures, a person who attempts suicide is considered mentally ill and is immediately hospitalized if, indeed, he is not already confined when the attempt is made. The individual states have enacted legislation which makes it possible for law enforcing and other persons to hospitalize an individual who makes a suicidal attempt for observation and treatment. In some cultures and subcultures, however, self-destructive behavior may not be looked upon as abnormal. There are accounts of Orientals who commit hara-kiri when failure in some life situation brings dishonor upon themselves and their family. Immolations by religious martyrs and stories of sea captains who remained with their sinking ships are some of the evidence that the teachings and expectations of the culture influence the interpretation and response made to self-destructive behavior.

PRECIPITATING FACTORS

What some people refer to as "reasons" why individuals make suicidal attempts are actually precipitating, motivating circumstances which trigger the suicidal act. These are the more immediate events or crisis situations preceding suicidal attempts which evoke recall of earlier, predisposing situations and feelings that have been repressed and retained in the unconscious mind. Feelings of apprehension, fear, and guilt are released and reactivated at the sensory level of behavior during periods of precipitating crisis. Predisposing factors may be thought of as the lifelong influential forces of personality development which may lead, in some persons, to a weakening of psychological defenses and disintegration of the personality. This process is comparable to that which goes on in people who become more susceptible to certain physical illnesses than other individuals exposed to the same organisms. Those persons who are able to adjust to life situations successfully have developed the psychological strength to face and cope with the reality, stress, and strain of living. This would explain why some individuals can endure emotional suffering and recover satisfactorily from a mentally traumatizing experience while others are crushed by its affective impact and forced to the edge of destruction.

When analyzed, precipitating factors are those events associated in one way or another with an individual's reaction to a deep personal loss of some kind, such as the following:

Loss through separation; separation from a close relative or friend owing to death, distance, rejection, divorce, long term hospitalization.

Loss of health owing to illness conceived of as being incurable, distorting to the body image, physically incapacitating, disgraceful.

Loss through social, economic circumstances; failures in scholastic, career endeavors, social and business ambitions.

CUES PRECEDING SUICIDAL ACTS

When a person is physically ill, we are on the alert for symptoms indicative of complications. Symptoms observed are investigated and treatment is started to arrest and prevent a more serious development of the condition. The same procedure should be followed when caring for the mentally ill. Persons who harbor suicidal impulses often manifest deviant behavior symptoms which may be warnings that the individual is contemplating self-destruction. Some of these are as follows:

The development of depression, self preoccupation, and withdrawal from social relations and communications.

Sudden changes in behavior, such as unusual restlessness, agitation, or a shift from depression to gaiety which masks the true, underlying emotional state.

Development of continuous early-morning awakening with feelings of deep depression between the hours of 3 to 7 A.M.

Talking directly or indirectly about suicide with such statements as "I might as well be dead." "What's the use of living?" "They won't have to worry about me much longer." "It's the end of the road for me."

Previous suicidal attempts made by an individual should be considered forewarnings of possible future attempts.

Sometimes the nurse just has an uneasy feeling about the patient, as if something is wrong, but she can't quite identify and explain her feelings beyond saying, "There is something wrong, but I can't seem to put my finger on just what it is that causes me to feel this way."

Giving away articles and personal possessions of more than ordinary significance and value.

Public health authorities stress that it is important for nurses going into homes in the community to be on the alert for suicidal clues in family members who may be depressed by the death of a close relative.

Sometimes distinct changes in the appearance and expression of the eyes of patients having strong suicidal impulses. Smallness in size, a glassy look, and vacant stare may be profoundly obvious.

THERAPEUTIC AND PREVENTIVE
NURSING APPROACHES

Establishing safe conditions in the physical environment is necessary and important, but the most effective preventive is the establishment of a relationship with the patient which causes him to feel that someone is interested, cares about him, and wants to help. The nursing aim is to develop in the individual the belief that he is worthwhile, the desire to live, and the conviction that others want him to survive. To do this requires nursing skill in being able to establish relationships which are emotionally supportive. While carefully observing in order to protect the patient, the nurse must be able to show attitudes of interest, trust, and encouragement which favor the development of interpersonal trust. Constant watchfulness of every move made by the patient and restriction of his movements and use of facilities can be very ineffective. Indeed, these approaches may cause the patient to feel that he is thought of by the staff as being unreliable and untrustworthy and lower his feelings of self-esteem.

The skillful nurse can often observe and protect the patient through companionate approaches. She may initiate and participate in social, recreational activities with the individual and encourage socialization with others. Acceptance in social relationships helps the patient to feel worthwhile. Activities help to divert the patient's interests and impulses into constructive channels.

Some readers may wonder how adequate individualized attention can be given by the nursing staff when the patient population is great. In general hospital wards having thirty to forty patients, the nursing staff identifies and concentrates their major efforts upon the sickest patients. The same can be done in mental hospitals where suicidal patients are in the sickest group. The nurse who cares for several patients would give the most attention to those who need it. Group activities would also be utilized.

Emotional support may be given when the nurse seeks out the patient, sits with him, and encourages verbalization as she listens. These patients often harbor feelings of hate, revenge, and hostility which they are unable to express by acting out owing to the anxiety of guilt. When feelings can be verbalized, the destructive power of the emotions is released through talking instead of self-infliction. The therapeutic effects of encouraging the patient to talk while the nurse listens should never be underestimated. It is an approach that may be as helpful when the patient experiences continuous early morning awakening as it is during the day. A warm beverage offered during sleepless, anxious depressive episodes is soothing and relaxing.

Suicide may be attempted in any environmental setting, including the home and all types of hospitals. Preventive measures may be taken to protect the individual in the physical environment. The individual institution's philosophy, policies, and facilities influence the implementation of preventive procedures. There is, however, a growing recognition by medical and nursing personnel that it is demoralizing as well as unhealthy to subject the entire patient population of a hospital ward to restrictions and deprivations intended for the protection of suicidal patients. Authorities maintain that overprotective approaches simply communicate ideas to the patient about how the staff expects him to behave. Some protective procedures are not as distressing to patients as others, because they can be integrated as part of nursing procedures. Care is taken to make certain that medications given to patients are swallowed and never left to accumulate at the bedside. The temperature and level of water drawn for tub baths is prepared by the nurse who remains in the bathing area to observe patients during the procedure. Sharp implements, such as scissors, knives, and arts and crafts tools used by patients are accounted for under the supervision of nurses and therapists. Suicidal statements made by a patient are reported immediately, recorded, and made known to members of the medical and nursing staff caring for the individual. When the plan of care permits the nurse to spend most of her time with patients in group and individual activities, there is opportunity to observe the patient indirectly instead of by timed rounds.

Helping the patient to recover is a process during which the nurse recognizes the patient's need for guidance in making some decisions and gives support as the individual gradually assumes responsibility for his personal actions. Evaluating and reporting to the medical staff on the patient's progress and readiness to be transferred to an environment which offers greater opportunity to develop self-reliance is an important nursing function.

Anxiety may develop in staff members when a suicidal attempt is intercepted. Fear of what may happen to the patient may concern the personnel as emergency measures to treat and keep the patient alive are implemented. When the critical circumstances have been attended to and the outcome is favorable, the staff's attention turns to making the required written reports. It is not unusual to observe among the staff a tendency to pinpoint the blame. At this time, when personnel are in need of emotional support, feelings of guilt may instead be projected upon them. Many patients who attempted suicide were saved through the timely interventions of nursing personnel. It is unfortunate that owing to our cultural concepts a suicide occuring in a mental hospital often makes dramatic news which evokes public criticism of the institution. This is in contrast to the reaction shown toward death in other accidental circumstances.

For the purposes of alleviating anxiety in the staff and preventing future attempts, the suicidal incident can be reconstructed and discussed. Reconstructing the attempt aids in discovering where a break in the technique may have occurred and what can be done to prevent the development of an attempt under similar conditions.

SUGGESTED REFERENCES

Bennett, A., and Evans, P.: Suicide prevention on psychiatric wards. Ment. Hosp. 16: 31 (Mar.), 1965.
Bodie, M.: When a patient threatens suicide. Perspect. Psychiat. Care 6: 76 (Mar.-Apr.), 1968.
Chapman, M.: Movement therapy in the treatment of suicidal patients. Perspect. Psychiat. Care 9: 119 (May-June), 1971.
Clemmons, P.: Role of the nurse in suicide prevention. J. Psychiat. Nurs. 9: 27 (Jan.-Feb.), 1971.
Farberow, N., and Palmer, R.: The nurse's role in prevention of suicide. Nurs. Forum 3: 93, 1964.
McLean, L.: Action and reaction in suicidal crisis. Nurs. Forum 8: 28 (Winter), 1969.
Shneidman, E.: Preventing suicide. Am. J. Nurs. 65: 111 (May), 1965.
Stevens, B.: A phenomenological approach to understanding suicidal behavior. J. Psychiat. Nurs. 9: 33 (Sept.-Oct.), 1971.
Tallent, N., Kennedy, G., et al.: A program for suicidal patients. Am. J. Nurs. 66: 2014 (Sept.), 1966.
The Los Angeles suicide prevention center (Editorial). Nurs. Outlook 13: 61 (Nov.), 1965.
Umscheid, T.: With suicidal patients: caring for is caring about. Am. J. Nurs. 6: 1230 (June), 1967.
Wallace, M.: The nurse in suicide prevention. Nurs. Outlook 15: 55 (Mar.), 1967.

For reviewing this chapter, grateful acknowledgment is made to Mrs. Gloria Matulis, R.N., Mrs. Rosemary Wynn, R.N., and Miss Nancy Fell, R.N.

CHAPTER 24

Recording Observations and Behavior

PURPOSES

The nurse is in an excellent position to observe the patient because she is with him several hours a day. Her notes can relay to the doctor a word picture of the patient's condition and progress and assist him in planning the most effective treatment and care for his patients. Situations frequently arise during the course of a day which would never be known to the physician if it were not for the nurse's observations and recording of them.

Secondly, hospital charts are sometimes subpoenaed into court as testimony. The nurse's notes may be very important to the outcome of a legal controversy.

Last of all, patient's records are an invaluable research aid. Important statistics may be compiled from them. Clues related to mental disorders and treatments may be detected in the nurse's notes by the researcher.

SYSTEMS OF CHARTING

Systems of charting vary according to particular hospitals and are based upon their individual interests and needs. A hospital devoted to research usually has specific types of records which call for information directly related to particular research projects being conducted. In addition, detailed daily notes on all patients are required. These hospitals are smaller in size and adapted to such requirements. Large state hospitals, which care for many chronically ill patients who remain year after year, may require only a weekly or monthly notation on each patient. There are exceptions, however, in these hospitals: daily notes are kept on patients who are acutely ill. These patients are cared for in the infirmary section of the hospital where the system of recording is more detailed than in the chronic wards.

Some hospitals record temperature, pulse, and respirations every four hours for three days following admission. A record of the cardinal signs is then discontinued. Other hospitals follow up the three-day period by charting these symptoms once each day. In all hospitals, however, nurses are instructed to take the temperature, pulse, and respirations of any patient who complains of physical illness.

Each hospital has its individual way of recording sleep. There are various types of sleep charts. Some institutions do not keep sleep records of patients who have been hospitalized over a period of years. Many record the catamenial period and weekly weight of the patient on the behavior chart. Some have individual weight and catamenial charts for each patient. The nurse, therefore, must necessarily learn the particular system of recording of her own hospital.

Recording may be done by one nurse during the daytime, or it may be done by one nurse assigned to a specific group of patients. It is always possible for a nurse to observe certain things about another nurse's patients. When this occurs, she should write up the situation clearly and concisely on a piece of paper and clip it to the patient's chart. Her name should be signed to the note. When the patient's nurse is ready to record, she will have this information to add to her own observations. When one nurse is assigned to do all of the recording, the other nurses, in the same manner, should make notes which are informative about the patients and clip them to the individual charts.

IMPORTANT ASPECTS TO RECORD

The three most important aspects to observe and record are the appearance, behavior, and conversation of the patient.

APPEARANCE OF PATIENT

The appearance includes everything one can see about the patient from his head to his toes: the hair, eyes, facial expression, skin, mouth, hands, clothing, posture, and movements. These are very obvious and reveal many things at a glance. Together they give the observer a general impression of the patient's entire appearance. Terms used to describe appearance are suggested in the following paragraphs.

Hair

The first thing one usually observes in scanning the person's appearance is the hair. The general appearance and condition of the hair and scalp are directly related to the person's state of health. One may observe hair which just naturally looks clean or unclean. It may be dry, oily, shiny, or dull. Perhaps the patient has not bothered to comb his hair, and it may appear to be stringy or straggly. If the person has long hair, snarls may be evident, an indication that little attention has been given the hair. This observation is frequently made about patients who have been bedridden. Lice may also be obvious. The hair may be generally attractive or unattractive, and either carefully or carelessly styled.

Eyes

It has often been said that the eyes reveal the state of the soul. Eyes may sparkle, move rapidly, appear sad, or seem empty. When the patient has been weeping, the eyes may be tearful and reddened. The suspicious person's eyes may have a questioning look. The disinterested, completely unaffected person may have a blank expression about his eyes.

Facial Expression

The facial expression is easily detected, and moods and attitudes are frequently reflected in the facial expression of the patient. The person may look happy, sad, angry, haggard, worn, bewildered, dissatisfied, interested, or disinterested.

Skin

The skin of the patient who is well nourished is firm and sufficiently moist in texture. The emaciated person's skin looks dry and flabby. The skin may be clear and clean-looking, or blemished. It may feel warm and comfortable, or cold and moist. Bruises, scars, and lacerations may be observed. The nurse must always record exactly how bruises, scars, and lacerations were obtained. The complexion may appear healthy, sallow, pasty, or ruddy.

Mouth

The expression about the mouth is indicated by the lips. These may be relaxed or firm. Lips may curl in resentment or separate in a pleasant smile. The membranes may be dry and cracked, or healthy in appearance.

Hands

The hands may be steady or tremble. They are frequently used in a demonstrative manner when the patient speaks. Hands may look clean or unclean. Fingernails may be beautifully manicured or chewed to the finger tips. They may be too long or unclean.

Clothing

Clothing may be clean or soiled; torn or ragged; wrinkled or carefully pressed; and well selected and fitted or improperly selected and fitted.

Posture

Posture may be excellent or poor. The patient may stand and walk erect, or his shoulders may droop and his body sag.

Movements

The patient may move slowly or fast. One may observe twitching or jerking movements of the person's head or extremities.

Use of Descriptive Terms

The over-all appearance which one sees from day to day may be indicative of the patient's progress or regression. The patient may assume or lose interest in part or all of his appearance. It is important, therefore, to use descriptive terms in writing of the person's appearance in nursing notes.

PATIENT'S BEHAVIOR

The patient's behavior constitutes all of his actions: spontaneous, required behavior, and habitual responses.

It is advantageous to have informative notes about the patient's behavior. The following self-directed queries may be helpful when recording notations about certain aspects of the patient's behavior.

Sleep

Does the patient retire willingly or have to be urged? Does he have difficulty falling asleep? Is his sleep restless or broken? Does he awaken in the early morning? Is he receiving sedation? What is the relation of his sleep to his sedation?

Appetite and Eating Mannerisms

What kind of appetite does the patient have? How does he eat (fast, slowly, by grabbing, by handling food with fingers, by taking other patients' food)? Does he refuse food? Does he seem afraid of food?

Hygienic Practices

Does the patient bathe, brush his teeth, comb his hair, and dress of his own accord? Do the nurses have to urge, assist, or supervise his hygiene? Does he accomplish these practices in the usual time or spend a great deal of time doing them?

Elimination

Is he incontinent and untidy? Does he have to be reminded to go to the toilet routinely? Is he unable to care for himself after elimination? Is he overly concerned about elimination?

Medications

Does the patient refuse medications? What does he say about them? Does he ever request particular medications? Is his physical response to medications usual or unusual? Does he appear afraid or suspicious of medications?

Treatment

Does he refuse or resent treatments? Do nurses have to urge or assist him in preparation for treatment? Is he afraid of treatment? Does he offer any excuses to avoid treatment? What ideas does he express about them?

Classes and Activities

What classes and activities does he attend? Does he have to be urged to attend? What remarks does he make about them? Does he appear cooperative, interested, or disinterested? Does he participate wholeheartedly or halfheartedly?

Rate of Accomplishment

Is he unusually slow or fast about everything he does? Does he worry if he cannot keep up with the rate of others? Is he easily provoked if he has to wait for others who are slower?

Actions

Any bizarre action should be recorded. *Example:* One patient stood in front of the clock each morning between 6 A.M. and 7 A.M. He would watch the hands of the clock and salute it at intervals. Any attempt to interrupt his action was completely ignored by him until breakfast was served.

CONVERSATION OF PATIENT

It is important to record conversation accurately and concisely. Direct quotations should be used rather than the narrative form. A conversation turned into narrative style never conveys the same impression and may be the cause of misinterpretation by those who read it. Some conversations are important enough to cause the transfer of a patient from one service to another or to place him on suicidal or elopement precautions. In all fairness to the patient, it is extremely important to quote his statements.

Conversation may be relevant or irrelevant. The patient may speak rapidly, or his thoughts may be entirely unrelated and disconnected. He may constantly repeat the same word or words so that immediately one thinks of his speech as being repetitious. Perhaps he may have difficulty in responding to questions so that his speech is noticeably retarded. Parts of his conversation may be inaudible, or there may be a hesitancy in the middle of his speech which indicates a mental blocking.

The nurse may, at times, detect the patient's mood or attitude in his conversation. The patient's tone of voice and mannerisms of speech, added to the words he uses, may be a reflection of his mood and attitude. It is not difficult to sense the patient's mood; sad, cheerful, irritable, impatient, or impulsive moods may be detected through the patient's conversation. Sarcastic, critical, aggressive, demanding, or domineering attitudes may likewise be quite obvious. His statements may indicate that he is cooperative or uncooperative. His mood may not be in keeping with the general situation.

The nurse must guard against projecting her own feelings and interpretations into the patient's record. She must learn to record facts exactly as she sees and hears them. The words she uses must enable the reader to quickly grasp a picture of the whole situation. Her grammatical construction must be good; short, well-worded, properly constructed sentences can be far superior to long-winded, rambling statements, which are oftentimes loosely connected and provoking.

Charting Aids

Quotation marks, parentheses, and short and long dashes are frequently helpful in charting conversation.

Quotation Marks. Anything written inside quotation marks signifies the exact words of the patient. *Example:* "I cannot stand any more of this. I might as well be dead."

Parentheses. Words inserted between parentheses are related to the term immediately preceding the parentheses. These insertions clarify the meaning of the preceding term. *Example:* "She must want my husband. I had a ring on he gave to me and she (nurse) took it away from me."

Short Dashes. Short dashes following part of a conversation may be used to indicate words mumbled by the patient which the nurse could not hear. *Example:* "I went into the house and while I was there I heard Mary saying - - - - - - -shouldn't have listened to her."

Long Dashes. Long dashes may be placed at the end of incomplete statements. *Example:* "Don't come near me Mr. because————."

Interpretation

Nurses should never record that the patient is hallucinating or has delusions. The correct way to convey this impression to the psychiatrist is to chart the attending situation, the patient's actions, and conversations so that the idea is contained in the record. *Example:* The patient stands at his window for long periods of time. Now and then he mumbles a few words and then presses his ear against the window screen. Soon he begins to nod his head as if in agreement. When he is approached, he appears irritable and shouts, "Get away from me! You are devils torturing me. God told me so." The words "You are devils torturing me" may indicate that the patient has delusions of persecution. "God told me so" may be an indication that the patient is hearing voices. However, the interpretation is made by the psychiatrist.

What to Chart

It is important to record normal as well as abnormal conversation, especially when the patient's conversation has previously been abnormal. This charting denotes the change which has occurred. It is also important to chart in detail any physical complaints that the patient makes. These complaints sometimes have organic or psychologic significance and must always be investigated. Three things must be uppermost in the mind of the nurse who is recording: appearance, behavior, and conversation.

Interpersonal Process Recording

In some instances, nursing students are being required to record in detail the events and actual conversation which took place between them and individual patients to whom the nurses are assigned. This is known as recording of the interpersonal process and there are various methods of writing these notes. The purpose of this type of recording is to make it possible to refer to the nurse's notes during an individual conference with the instructor. The nurse has an opportunity to discuss with the instructor the events and conversations recorded. Through this discussion she often develops a better understanding of the patient's behavior and conversation. The nurse also may receive valuable assistance in understanding her own behavior in the interpersonal situation, as well as become aware of positive and negative approaches made by her toward the patient.

NURSING CARE PLANS

The nursing care plan is an ongoing record of information concerning the patient and his care that commences with the admission of the patient. It is designed to give goal-directed, patient-centered individualized care. When properly utilized, the nursing care plan enables nursing personnel to gain an orientation to the patient, his needs, and the treatment plan. Communication between staff is facilitated through the use of the plan. It serves as a basic instrument for sharing information with team members as well as promoting consistency in maintaining individualized nursing care and psychological approaches.

In the psychiatric setting nursing care plans are usually initiated by the nursing team leader. They are kept up to date through discussion that takes place during regularly scheduled team conferences. The information appearing on the plan is obtained from the patient's history, observations of the individual's behavior, suggestions contributed by staff members, and written doctor's orders.

Nursing Care Plan

Medication	Start	Stop	Activities
1) Serax 15 mg. tid 9-1-6	2-10-72		O.T.
2) Chloral Hydrate 3 3/4 gr—H.S.	2-10-72		Has a stamp collection
3) Milk of Magnesia 1 oz. H.S. P.R.N.	2-13-72		Full ward privileges with assistance

Treatments			Family Relationships

Inhalation Therapy Daily a.m.	2-15-72		Widowed
			Son—Earl Simpson
			   910 East Road
			   Corning, Florida
			   (Lives 500 miles away)

Name: Thomas Simpson Birthdate: 2-7-1900 Religion: Prot. Diet: Reg. Adm. 10-17-71

Description of Appearance and Behavior: Mr. Simpson is a white-haired Caucasian male aged 71. He is disoriented at times, somewhat unsteady. Is lonely, irritable at times and has some incontinence. Wears dentures and eyeglasses. Eats well. May strike out if frustrated.
Goal(s): Keep Mr. Simpson as productive as possible at his functioning capacity. Encourage him to show his collection of stamps.

Needs	Suggestions for Nursing Care
Orientation	Have a clock and calendar in convenient place.
Security	Have consistent ward routine. Have him eat at same place and table in dining room. Don't change his room or move his bed.
Attention	Refer to him as Mr. S. not Tom.
Respect	Spend time with him a.m. & p.m. daily.
Feeling of usefulness	Encourage socializing with other patients.
	Encourage him to care for his own needs as much as he can.
	Help with letter writing.
Walking	Don't place throw rugs in room.
Elimination	Encourage fluids.
	Record intake and output.
	Toilet at regular intervals during waking hours.

Goals set by the staff should be based upon observations of the patient's needs. They should be realistic and attainable. Goals are sometimes influenced by the philosophy and treatment plan of the particular facility as well as the anticipated length of hospitalization of the patient. That is, whether the facility is a crisis intervention unit, a short term service, or an extended care facility.

In some large mental hospitals it is extremely difficult for the staff to accept the value of a nursing care plan and the need to become an involved contributor to its development and use. A nursing care plan is shown here that may be helpful in assisting readers to develop a plan and participate in its continuity.

SUGGESTED REFERENCES

Bloom, J., Dressler, J., et al.: Problem oriented charting. Am. J. Nurs. 71: 2144 (Nov.), 1971.

Davitz, L.: Interpersonal Processes in Nursing Case Histories. Springer Publishing Co., Inc., New York, 1970.

Fuerst, E., and Wolff, L.: Fundamentals of Nursing. J. B. Lippincott Co., Philadelphia, 1969, p. 42.

Gragg, S., and Rees, O.: Scientific Principles in Nursing. C. V. Mosby Co., St. Louis, 1970, p. 59.

Kron, T.: The Management of Patient Care. W. B. Saunders Co., Philadelphia, 1971, p. 95.

Maddison, D., Day, P., and Leabeater, B.: Psychiatric Nursing. E. & S. Livingstone Ltd., London, 1968, p. 403.

UNIT 7

Treatments for the Mentally Ill

CHAPTER **25**

Somatic Therapies

Although the tranquilizing and antidepressant drugs have largely replaced other somatic therapies, some patients may not respond as quickly or favorably as others to drug therapy. Electrotherapy and Indoklon inhalation therapy are being used on a selective basis and have been especially useful for patients receiving treatment in outpatient facilities. Insulin treatment is administered in a relatively small number of hospitals. Individual hospitals have printed procedures for each somatic therapy to which the nurse should refer.

PREPARATION OF THE PATIENT

Certain general preparation of the patient is essential for all types of somatic therapies. Written permission to administer treatment is obtained from someone having legal responsibility for the patient. A complete physical examination, electrocardiogram, x-rays of the chest and thoracic spine, urinalysis, and blood studies are done before therapy is commenced to rule out the possibility of contraindications. Immediately preceding treatment, the patient's temperature, pulse, and respiration rate are taken, and treatment is omitted if the temperature is elevated. Hairpins, bobbie pins, and dentures are removed, and the patient is encouraged to void. It is the nurse's responsibility to see that all reports and treatment permission are on the patient's chart before treatment is started.

ELECTROTHERAPY

Doctors Ugo Cerletti and Lucio Bini of Rome, Italy, introduced electrotherapy in 1937. It is most beneficial for persons afflicted with various types of depressive states. The method of Cerletti and Bini is known as the "classical" technique.

The treatment may be given in a special treatment unit of the hospital or in the patient's room on the ward. The regular meal preceding treatment is omitted. The patient may be dressed in sleeping garments or wear civilian clothing which is loosened at the waist and neck. A team composed of the doctor and usually two or three members of the nursing staff conduct the treatment. In general, the procedure is as follows:

The patient's vital signs are checked and recorded on the chart by the nurse. Atropine sulphate 1/60 grains is given by hypodermic injection one hour before treatment is started to dry secretions and to prevent vagal stimulation of the heart. In most hospitals, muscle relaxant drugs are given by the doctor at the beginning of treatment. An intravenous injection of 1 per cent Brevital Sodium (methohexital) in an average dose of 8 to 10 cc. is given and followed immediately by a small dose of Anectine (succinylcholine chloride). The amount used depends upon the muscular development of the patient and may vary from 10 to 20 mg. for a woman of average weight to 20 to 40 mg. for an average weight man. Separate syringes are used for each drug administered. After rubbing the patient's temples with electrode jelly, the padded electrodes which have been soaked in a 20 per cent physiologic-saline solution are applied. A soft, absorbent mouth gag is placed between the patient's upper teeth and tongue. After a brief testing of the apparatus, the doctor sets the automatic timing device of the machine. Dependent upon the individual patient, from 70 to 150 volts of electricity may be used, requiring from 0.1 to 1.0 seconds to be administered. A grand mal convulsive seizure of the tonic-clonic pattern develops (see p. 412). The patient usually sleeps from 5 to 10 minutes following the seizure and upon awakening does not remember the period of treatment. It is usually helpful to administer a few breaths of oxygen following treatment. If respiratory difficulty occurs, the patient is given artificial respiration. Close observation by the nurse is essential until the patient is fully oriented, steady on his feet, and able to be out of bed. A series of treatments consists of 8 to 15 treatments, given on alternate days three times a week. If the individual does not respond well to a series, another series may be started within a short period of time. Cathartics, when needed, should be given the evening before a day when treatment is omitted.

BRIEF-STIMULUS ELECTROTHERAPY

Brief-stimulus electrotherapy is a modified, or refined technique of the original classical method. Premedication is given as prescribed. The amount of electric current used is reduced. The individual experiences a dazed mental reaction and there is only minimal muscle activity instead of

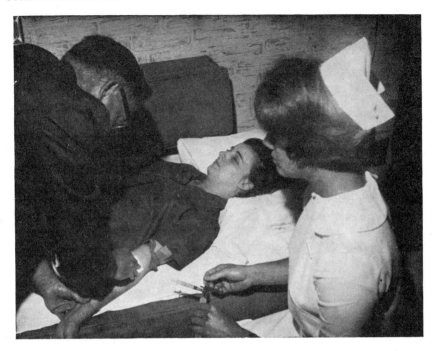

Fig. 1 Premedicating the patient for Indoklon inhalation therapy. (Courtesy of Swedish-American Hospital, Rockford, Ill.)

a grand mal seizure. Patients may be fully oriented 2 minutes after treatment is administered. The main advantage of brief-stimulus electrotherapy is that the patients do not develop marked amnesia as is observed in persons receiving the classical technique.

COMPLICATIONS

Although muscular and joint pain complained of by the patient is not always indicative of a fracture, complaints of facial, back, and extremity pain should always be reported so that x-rays can be considered. Treatment is discontinued if a fracture is detected. Aspirin (acetylsalicylic acid) is usually prescribed for headache.

INDOKLON INHALATION THERAPY

Indoklon (flurothyl), a colorless, volatile liquid which is administered with oxygen inhalation, is being used in some hospitals for the treatment of mentally-ill patients in whom convulsive therapy is indicated. The technique may be used by itself as a replacement for electrotherapy or in combination with selected tranquilizing drug therapy. It is a treatment that, once started, may be given daily without interruption, when the patient's condition is satisfactory, until a series of 8 to 15 treatments is completed. For those patients who fear electrotherapy, Indoklon offers an alternative which is usually more acceptable. The most beneficial results have been achieved in psychotic depressed persons. Although the seizures induced by Indoklon are similar to those produced by the classical type of electrotherapy, their outset is more gradual. The tonic phase lasts for 10 seconds, but the clonic phase lasts approximately one minute. Only minimal amnesia may develop after treatment, therefore Indoklon may be useful in outpatient facilities.

Indoklon therapy is given only after the required physical examination, laboratory procedures, tests, and x-rays are completed for the purpose of ruling out contraindications which are similar to those for electrotherapy. The patient's vital signs are checked twice a day for two days before treatment is commenced and twice a day thereafter during the series, including being recorded before individual treatments. The patient is not permitted to ingest anything by mouth on the morning of treatment.

The following procedure is used to administer treatment. A 5-liter bag attached to an oxygen supply tank is connected to the Indoklon vaporizer. The vaporizer is connected to the face mask. About 0.5 cc. of Indoklon is put into the vaporizer and the bag is partially inflated with oxygen. Connection to the oxygen supply is maintained during therapy.

Some physicians administer Indoklon therapy without giving the patient premedication. Others prefer to prescribe atropine sulphate 1/60 grains by hypodermic injection 1 hour before treatment in order to dry secretions and to prevent vagal stimulation of the heart. The alternative may be to give atropine sulphate 1/75 grains intravenously as treatment is started. An intravenous injection of 1 per cent Brevital Sodium (methohexital) in an average dose of 8 to 10 cc. is given and followed immediately by a small dose of Anectine (succinylcholine chloride). The amount used depends upon the muscular development of the patient and may vary from 15 to 20 mg. for a woman of average weight to 20 to 40 mg. for a man of average weight. Separate syringes are used for each drug administered. An adult rubber Guedel oral pharyngeal airway is then inserted through the patient's mouth. The face mask is placed tightly on the patient's face and the bag is squeezed gently, forcing the oxygen-Indoklon mixture into the lungs at the rate of one inhalation every 5 seconds. The patient breathes into the bag. The usual number of inhalations required to cause a convulsion may vary from three to six. A seizure usually occurs within 40 seconds.

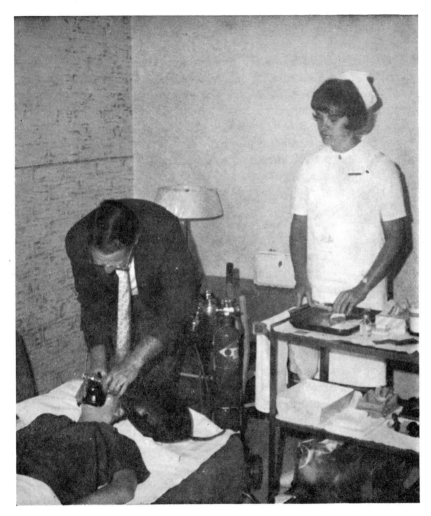

Fig. 2 Treatment is implemented as the patient commences to inhale the Indoklon-oxygen mixture. (Courtesy of Swedish-American Hospital, Rockford, Ill.)

In most patients respiration starts at the termination of the clonic phase, as the patient is, in effect, being resuscitated during the inhalation. Some investigators have found it unnecessary to continue resuscitation following termination of the seizure. Others continue resuscitation until the effects of the Anectine (succinylcholine cloride) have completely disappeared. Indoklon is eliminated from the body through the lungs. Observation of the patient following treatment is the same as that carried out following electrotherapy.

INSULIN THERAPY

Doctor Manfred Sakel of Vienna introduced insulin therapy in 1933. It is used chiefly in the treatment of schizophrenia.

When large doses of insulin are given to patients, they develop a marked hypoglycemia which, when prolonged, leads to a state of coma. Many theories have been advanced as to how insulin produces beneficial results, but the exact effect is not really known. The same general preparation of the patient outlined in the beginning of this chapter is followed when therapy is commenced.

Dressed in sleeping attire, the patient is taken to the insulin treatment department in the early morning. Breakfast is omitted. He is put to bed and the nurse checks his temperature, pulse, respirations, and blood pressure. Treatment is not given if abnormalities in the vital signs are detected. The patient voids before receiving a deep intramuscular injection of insulin. The initial dose is small and varies usually from 5 to 10 units of insulin, dependent upon the person's age, weight, and physical condition. When the first injection is given, careful observation is made for signs of hypersensitivity or allergic reactions to the drug. Raised welts around the injection site or an itching sensation experienced by the patient and scratching of the affected area are indications to terminate treatment for the day. Another brand or type of insulin obtained from a different animal species is given for the next treatment. If the patient is sensitive to all types of insulin, an antihistamine drug is given in combination with the insulin. Hyaluronidase (Alidase) is sometimes injected in conjunction with insulin to facilitate the rate of insulin absorption by the body, making it possible to reduce the dosage.

A series of treatments consists of 50 to 60 treatments. One treatment is given each day, five days a week. The amount of insulin is increased daily until the coma stage is reached. Coma may not develop for several or more days. When it is reached, the insulin dose producing it is maintained as long as the depth of the reaction remains the same. In some instances it may be necessary to increase the dosage, in others it is possible to produce coma by decreasing the maintenance dose. The chief characteristics of coma are loss of consciousness, profuse perspiration, and flushing of the face. When deep coma is reached, the patient cannot be aroused, superficial reflexes disappear and other pathological reflexes appear. If coma is continued for too long a period, there is a complete absence of body reflexes. The patient must be closely observed in order to recognize the onset of coma so that it can be terminated within proper time limits. Cathartics, when necessary, are given the night before rest days.

NURSING OBSERVATIONS

Some patients become increasingly drowsy and gradually lapse into coma. Others may appear mildly excited and confused for a short period, then become drowsy and develop coma. If the patient becomes unduly excited, treatment should be terminated. When perspiration is profuse, the nurse may dry the patient's face and body with a towel, turn the pillow, change the gown, but the patient should not be disturbed to have the bedding changed. If the swallowing reflexes are present and the individual complains of thirst, cracked ice may be given. Sips of water will sometimes relieve hunger excitement, but if given and ineffective, treatment is terminated. The patient should be turned on his side to promote drainage of saliva. Electric suction may be used to drain excessive flow of saliva. Pulse and respirations should be counted and their characteristics observed frequently. Unusually slow, weak, rapid, thready, or irregular pulse should be reported immediately to the physician for consideration of treatment termination. Shallow respirations may be deepened by turning the patient on his side with his head raised and mouth opened. Chindrop, resulting in labored respirations, may be relieved temporarily by holding the patient's jaw in its proper position. Hypoglycemia may have to be terminated if respiratory embarrassment is severe. Laryngospasm occurs very rarely and may be relieved by passing a nasal-gavage tube. Treatment is terminated if this procedure fails. If the patient's temperature is elevated above 103° F. when treatment is ended, an alcohol sponge may be ordered and fluids forced. If the temperature is subnormal, the patient is kept in bed covered with extra blankets. Hot water bags may be placed along the side of the top blanket. During treatment there may be spasmodic twitchings and stretchings of the muscles which may subside, or the patient may become restless. The development of a convulsive seizure is an indication to terminate treatment immediately.

TERMINATION OF TREATMENT

Coma is usually allowed to progress for about one hour before hypoglycemia is terminated with sugar water or glucose solution. When the patient does not develop coma and can swallow, he is given 400 cc. of 40 per cent sugar water to drink. Patients in coma may be terminated with a nasal gavage of sugar solution, the prescription of which is based upon the dose of insulin given to the individual patient. In some hospitals, hypoglycemia is terminated routinely with an intravenous injection of glucose. When complications lead to termination of treatment, an intravenous injection of 50 cc. of 50 per cent glucose is administered rapidly. When the patient awakens, his vital signs are checked, his body dried, gown changed, and he is permitted to rest in bed between two dry blankets. A meal is served to him about one-half hour later. When he returns to the ward the patient is put to bed for a two-hour rest period. He bathes, dresses, is given nourishment, permitted to socialize and partake of the regular evening meal. Later he is given 200 cc. of 40 per cent sugar water and a glass of fruit juice to drink.

Patients receiving insulin therapy must be carefully observed to make certain that they eat their meals and drink beverages served. If the patient does not consume sufficient food and nourishment offered, he may develop a later secondary insulin reaction. This may occur at any time during the day or night. The most outstanding symptoms of a delayed reaction are weakness, drowsiness, unsteady gait, profuse perspiration, and hunger complaints. The patient should be given 200 cc. of 40 per cent sugar solution by mouth or a glass of pure orange juice. If coma develops, the individual will be unable to swallow. A physician should be called to give the intravenous injection of 50 per cent glucose. A light lunch should be fed to the patient following termination of a secondary reaction by either of these methods. Whenever the patient leaves the ward for any activity, he should be escorted and closely observed for secondary reaction symptoms. A bottle containing 400 cc. of sugar solution should be carried by escorting personnel so that it is readily available.

COMPLICATIONS

Most of the complications which occur during treatment can be dealt with successfully. Circulatory failure, convulsions, fractures, and aspirations of saliva and fluid into the lungs, resulting sometimes in lung abscess, are the most commonly observed. The physician should be notified immediately. A nasal gavage tray having the necessary equipment and a prescribed sugar solution should be kept immediately available during treatment to terminate hypoglycemia when indicated. There should also be an emergency tray having sterile equipment for giving injections as well as ampuls of 50 per cent glucose solution and other stimulating drugs.

COMBINED THERAPY

Combined therapy may be used when the patient fails to respond to one specific type of therapy. Insulin may be combined with electrotherapy. Treatment may be given on the same day. Electrotherapy may be given at the close of the patient's insulin treatment before hypoglycemia is terminated.

NURSING CARE DURING SOMATIC THERAPIES

During somatic therapies the nurse may be helpful in promoting recovery. Her chief aim should be to assist the patient in focusing his attention on external influences and preventing him from experiencing a relapse. When the nurse observes personality changes, such as reduced overactivity, increased interest in surroundings and activities, and a desire to converse with others, she should recognize these as an indication that the patient is attempting to attach himself to healthful, sustaining interests.

The nurse should encourage the patient to participate in social and recreational activities which help to strengthen his hold on reality and adjustment.

When the patient is ready for group associations, the nurse can gradually bring him in contact with other patients by card games, checkers, radio programs, entertainment, and small parties during unoccupied ward periods.

If the person has regressed considerably during the illness, the nurse will have to help to reeducate the patient.

Oftentimes patients suffering from amnesia become distressed when recent events are difficult to recall. They may seek reassurance from the nurse. The nurse may explain that amnesia is a usual reaction which subsides gradually after treatment is terminated.

Daily notes on the patient's behavior should be made throughout the course of therapy. This will help to guide both the physicians and nurses concerned with the patient's care. Notations on the following observations are important:

Degree of interest and effort shown in activity.
Level of ability to carry out personal hygiene measures.
Kind of appetite.
Type of sleep.
Any symptoms of amnesia.
Reassurance sought from nurse.
Noteworthy personality changes.

SUGGESTED REFERENCES

Cohen, R.: EST + group therapy = improved care. Am. J. Nurs., 71: 1195 (June), 1971.
Freedman, A., and Kaplan, H. (eds.): Comprehensive Textbook of Psychiatry. The Williams

& Wilkins Co., Baltimore, 1967, pp. 558, 795.

Gilmore, B.: Advances in insulin coma therapy. Am. J. Nurs. 60: 1626 (Nov.), 1960.

Indoklon (Flurothyl)—A Convulsant Agent for Psychiatric Use. Ohio Chemical and Surgical Co., Madison, Wisconsin.

Kolb, L.: Noyes' Modern Clinical Psychiatry, ed. 7. W. B. Saunders Co., Philadelphia, 1968, p. 590.

CHAPTER 26

Social, Recreational, Art, and Music Therapies

by BERTHA E. SCHLOTTER*

Every good psychiatric hospital conducts activities such as recreational, occupational, musical, educational, and industrial therapy. Bibliotherapy is also utilized.

The mentally ill patient is often unable to participate acceptably or with satisfaction in the prevailing social order. His illness is usually the result of an accumulation of social maladjustments rather than a single great catastrophe. As a result, the patient's home and community environments have become burdensome. He has come to live, to a large extent, in a world of his own making, which may or may not include reality. Therefore, it is the hospital's responsibility to provide treatment which will help him to accept his social obligations and become a contributing member of society. To provide this treatment, psychiatric hospitals include in their programs therapeutic activities which help the patient to accept his environment and contribute to his own and other persons' well being. Thus, an acceptable social adaptation brings about in the patient better personality integration.

Spontaneous diversional or medically prescribed therapeutic activities may be administered by professionally trained therapists, volunteers, nurses, aides or by the patients themselves. The benefits derived from these activities depend upon the wisdom exercised in their administration.

THERAPEUTIC RELATIONSHIPS

Warmth and friendliness toward the patient from the therapist and

*Formerly Institutional Therapy Consultant, Illinois Department of Public Welfare.

other persons engaged in planning and carrying out these activities affect not only the relationship between the therapist and the patients but also the relationships between the patients themselves. When the association of a particular group extends over a considerable period of time, and when the patients engage in activities which may be carried out only through cooperative interaction, friendly helpfulness tends to develop to a higher degree than when personal relationships are less close.

SELECTION OF ACTIVITIES

Selection involves planning for and anticipating favorable developments in the patient's condition as a result of planned therapeutic activities. Selection of activities is made not only to develop the native abilities of the patient but to motivate new interests in him. For effective treatment, activities should be selected which coordinate the patient's impulse of the moment with the more stable aspects of his behavior. Experimental methods of selecting activities are necessary, in so far as possible, to hold the patient's interest and to find increasingly better ways of using these activities to achieve beneficial results. Furthermore, experimentation keeps the activity from becoming monotonous, static, and repetitious, all of which have little or no therapeutic value. Beneficial results are best achieved through spontaneous and voluntary participation of the patient. Every possible device should be used to induce active, voluntary participation. When attempting to interest a resistive patient, this may be exceedingly difficult, but patience, kindness, friendliness, and repeated invitations to join the activity are difficult for the patient to resist, particularly if the gesture is made when the group is in a happy mood. Although the patient may not participate immediately, repeated exposure to the activity tends to break down his fear and disinterest. Rightly used, therapeutic activities help to reduce patients' reactions of resistance, fear, and hostility, and stimulate more positive responses from the patient.

Therapeutic activities are most successful when patients are given new and challenging projects which require constant mental and physical reorganization in accordance with the patient's level of ability performance. New projects assist in reviving a patient's old healthy pattern of behavior, as well as in stimulating new patterns which are essential for the reintegration of the patient's personality. Persons who engage in the administration of therapeutic activities also need the stimulation which comes from experimentation. Actually, it is difficult to separate the personnel's satisfactions and success from those of the patient. Both need problems to solve if the patient's rehabilitation is to be successful.

PLANNING THERAPEUTIC ACTIVITIES

Basic in planning a therapeutic activity program for the mentally ill are two concepts. First, setting up a stimulating situation which will induce spontaneous problem-solving behavior provides an organizing medium of expression. Second, the greatest stimulation for an individual comes from relationships with other persons. Therefore, patients should be organized, when possible, into congenial groups so that cooperation and integration may develop as they participate in activities over a considerable period of time. Common interests and shared experiences are the means by which patients learn to function with others.

When promoting therapeutic activities, every effort should be made to create situations in which the members of the group will be able to participate physically, mentally and socially. Therefore, it is necessary that many activities, varying in complexity, be provided to interest patients so that they may participate in them with some degree of ease and spontaneity. For example, very regressed male patients should not be expected to play a game of baseball or basketball involving a need for alertness, multiple mental responses, and a high degree of social awareness. Simple ball-tossing games should be introduced for such patients. During simple activity of this type, the patient is largely participating as an individual. Little social interaction and physical and mental exertion are required. It is important to observe patients carefully and introduce more complex activities only when it is obvious that the patient is able to respond and participate on a higher performance level. Progress toward the more complex level is gradual.

TYPES OF GROUP ACTIVITY

The first type of group activity is the spectator activity in which the individual has little or nothing to do with other members of the group. Motion pictures, stage shows, concerts, radio, television, ball games, and other amusements are examples of spectator activities. The patient observes or listens to the program but does not assume an active part in its production. Spectator group activities require very simple relationships. Each individual may participate without having to exert himself to the point of feeling socially uncomfortable or inadequate. These activities continue whether or not the individual patient loses interest, observes, or listens.

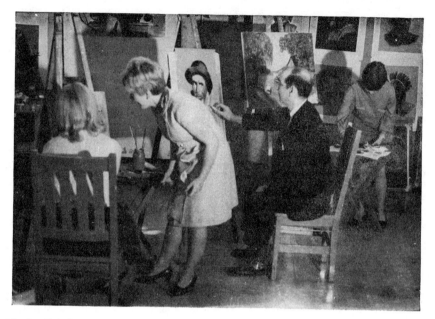

Fig. 1. Painting helps to express creative talents and free the emotions. (Courtesy of Essex County Overbrook Hospital, Cedar Grove, N.J.)

A second type of group organization is the casual coming together of persons to carry on individual patient activities. A sufficient amount of cooperation is necessary to permit the members of the group to use the equipment and facilities with a minimum of friction. Roller skating, swimming, painting and certain hobby classes are examples of this type of group activity.

Higher development in group interaction is inherent in such activities as community singing, rhythm bands, calisthenics, and certain craft projects. Each patient works on a part of the total project. In this third type of social organization, patients are required to participate with a fairly high degree of concentrated cooperation. Each person taking part in community singing sings as an individual, but he must sing the same song, in the same tempo, in the same key. He must commence and stop on time if singing is to be a happy experience. Individual patients do sometimes lose interest in something else for the moment, but the song is carried by other members of the group. The patient may rejoin the singing when he desires. Generally speaking, the patient's lack of complete participation does not cause this type of activity to fail.

A fourth, higher ability level of group activity requires continuous cooperation and interaction between patients over a relatively short period

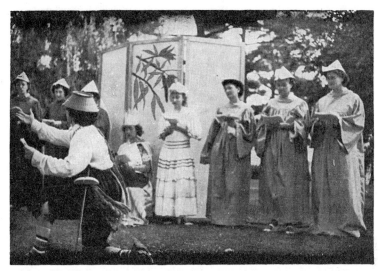

Fig. 2.   Dramatic group. (Courtesy of Illinois Department of Public Welfare.)

of time; namely, for the duration of the activity. Active participation in basketball, baseball, bridge, pinochle, and square dancing are examples of this type of group activity. A high degree of mental, physical, and social interaction is required of patients during such activities. Success is dependent upon each participant assuming his responsibility and role in the diversion; otherwise, the activity ceases until reorganization occurs through the replacement of nonparticipants with active participants.

A fifth type of group organization is that in which the patients must be able to engage in creative interaction of an intensive, cooperative nature during the entire progress of the activity. A dramatic production is a fine example of this type of group organization. Patients rehearsing the drama must be able to work harmoniously together and to develop the roles they are portraying in relation to each other. Such activities may extend for a period of weeks or months. Participants must concentrate upon and cooperate toward the successful development of the drama. Each patient must accept responsibility for his share in the production and be ready to assume this responsibility according to the set practice schedule and in relation to the other participants.

The sixth type of group organization is seldom found in a psychiatric hospital. It is the social club which requires considerable homogeneity. For full development of the social club there must be a long period of sharing mutual responsibility and a concern for the common good of the group. Many groups of this type meet together for years. Members plan their own activities, which change from time to time as the members mature and their interests change. Activities chosen by the group might include individual and committee assignments to develop a project such as a flower show, an art exhibit, or a literary publication. Other activities might include group perfection of a skill or art, such as photography; also the development of special-interest groups to study such subjects as the history of art and music.

The last development is group federation. Patients function collectively and undertake activities which cannot be carried on by single groups or clubs. Delegates are sent to the federation and must be able to report the wishes of their group to the federation. Upon their return they must be able to report the thinking of the federate group and receive further instructions from their own group. This type of activity requires a high degree of social control and intenseinteraction. It involves sharing and cooperating with a single group as well as a large group and an additional ability to compromise and help solve problems involving several groups (see p. 282).

Psychiatric hospitals function quite successfully today in engaging patients in therapeutic activities involving the first four or possibly five types of social organization and interaction described above. To participate satisfactorily in social and federated types of activities, the patients must be stable, homogeneous, and able to meet over a long period of time. Patients who are able to function in such highly complex social activities are usually ready for discharge from the hospital.

It has been observed that a large part of the psychiatric hospital's therapeutic-activity program is at the amusement or entertainment level. While these programs are to be commended, it should be borne in mind that they are a first step in bringing groups together. For maximum therapeutic benefit, the patient should be encouraged actively to participate in progressively more and more complex activities which challenge his interest, ability and imagination.

PRESCRIBING THERAPEUTIC ACTIVITIES

The psychiatrist's role in prescribing therapeutic activities is of the utmost importance. A written prescription for each patient should be obtained. Knowing and understanding his patient's illness, the doctor prescribes a course of treatment which includes not only medical treatment but also a program of activity based upon the individual patient's interests, needs, and abilities. Although the psychiatrist may not always prescribe the specific projects, hobbies, recreation, and so on, his general plan and guiding suggestions are extremely helpful to those who administer the activity program. Maximum therapeutic results are achieved when the therapist has a knowledge of the attitudes, precautions and types of relationships suggested by the psychiatrist.

Conferences between the therapist, psychiatrist and other members of

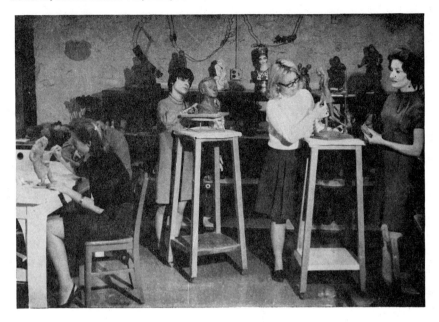

Fig. 3. Moulding clay helps to stimulate the imagination and release the creative impulse. (Courtesy of Essex County Overbrook Hospital, Cedar Grove, N. J.)

the clinical team are invaluable. During these meetings the patient, as an individual, is considered. A planned program is outlined. Later when evaluation conferences are held, a need may be revealed to revise the original planned program in accordance with observations made about the patient's behavior and attitude.

TYPES OF THERAPEUTIC ACTIVITIES

RECREATIONAL THERAPY

The old adage, "All work and no play makes Johnny a dull boy," is applied in the consideration of a recreational program. In its broadest sense, the term "recreation" applies to any activity which revitalizes the patient's interest and helps him to relax and feel refreshed. Recreation must necessarily be an activity which is different and provides a change from the patient's usual routine. What might be considered vocational for one patient might well be recreation for another. For instance, a concert pianist would have a professional interest in a piano recital and might actually become more tense instead of relaxed during such a performance. The same reaction might be anticipated from a professional baseball player observing a baseball game. In fact, psychiatrists have been known to prescribe complete avoidance of activities which are concerned with the patient's past indulgences or accomplishments. Therefore, recreation should be planned in accordance with knowledge concerning past and present interests, individual abilities, and needs.

Dependent upon the particular patient, recreation might be found in practically all of the therapeutic activities. Some of the common forms of recreation observed in psychiatric hospitals are listed here:

Motion pictures
Concerts
Recitals
Plays
Radio
Television
Recorded music
Motoring
Holiday celebrations
Dancing
  Social
  Square
  Folk
Parties
Picnics
Instrumental Music
  Individual
  Rhythm band
  Orchestra
Dramatics
  Musical comedies
  Plays
  Charades
  Operettas
  Socio-drama
Singing
  Individual
  Choral
  Community
Special interest
  Stamps
  Photography

Designing
Arts
Crafts
Dressmaking
Woodcraft
Literary groups
Nature lore
Forums
Reading
Swimming
Games
Complex: Such as, Bridge, Pinochle, Basketball, Football
Less Complex: Such as Cat and Rat, Checkers, Simple card games

OCCUPATIONAL THERAPY

Occupational therapy is described as any activity, mental or physical, prescribed and guided to aid an individual's recovery from disease or injury.

In some psychiatric hospitals all of the therapeutic activities are categorized as occupational therapy. In other hospitals these activites are departmentally categorized. Recreational, musical, educational, occupational and industrial therapy all constitute separate departmental therapies. In this discussion, occupational therapy will be limited to a consideration of the arts and crafts. The following list provides some idea of the arts and crafts herein considered:

Painting	Modeling
Sketching	Toymaking
Ceramics	Sewing
Leatherwork	Knitting
Basketry	Woodwork
Weaving	Jewelry
Metalwork	Needlework
Plastics	Bookbinding

Many patients enjoy the arts and crafts because these exclude competition and pressure from the activity. There is opportunity for individual creativeness, to harmonize colors and produce something tangible out of

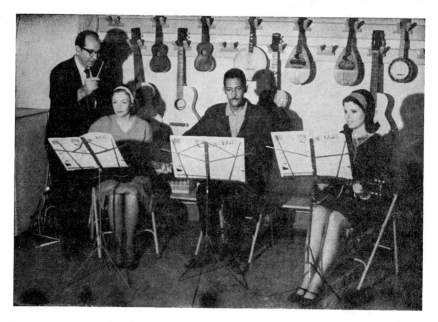

Fig. 4. Taking a guitar lesson in music therapy. (Courtesy of Essex County Overbrook Hospital, Cedar Grove, N. J.)

the patient's own thinking and imagination. New interests may emerge or be combined with the old. Self-confidence and personal achievement frequently evolve from these activities. The relaxed, informal atmosphere in the hospital studio shop helps to reshape attitudes and foster relationships which aid in the patient's recovery.

A sincere demonstration of genuine interest and enthusiasm in whatever the patient undertakes will assist the therapist to inspire faith and confidence in the patient. Suggestions, encouragement and deserved compliments are all helpful approaches toward breaking down the patient's timidity or resistance toward activity. Happy and successful experiences with the arts and crafts may help the patient to reorganize his bewildered and sometimes chaotic thinking. For the patient who is a perfectionist, such a dynamic experience in a friendly environment may help him to become more flexible, spontaneous and better adjusted.

MUSICAL THERAPY

Singing and dancing are probably the oldest arts. From the standpoint of racial development, music as a means of communication probably

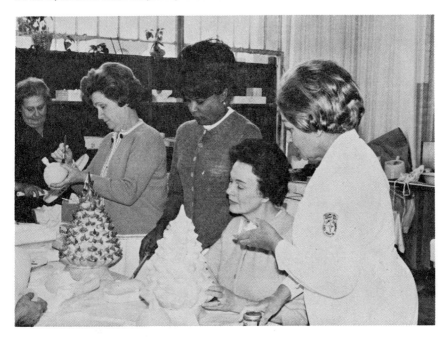

Fig. 5. A class in ceramics making Christmas trees and other articles. (Courtesy of Essex County Overbrook Hospital, Cedar Grove, N. J.)

preceded conversation. When the pattern of the song or dance is fixed in a rhythmical form, there seems to be a sort of contagious compulsion which motivates the observer to imitate the pattern. It is probable that singing and dancing were the strongest factors in bringing group strength, harmony, orderliness and unity into the lives of primitive peoples. With musical accompaniment and chanting, these early inhabitants shared sad, religious or joyful experiences which made them one people. These associations were not on a verbal or spectator level. Primitive peoples actually made the music and dance. It was a part of themselves. Emotions were expressed and shared with others through these media. Music, therefore, was not only a creative expression but an emotional stabilizer—a means of enriching their lives.

Why it is that a group of people engaged in a musical activity seem to be drawn together and function happily with less friction than in many other pursuits almost defies analysis. Lack of competition may be one explanation. The pleasing and soothing effects of music upon humans may be another, as well as the outlet music provides for emotional release.

Musical therapy is rapidly developing as a therapeutic medium in psychiatric hospitals. Patients engage in various forms of musical expres-

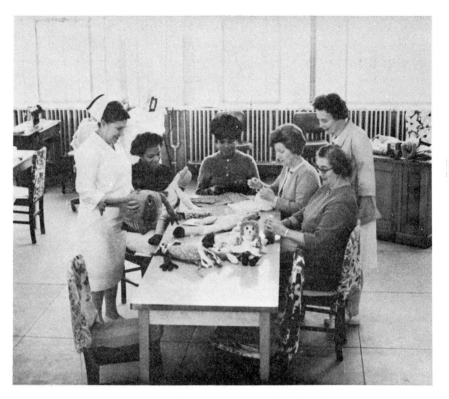

Fig. 6. Making stuffed toys and dolls for the children's party. (Courtesy of Essex County Overbrook Hospital, Cedar Grove, N. J.)

sion according to their interests, needs, and mental and social abilities. Music, in some form, makes it possible for the patient to participate spontaneously with others. As the patient improves, the therapist may introduce musical activities on progressively higher levels. New experiences, however, should not be introduced at the expense of spontaneity and free experimentation in the activity of the patient who is participating.

When introducing musical activities, it is important to bear in mind that most patients in psychiatric hospitals are adults and should be treated accordingly. Although the adult patient may demonstrate childish behavior, children's dances and singing games should be avoided. Rhythms composed of a few simple dance steps accompanied by music considered to be on an adult level should be encouraged. For instance, one should not expect the adult patient to exhibit the glee and merriment of a child and introduce such an activity as singing and dancing to the tune of "Mulberry Bush." Clapping, stamping, and rhythmic movements to the tune of

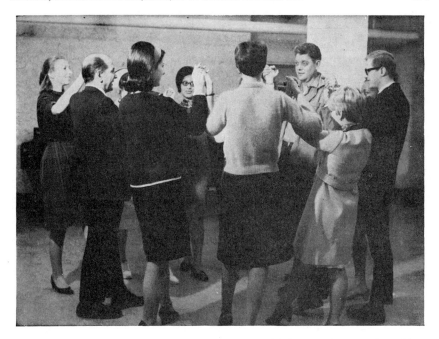

Fig. 7. Dancing promotes togetherness in a group and helps to release tensions. (Essex County Overbrook Hospital, Cedar Grove, N. J.)

"Camptown Races" would be more suitable and would be enjoyed by the adult. The fox trot and waltz may be very pleasurable for many adult patients.

Rhythm bands afford happy musical expression for more regressed patients. Selection of instruments for the band should be based upon a consideration of the patient's age and experiences. Large triangles, bells, tambourines, drums, and cymbals used in dance orchestras are appropriate instruments which may be surprisingly pleasing to listeners who observe obviously very ill patients making music with these simple instruments. Tiny instruments used in children's rhythm bands are not socially acceptable to the adult patient. Patients who are in good contact and capable of extended concentration may play more complex orchestral types of instruments, such as the piano, violin, drums, saxophone, trumpet, and so on. Each patient may have some individual preferences. A survey of the various patients' choice of music helps to alternate preferences and provide enjoyment for all.

Music appreciation may be provided for those patients who are unable to participate actively in musical activities. A variety of selected recordings are always enjoyed by patients. Television and radio programs may be reviewed in advance and particular programs selected according to patient preferences. Perhaps a professional orchestra would welcome suggestions from the patients in the audience.

EDUCATIONAL THERAPY

Generally speaking, the time spent in a psychiatric hospital should be a worthwhile, continuous learning experience for the patient. Incidental knowledges may be subtly achieved through any of the therapeutic activities and the realtionships inherent in group association. More specifically, courses of instruction are planned by qualified teachers for the school-age patient as well as the individual who is desirous of extending his previous education or attaining skill and efficiency in an entirely different field of endeavor. The school-age patient who is in good contact and able to concentrate sufficiently should be encouraged to continue study and complete his formal education. University extension courses are available in many special subjects and more recently have been introduced into psychiatric hospitals for adult patients. To achieve success in a new or university-extended course of instruction, the patient must possess certain background preparation, a genuine interest and the intellectual capacity to succeed. Some supervision and assistance may be required with these higher-level courses of instruction.

Planning for vocational-education experiences should be based upon intelligence quotient and aptitude and interest tests as well as on conferences with the patient. Individuals are endowed with native abilities, and the capacity for achievement in certain vocations may be revealed through scientific testing and assistance. Some of the subjects which may be taught in a psychiatric hospital are as follows:

ELEMENTARY:
   Arithmetic, Geography, History, English, Reading
SECONDARY:
   Mathematics, Sociology, English, Typewriting, Shorthand
ADVANCED INSTRUCTION:
   Business Administration, Hotel Management, Scientific Farming, Salesmanship, Political Science

Of course, this list includes only a few of the many subjects which might be taught to the patient. We recognize that the chief objective of the psychiatric hospital is to help reeducate and rehabilitate the patient so that he may return and successfully live in the community. One of the important avenues of return is educational therapy.

INDUSTRIAL THERAPY

The statement that satisfactory, gainful employment is nature's best medicine and is essential to human happiness is as true today as when it was made by Galen in 172 A.D. Therefore, meaningful, therapeutic employment plays an important part in the treatment of the mentally ill. No better laboratory may be provided than the realistic experiences embodied in active employment where practice opportunities exist. Patients may be employed in certain hospital or community industries, dependent upon their individualistic abilities, degrees of self-sufficiency, and needs for guidance and supervision.

Therapeutic industrial assignments should be prescribed by the patient's doctor. Their value lies in serious consideration and is lost when the assignment is lightly made in terms of providing something for the patient to do to while away time. Job analysis, training, and supervision help to ensure therapeutic results.

An industrial therapist must be aware of the patient's abilities, possible achievement levels, and interests when attempting to secure employment for the patient. Proper orientation, instruction, and guidance must be provided for the patient by those who are guiding, supervising, and observing his adjustment. Patience, understanding of human failings, flexibility, and the ability to encourage and inspire are absolute requisites for those persons who supervise employed patients.

A successful industrial therapy program must be well organized. Working conditions, possible hazards, and physical and psychological effects upon the patient must be anticipated in advance, so that detrimental industrial therapy assignments may be avoided.

BIBLIOTHERAPY

The printed word may be a means of modifying or stimulating the emotions. Reading may help to lift the spirits of the depressed patient, improve the attention span of the individual with limited powers of concentration, educate the student, relieve insomnia, stimulate the imagination, and foster desirable attitudes and ideals in patients.

Modern printing methods have increased the amount of literature available today. Our educational system is so highly developed that practically all persons except the extremely illiterate are able to read and enjoy and enrich their lives through the many books, periodicals and newspapers published. The development of Braille has enabled the blind to enjoy literature, and recorded literature (the talking book) is another means of providing bibliotherapy for those patients who are unable to read.

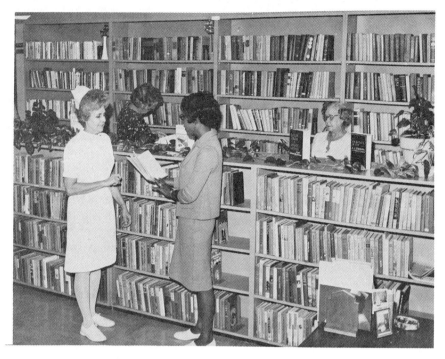

Fig. 8. Bibliotherapy is most successful when the hospital is well stocked with a wide selection of literature. (Courtesy of Arkansas State Hospital, Little Rock, Ark.)

Certain principles are helpful when selecting literature for the mentally ill.

1. Select literature in accordance with the patient's educational preparation, intellectual capacity, and interests.

2. Size up the personality of the patient and attempt to select material which you think may be interesting.

3. Avoid literature of a controversial nature or the type which appears to stir up feelings of distress within the patient. Literature concerning medicine, psychology, psychiatry, politics, and tense murder mysteries may do patients more harm than good. In some hospitals a careful review of all literature is made by a librarian before it is made available to the patients.

4. For educational reading, choose books recommended by reliable authorities. Special subject matter may be referred to the librarian. If the literature is not available in the hospital, it may be possible to secure it through the community library.

5. History, travel, art, science, biography, and literature concerning hobbies are usually interesting subjects for most patients.

To motivate an interest in bibliotherapy one must first arouse the patient's interest. Impromptu discussions frequently stimulate a patient's interest. Sketching the highlights of certain literature may be enough to stimulate the patient's interest to read the particular book or article. Book reviews published in the hospital newspaper help to interest the patients and keep them up to date with desirable current literature; patients frequently assist in publishing these reviews. Literary groups are stimulating because they provide an opportunity for the individual patient's self-expression. In addition, the members of these groups absorb considerable knowledge and frequently exchange worthwhile ideas.

Bibliotherapy is most successful when the hospital is well stocked with a wide selection of literature. Books and magazines should also be plentiful on all of the wards where patients who cannot go to the library are confined. Some system of exchange should be instituted so that the ward library is kept up to date.

It is interesting as well as helpful to observe the types of reading material selected by patients who are allowed free selection. A variety of interests from the romantic fiction to literature concerning the serious, realistic side of life may be detected. Some patients seem to be seeking in literature a knowledge of the past or a better way of life through the written experiences of others. And there are those patients who enjoy literature which fires their imaginations or gives them a lift.

One may also observe differences in the patient's reading habits which may be attributed to his illness. The preoccupied patient may read spasmodically, as if shifting his attention from the literature to himself and to things afar. Others appear to be such fast, avid readers that one feels prompted subtly to discuss the material with the patient to determine just how much has actually been absorbed. Sometimes it is surprising to discover how little or how much has been retained. It is just as possible to discover a patient who has been challenged by the literature and is anxious to discuss certain viewpoints with you.

SUGGESTED REFERENCES

Dreikurs, S.: Art therapy for psychiatric patients. Perspect. Psychiat. Care 7: 102 (May-June), 1969.

Fidler, G., and Fidler, J.: Occupational Therapy. The Macmillan Co., New York, 1963.

Freedman, A., and Kaplan, H.: Comprehensive Textbook of Psychiatry. The Williams & Wilkins Co., Baltimore, 1967, p. 1215.

Knesh, T., et al.: Using community classes for outpatient occupational therapy. Ment. Hosp. 16: 29 (May), 1965.

Roehler, S.: The therapeutic milieu of the art department at the Allan Memorial Institute. J. Psychiat. Nurs. 5: 545 (Nov.—Dec.) 1967.

Wearne, R.: Work therapy programs in psychiatric hospitals. Perspect. Psychiat. Care 5: 141 (May-June), 1967.

CHAPTER 27

Psychotherapeutic Techniques

The psychotherapeutic techniques being used considerably today are individual and group psychotherapy, psychoanalysis, narcotherapy, hypnotherapy, and play therapy. Sometimes one technique is used in conjunction with another; for example, hypnotherapy may be used during individual psychotherapy or during psychoanalysis. The particular techniques selected by the psychiatrist in each instance are dependent upon his clinical judgment as to which will be most effective.

REQUISITE

The most important requisite for success in the use of any technique is the establishment of a favorable rapport between the psychiatrist and the patient. When this occurs, it is much easier for the patient to discuss his difficulties, thereby permitting the physician to gain information concerning the patient's conflicts.

The physician-patient relationship is commonly referred to as a "transference." Dr. Sigmund Freud studied the reaction of the patient toward the physician and described the patient's feelings toward the physician as "emotions felt for other persons in other experiences and now transferred to the physician." He contended that the psychiatrist could analyze the patient's feelings toward him and interpret them with helpful therapeutic effects. In some instances, there is a transfer of negative feelings toward the psychiatrist. When this happens, the patient is usually placed under the treatment of another psychiatrist. Dr. Freud also revealed that a "counter transference" occurred during these relationships, that is, he believed the physician reacted emotionally toward the patient. He advised physicians to study these two aspects of human relationships in order to treat a patient successfully and to avoid the detrimental influence of their own feelings. These theories have been studied and found helpful by physicians in general as well as by those in psychiatric practice. Nurses, too, have recognized the applicability of these theories in nurse-patient relationships. When a positive rapport, or transference, is not achieved between the psychiatrist and patient, it becomes impossible for the physician to gain access to the repressed mental content. The patient does not feel at ease, remains strongly inhibited, and will not freely discuss himself or his illness.

INDICATIONS

It is said that there is not a single psychosis or neurosis in which some form of psychotherapy cannot be employed. The advantageous use of a technique, however, is gauged by the stage or severity of the illness. For example, many persons who are considered mildly ill can be successfully treated during periodic visits to a physician's office or a psychiatric outpatient clinic. These patients manifest good control of their mental faculties and insight into their illnesses. Other mentally ill persons who are completely out of contact and unable to demonstrate logic or reasoning require hospitalization. Psychotherapy cannot be utilized unless there is a sufficient amount of reasoning intact. Therefore, these patients are treated first by other methods. When it is obvious they are in good enough contact to participate in some form of psychotherapy, the method is then employed. The usual primary treatment in such instances is the administration of tranquilizing drugs or one of the somatic therapies, along with an appropriate schedule of rest, recreation, and diet.

PSYCHOTHERAPY AS A SKILL

While the psychiatrist is very much aware that psychotherapy is a skilled technique, accomplished effectively through understanding of the principles of dynamic psychology, there are so called "quacks" and "fakers" attempting to practice psychotherapy who do not possess such understanding or skill. This unfortunate situation has led to serious handicaps and sometimes tragedy for mentally ill persons. Patients who might have been helped have been easy prey for these "mind meddlers" as one prominent physician termed them. Psychotherapy had a crude beginning, partially derived from unscientific sources, such as primitive magical and medical practices, religious rites, mysticism, and common-sense advice of friends and quacks. It has, however, developed gradually along scientific principles through study and research.

ROLE OF NURSE

The nurse assuming a role in a community mental-health program should be aware of the dangers and consequences involved when a person who is on the verge of mental illness is exposed to treatment by incompetent individuals. She should guide the person to a competent psychiatrist for proper assistance.

The nurse who is caring for the patient undergoing psychotherapy can be of assistance to both patient and physician. Her behavior will influence a good or poor rapport between the physician and patient. Her attempts may be directed toward instilling confidence in the patient toward his physician. She will, at the same time, effect in the patient a feeling of confidence toward her. This aids in establishing a necessary feeling of security and faith. When the nurse is in poor rapport with the patient, the relationship tends to aggravate the patient and may make it more difficult for the physician to gain access to the desired information. Should the patient feel secure in the nurse's presence and attempt to seek counsel from her or to discuss his association with the physician, the nurse may listen attentively to the patient but not commit herself to counsel. Such counsel may interfere with the physician's advice. She can, however, relay any pertinent information to the psychiatrist, who will know what approach is best and advise her accordingly.

INDIVIDUAL PSYCHOTHERAPY

Individual psychotherapy, sometimes referred to as "direct-interview psychotherapy," is conducted through interviews or talks between the physician and patient. This type of psychotherapy is the foundation upon which all psychiatric treatment rests.

The patient may seek help from the psychiatrist because he is experiencing discontent, general unhappiness, feelings of anxiety, or frustration. He may be going through an emotional crisis which makes it extremely difficult for him to carry on with a normal, happy life.

This type of psychotherapy does not require the physician to delve into the deep causative forces in the unconscious mind. The patient merely discusses his immediate symptoms with the psychiatrist on a conscious level. Although the psychiatrist may have an understanding of the relationship between the patient's symptoms and unconscious motivation, he does not probe deeply into the unconscious. He may, and very often does, however, arrive at conclusions regarding the relationship between the patient's symptoms and his repressed mental content. The psychiatrist then makes use of this knowledge in alleviating the patient's symptoms. This constitutes the main difference between individual psychotherapy and psychoanalysis: Psychoanalysis requires deep probing of relative unconscious causative factors.

PROCEDURE

During the interviews, the physician's objective is to gain an understanding of the patient's personality and problems. He learns all he can about the patient's early development: his adjustment to family, school, friends, and vocation, and all factors which have contributed to development of the patient's personality and conflictual situation.

The psychiatrist utilizes several techniques while conducting these interviews with the patient. He may find it necessary to desensitize certain incidents in the patient's life which have had a mentally traumatizing effect. It may be necessary for the physician to reassure or encourage a patient who has little faith, hope, or courage about himself or the future. The psychiatrist may recognize certain behavior patterns in the patient which require a change. He may be able to help the patient change his behavior through the use of persuasion and suggestion.

Perhaps the patient's ideas may have to be revised. He may be in need of some type of reeducation or have to be taught to face something he fears. Through such teaching, he will learn that doing the thing he fears is the very treatment he needs. Perhaps he will have to be taught how to maintain stricter control of his impulses so that he will be the master of them. The patient may be in need of guidance and advice in social relationships. A timid person who has always shied away from social activities may have to be shown how to make a success of social relationships. The aggressive person who has experienced rejection from the group may have to be taught how to make a more acceptable approach socially. Permitting the patient to talk freely about himself and anything which is emotionally distressing to him may be utilized by the psychiatrist in these interviews. Purging, or catharsis, of the mind sometimes brings great relief to patients. Any of these techniques may be used separately or together during the course of individual psychotherapy, dependent upon the need, in bringing about successful amelioration of the patient's symptoms and suffering.

INDICATIONS

Individual psychotherapy may be used as a treatment in itself, as a primary step to other psychiatric treatment, or in conjunction with tranquilizing drugs or somatic therapies.

GROUP PSYCHOTHERAPY

Group psychotherapy came into prominence during World War II. The limited number of trained psychiatrists available to administer individual psychotherapy was responsible for the impetus this form of therapy received.

The object of group psychotherapy is to help the patient understand the causes of emotional difficulties and resolve problems associated with living experiences. The method differs from individual psychotherapy because it is an indirect way of helping a person to gain insight into his problematical situation and the resolution of conflict.

PROCEDURE

The groups may vary in number from a few to a great many, but the ideal number is from four to six persons. The psychiatrist interviews each patient individually several times before group association is started. He becomes familiar with each one's history, personality development, and symptoms before forming the group. The members are varied in type: there are the aggressive, leader types, as well as the shy, retiring personalities. The leader types enter more readily into the discussions and gradually lead the more retiring patients toward participation.

These sessions are held regularly once or twice a week for about one hour at a time. During the first meeting, the members may feel uneasy and remain uncommunicative. As the members get to know each other, a feeling of friendship, closeness, and understanding develops among them.

The psychiatrist may choose one of several ways to start these meetings: he may ask each member to introduce himself; he may invite each one to drop an unsigned question into a box for him to answer; or perhaps he may simply discuss the weather, current events, or things in general; anything to get the discussion under way. Another method is that of lecture and case history. The psychiatrist devotes the first one or two sessions to an explanation of the structure of the mind, how primitive drives are repressed, and how conflicts develop between the conscious and unconscious mind. Then he may discuss a patient's case history. This case history may be very similar to the case history of one group member, or he may actually use a history of one member, being very careful to shield the identity of the person involved from the patient himself. He may proceed to tell the group just how this particular patient's conflicts might be solved, or he may ask for solutions from the members.

It is surprising how members in the group may offer suggestions to solve a conflict similar to their own problems and yet be quite unaware of this example's significance. Some of the more retiring persons may listen attentively and be timid about joining in the discussion, but it is obvious that they are deriving help from the group by making quiet, inward applications to their own difficulties.

Once the psychiatrist has the group spirit developed and the discussion well under way, he assumes a more or less passive role. His part, then, is limited to occasional clarifications, suggestions, and guidance. He purposely avoids the spotlight but attempts to encourage free association among the members. Occasionally, he may have to intervene if one or two persons tend to dominate the discussion.

The airing of members' problems helps to release their tensions and anxieties. As the discussions proceed, they learn that people are much the same the world over; experience the same feelings of shame, guilt, and inferiority; and attempt to shroud these feelings in secrecy. By sharing the problems of others, each is able to discover solutions to his own conflicts.

INDICATIONS

Group psychotherapy has not been found to be successful with patients who are extremely depressed, mentally dull, or suffering from disintegrating types of mental illness. The persons participating in group psychotherapy must have enough reasoning and judgment to understand what is being discussed if they are to make applications to their own problems.

PSYCHOANALYSIS

Psychoanalysis is the most widely discussed and least understood of the psychotherapeutic techniques. It has been both glorified and ridiculed in modern literature. Because of this fact, the general public, at large, has a distorted conception and understanding about the application of this method. Many have interpreted it as a cure-all for mental illness.

Psychoanalysis is helpful in the treatment of the neuroses. These disorders have been linked to anxiety associated with repression of early childhood experiences. When these experiences can be brought to the conscious level and analyzed the patient may be helped.

Dr. Sigmund Freud, the founder of this method, is known as the "Father of Psychoanalysis." Dr. Freud, a Viennese neurologist, was treating, by means of hypnosis, a young woman patient suffering with a hysterical paralysis. He discovered that while the patient was under the influence of the hypnotic trance, she recalled incidents in her early life to which she reacted painfully. When she was out of the trance, she could not remember these same painful experiences. In his determination to find some way to help her recall these incidents on a conscious level, Freud developed the method of free association, the basis of psychoanalytic treatment.

PROCEDURE

There are three phases, or stages, of psychoanalytic treatment: free association; interpretation of the patient's symptoms and behavior as related to earlier experiences; and the development of independence by the patient, with a willingness to accept his limitations and face the inevitable frustrations of life.

During the first stage, the patient lies on a couch in a dimly lighted room. The analyst sits behind the patient. This position, though often resented by the patient, is necessary in order to reduce external stimuli. The psychoanalyst encourages the patient to discuss anything and everything that comes into his mind during these sessions. The patient is advised to hold nothing back. Ideas, impressions, feelings, reactions to previous situations, incidents of any nature, dreams, and so on, are all expressed freely by the patient. Throughout these sessions, the analyst makes a careful observation of the patient's emotional reaction toward him. He aims during these periods to achieve a favorable rapport with the patient in order to instill in him a feeling of trust, which is necessary for free association.

The second stage is filled with a charged emotional reaction which changes from a positive to a negative feeling of the patient toward the analyst. When the patient realizes that he must do something about his problems, he leans toward the analyst for guidance, love, and help. As soon as the analyst does not react according to the patient's desires, the patient develops feelings of resistance, and hostility toward the analyst. The physician constantly reviews the patient's behavior and connects his present attitude and actions with his attitudes and behavior toward people in the past, especially those persons whom the analyst has replaced in the patient's mind throughout the course of treatment. All of these facts are interpreted to the patient by the analyst, who attempts to show the patient that he is still reacting to situations as he did in his childhood. The chief objective is to get the patient to reach emotional maturity under the guidance of the analyst.

During the third stage, there is a slow weaning of the patient from the analyst. The patient attempts to achieve independence and solve his conflicts on a mature level.

PREPARATION OF PSYCHOANALYST

Every psychoanalyst must undergo a rigid preparation before he is permitted to practice psychoanalysis. He must be graduated from an accredited medical school and intern in both general and psychiatric hospitals. The analyst must place himself under psychoanalytic treatment. A successful analyst must experience firsthand the feelings of anxiety that first surround free association, the security established in the patient through favorable rapport with the analyst, the defenses the patient will make to justify his actions, the letdown that comes when the analyst rejects the person's desires, the pride of the ego in his determination to become independent and self-reliant, and the relief which comes when the patient's problems are solved.

TIME REQUIRED AND COST

Psychoanalysis is a long, drawn-out, expensive form of treatment. The time involved and the financial requirements are not within the means of the average person. It may require from one to three years or more and cost a few thousand dollars to psychoanalyze a person. Psychoanalysis is not so widely practiced, therefore, as it might be if these two barriers did not exist. However, the basic principles employed with this technique have been incorporated in other forms of psychotherapy widely practiced in the treatment of mentally ill persons.

NARCOTHERAPY

Narcotherapy is also known as "narcosynthesis" and "narcoanalysis." It is the production of a drowsy, yet not an actual sleeplike, state by means of sedative drugs. During this period, the psychiatrist interviews the patient about his problems. He attempts to uncover and analyze emotional conflicts buried in the unconscious mind and not accessible to him when the patient converses on a conscious level. Lay persons often refer to narcotherapy as the administration of "truth serum." Actually this latter term is a misnomer. A determined person who does not want to reveal facts can hold back information while under the influence of the drugs administered.

The technique was first used in 1936 by Dr. J. S. Horsley. During the African campaign of World War II, narcotherapy was used extensively and came into prominence through the efforts of Drs. Roy Grinker and John Spiegel. It is commonly believed that its success at this time was owing to the fact that the disorders being treated involved conflicts of short duration, the result of combat and warfare, and were not too deeply repressed.

The chief value of narcotherapy lies in the ability of the drugs used to relax a previously tense, hardly communicative person to the point where he wants to talk freely about himself, thereby releasing tension and anxiety.

From the economic standpoint, it helps to reduce the time and cost of treatment and conserves the time of psychiatrists who must treat a great number of patients.

The two drugs used extensively are Pentothal Sodium (thiopental sodium) and Amytal Sodium (sodium amobarbital). Many doctors prefer Amytal Sodium because it is very simple to administer. The entire dose can be injected at once, thereby permitting the doctor to move out of the visual range of the patient and conduct the procedure in an analytic type of atmosphere. Pentothal Sodium cannot be injected in one dose. The needle must be left in the vein and small amounts of the drug must be injected at intervals in order to keep the patient relaxed.

PROCEDURE

Before therapy is commenced, the psychiatrist interviews the patient to obtain a history and explain the treatment to him. He encourages the patient to cooperate and tells him the drug will relieve his symptoms and bring about recovery.

The nurse prepares a treatment tray containing an intravenous syringe, a 20-gauge needle, alcohol swabs, a tourniquet, and the prescribed drug. In addition, an ampul of Adrenalin Chloride (epinephrine), 1:1000 solution, a hypodermic syringe and needle, and a tank of oxygen should be on hand to counteract any respiratory difficulties encountered. Atropine sulfate, 0.45 mg. (1/150 grain), is sometimes given subcutaneously beforehand to prevent spasms of the larynx. Benzedrine Sulfate (amphetamine), 10 mg. (1/6 grain), may also be given by mouth just prior to treatment. This reduces the marked effects of drowsiness sometimes observed following the use of Amytal Sodium. When Amytal Sodium is mixed with sterile water, the color of the mixture must be closely observed. If it is not entirely clear, but appears cloudy or brownish in appearance, it should never be used. Another fresh ampul of the drug must be prepared.

The patient lies on a bed in a darkened, quiet room and the tray is brought to the bedside. The doctor may or may not desire the presence of the nurse. Some patients relax more readily in the nurse's presence, while others experience tension with the thought of another person's presence during these interviews.

If Pentothal Sodium is given, the psychiatrist injects the needle and then tells the patient to start counting backwards from one hundred. As soon as the patient's counting becomes confused, it is obvious that he is relaxed, and the doctor proceeds to interview him. When Amytal Sodium is used, the patient appears generally relaxed and drowsy in a few minutes and may begin to talk spontaneously. The psychiatrist listens to the patient's revelations. He interrupts the patient now and then to ask questions which will clarify some of the statements made by the patient. The patient's reaction, in general, is very much like that of a person who has ingested alcohol: he feels very warm, friendly, talkative, and wants to share his experiences. When the effects of the drug appear to have worn off, the doctor may terminate the interview, or he may begin to discuss, on a conscious level, the material that the patient has revealed.

When the patient is hospitalized, the treatments may be administered two or three times a week, or oftener, until a desirable result is achieved. In outpatient clinics or doctors' offices, the patient usually returns for a second interview on the second day; the third session is usually conducted on the fourth day; and the patient may return for an interview at the end of the first or second week.

The nurse must closely observe these patients directly following treatment to detect any signs of respiratory difficulty. If the interview is not continued on a conscious level, the patient may fall asleep. He should be watched to make certain that he does not fall out of bed and injure himself.

Some very significant changes in the patient's behavior may be noted and should be recorded by the nurse. A person who has been unresponsive may begin to talk more freely and engage in contact with others. A disinterested patient may show interest in his surroundings and enjoyment in regular activities. There may be an increase in the patient's appetite and marked disappearance of apprehension and fear.

INDICATIONS

Narcotherapy has been found particularly helpful in treating certain types of hysteria and anxiety states. It is not believed to be helpful in treating deep-rooted neuroses or psychoses which have been in progress for a long time.

HYPNOTHERAPY

Hypnotherapy is as old as the sages. The ancient Egyptians, Hindus, and Persians practiced the divine trance. It is believed that the supernatural healing powers claimed by these peoples were actually achieved through the suggestive powers of hypnosis. The so-called "healing temples" of the ancients became popular and spread through Greece and Asia Minor. With the coming of Christianity, hypnotherapy was considered to be a form of witchcraft. Those who practiced it did so only in secrecy for fear of church reprisals.

During the eighteenth century Franz Anton Mesmer made the first attempt to bring hypnotherapy within the realm of science. A group of his followers, known as the "mesmerists," carried this technique into England and France. At the Salpêtrière Clinic in France, Jean Martin Charcot, neurologist, revealed some interesting studies and results on 12 patients treated by means of hypnosis. Within recent years, there has been a reawakening of interest in hypnotherapy by present-day psychiatrists.

PROCEDURE

Hypnotherapy is a technique wherein the psychiatrist induces a marked state of relaxation in the patient. Sometimes the patient appears to be in a sleeplike state. He is very prone to suggestion, answering the physician's questions freely or reenacting deep, emotional, painful, earlier experiences difficult to recall on a conscious level.

Before the physician makes use of hypnotherapy, he attempts to establish a good prehypnotic state in the patient. He discusses the technique with the patient in order to learn how much the patient knows about the procedure and how he feels about the treatment. He assures the patient that he will not lose consciousness at any time, that he will simply feel very sleepy and unable to move about freely or open his eyes. He further reassures him by telling him that he will not be forced to say or do anything humiliating, and that he will not be exposed as a weakling or run the risk of remaining in a hypnotic state forever. The psychiatrist encourages the patient to relax and attempt to concentrate as fully as possible with him in order to achieve the best results.

To induce a hypnotic state, the physician directs the patient to fix his attention on some illuminated object, such as a ring or a light. He repeatedly says to the patient in a soothing voice, "You are relaxing. You are beginning to feel very sleepy. Soon you will be asleep," and words to this effect. When the patient is completely relaxed and in a sleeplike state, the psychiatrist begins to carry on a conversation with him. He may be able to get the patient to talk about things he could not discuss during a direct interview, or he may strongly suggest the disappearance of symptoms, such as pain, headache, or paralysis of some part of the body. Sometimes the patient is given a light sedative drug about an hour before the hypnotic session in order to make him more calm and relaxed.

Although it is agreed that significant changes take place during a hypnotic session, it has never been decided whether the technique is just an altered state of consciousness, a highly charged, emotional relationship between two persons, or the combination of both.

One of the chief difficulties in employing this method is that there are some patients who fear the technique. Some believe they will be forced to do things they do not want to do while in the hypnotic state; others fear that the psychiatrist will be unable to take them out of the trance.

INDICATIONS

It is generally agreed that this method is most effective in treating patients having hysteria. Most authorities believe that a paranoid type of personality should not be hypnotized because this type of person commonly has the belief that he is under the influence of another person, and some medical authorities believe the technique might stimulate a latent paranoid trend, which might develop into a full-blown psychosis.

PLAY THERAPY

Play therapy is used in the treatment of children suffering from maladjustment or behavior disorders.

The average adult can discuss an inner conflict quite intelligently with a psychiatrist, but the child lacks the education, experience, insight, and judgment necessary to accomplish this act. The object of play therapy, therefore, is to discover the causes of the child's conflicts through observation of his play and to interpret it to the child in language which the child understands. Through play, the psychiatrist, especially trained in this technique, may discover a need to counsel the child's parents and others who have an influence on his behavior. Most frequently it is necessary to treat not only the child, but also other persons who may be able to alter the troublesome environmental situations which may be the root of the child's conflicts.

Anyone who has observed children playing is aware that they often imitate their parents, sisters, brothers, teachers, friends, and other persons. Children reconstruct past experiences in their play and carry out action which they would like to express in real life but may be fearful of doing because of the possibility of punishment. Perhaps the child holds back action he would like to take in a real situation because he senses his inferiority in size to the adult. He does not feel this restraint in play, and it is a means of releasing his tensions and anxieties.

PROCEDURE

A special room, equipped with play materials, is necessary for play therapy. Sand, water, clay, pencils, charcoal, chalk, crayons, paper, and figures of men, women, children, and animals are essential materials.

The psychiatrist brings the child into the room and invites him to make use of the materials, or the child may instinctively turn to them upon sight. The psychiatrist closely observes the child's behavior. Sometimes he enters actively into play with the child by moving some of the figures about, introducing new persons, or removing certain ones in order to observe the child's reactions. There may be times when the child's actions will cause the psychiatrist to question him as to why he has behaved as observed. The child's behavior may reveal his desires, likes and dislikes, fears, frustrations, resentment toward others, feelings of inferiority, and so on. One child, during play therapy, acted out a scene between two adults, a male and female. The male staggered into the room and began to beat up the female figure. Finally, the boy pushed the male figure over and sat the female figure down in a chair. When the psychiatrist asked him why he had done this, the child said, "That's the way my father does when he comes home drunk." The boy had released his tensions by pushing over the father figure, though the psychiatrist knew that in the real-life situation, he had never dared to do this; in reality, however, the child had a strong desire to carry out this sort of action. This helped the psychiatrist to understand the child's difficulties. It was obvious that the home situation was the causative factor and in need of investigation and remedy.

INDICATIONS

Play therapy has proved valuable in helping the psychiatrist establish rapport with the child and serves as a means of establishing communication between the psychiatrist and child. This form of psychotherapy is a path of investigation by which a wealth of information can be obtained about the child and his environment. It must be stressed, however, that in addition to these sessions, the psychiatrist works closely with a prepared psychiatric social worker. The social worker visits the child's home and school and plays an important part in helping the persons she contacts to understand the child's difficulties and to assist them to make the environment to which the child must return free from previous conflicting factors.

This form of therapy has also been used with small groups of children in child-guidance clinics when it has been necessary to observe the behavior of some children in group association.

SUGGESTED REFERENCES

Bellak, L., and Small, L.: Emergency Psychotherapy and Brief Psychotherapy. Grune & Stratton, New York, 1965.
Bueker, K., and Warrick, A.: Can nurses be group therapists? Am. J. Nurs. 64: 114 (May), 1964.
Coe, W., Curry, A., and Huels, M.: A method of group therapy training for nurses in psychiatric hospitals. Perspect. Psychiat. Care 5: 231 (Sept.-Oct.), 1967.

Cohen, R.: EST and group therapy give improved care. Am. J. Nurs. 71: 1195 (June), 1971.

Donelson, L.: The nurse as a sanctioned representative of the healing arts. Perspect. Psychiat. Care 5: 214 (Sept.-Oct.), 1967.

Eisenberg, J., and Abbott, R.: The monopolizing patient in group therapy. Perspect. Psychiat. Care 6: 66 (Mar.-Apr.), 1968.

Farberow, N.: Taboo Topics. Atherton Press, New York, 1966.

Hedman, L.: More than custodial care. Experiences in group therapy in five state mental institutions. Perspect. Psychiat. Care 4: 22, 1966.

Hyde, N.: Play therapy—the troubled child's self-encounter. Am. J. Nurs. 71: 1366 (July), 1971.

Reres, M., Sack, D., et al.: Individual psychotherapy by nurses. Nurs. Outlook 13: 63 (July), 1965.

Suarez, R.: The silent patient in group therapy. J. Psychiat. Nurs. 8: 10 (Jul.-Aug.), 1970.

Werner, J.: Relating group theory to nursing practice. Perspect. Psychiat. Care 8: 248 (Nov.-Dec.), 1970.

CHAPTER **28**

Family Therapy

GEORGE OSTER, M.S.W., A.C.S.W.
Psychiatric Social Worker and Family Therapist
Department of Psychiatry, Swedish-American Hospital
Rockford, Illinois

WHAT IS FAMILY THERAPY?

Family therapy is a psychotherapeutic technique in which the therapist focuses on the behavior of the entire family as a system instead of focusing on the pathology of one individual. The aim is to try to help them to understand and find new ways of coping with problems within the family system. My own observation is that frequently families who are in serious difficulty are utilizing very infantile methods of trying to cope with problems. Today we recognize that there are many systems in our society that affect human behavior. However, the family still appears to be the primary system influencing that behavior. Therefore, any therapeutic effort made to assist psychiatric patients should involve the family.

For many years the author has been presenting lectures to nursing and medical students relevant to social work and the impact of the environment on a patient. It is important to consider the effect of environmental influences upon psychiatric as well as general medical patients. Social workers have long been concerned about the effect of the environment and have developed many techniques for modifying environmental stresses on patients. Because they possessed these skills, social workers were brought into general medicine and psychiatric treatment teams.

IMPLICATIONS FOR NURSING

Medical science, including psychiatry and general medicine, recognizes the importance of understanding the patient and his relationship to his family. Thus, the physician and nurse will enhance their understanding of the patient through better understanding of the individual's family. Because nurses are taking the responsibility for the 24-hour care of patients, it is the nursing staff to whom the family frequently turns in times of stress and anxiety. It is the purpose of this chapter to deal primarily with family therapy as provided within the framework of a psychiatric setting. However, it is the author's belief that nurses need to understand and relate to families not only in psychiatric but also general medical settings. A warm responsive nurse can provide immeasurable support to an anxious family.

Dorothy B. Anderson, R.N., points out that nurses are skilled observers and have ample opportunities to meet the families of their patients. However, she also remarks that nurses generally fail to make the most of these contacts. They often tend to underestimate their abilities as well as their influence on families.[1] As part of her education the nursing student needs to be made aware of the importance of her role in relating to and understanding not only her patient, but her patient's family. Perhaps as nursing students become involved in family therapy sessions during their psychiatric affiliation they will gradually feel more comfortable in relating to families in general medical settings. It is my hope that all nursing students will eventually be given opportunities to participate as observers in family therapy during their psychiatric experience in order to relate better to patient's families.

HISTORY OF FAMILY THERAPY

Because of their concern with the influence of the environment on a patient, social workers have traditionally been involved in working with families. However, it is interesting that while social workers were prepared to deal with family problems they nevertheless followed the psychoanalytic model in terms of a one-to-one relationship with their patients. Historically, it appears that all psychotherapists, including psychiatrists, psychologists, and social workers, were pretty much bound to the one-to-one type of relationship approach in psychotherapy. In the early 1940s psychiatry recognized the importance of the influence of the family on the patient. Social workers were employed on the treatment team to provide therapy for the patient's family.

The early child guidance movement in this country recognized the importance of the family as it related to psychopathology in the child. They did involve the parents in treatment, but it was always on a one-to-one type of therapy basis. In the child guidance clinics the child was usually seen by

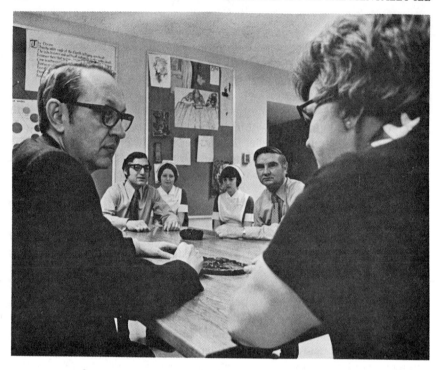

Fig. 1.   A family therapy session. (Courtesy of Swedish-American Hospital, Rockford, Ill.)

the psychiatrist. The social worker assisted by interviewing the parents to obtain the social history and to evaluate family relationships. Following the diagnostic study, the social worker continued to see the parents individually if therapy appeared to be indicated for them. Thus, psychoanalytic theory was probably largely responsible for most therapists continuing to practice the one-to-one type of therapeutic relationship. Psychotherapy, based on the psychoanalytic theory of behavior, focused primarily on the intrapsychic conflicts of the patient. Treatment was carried out in psychotherapy through the development of a relationship between the patient and his therapist. This type of treatment was based on a very personal therapist-patient relationship whereby family members were excluded completely. A step in the direction of involving families in therapy was made when social workers were brought in to work with the families. Up to this time, the therapist-patient relationship was held to be inviolable. Therapists were concerned that any contact with the patient's family would break down this relationship. The technique of treating a patient according to an approach based on the psychoanalytic model involved the development of a transference relationship between the patient and his therapist. Through the transference approach the patient was expected to develop insight into and modify his behavior. Much time was spent with patients exploring their early relationships with parental figures. At no point was any consideration given to having the parental figures involved in therapy for the purpose of providing an opportunity to observe the live family relationship that existed. Much of the material dealt with in the traditional one-to-one psychotherapy involved a great deal of historical material concerning the patient's early relationships. With the advent of family therapy whereby all family members were present, this suddenly became a live therapeutic situation in which the therapist could observe the intensity of the relationship between the patient and his family. When the patient presents material in the family's presence, the situation becomes more emotionally charged for the patient. For the therapist it becomes more meaningful in terms of analyzing what is going on and planning therapeutic approaches.

With the tremendous influence of the psychoanalytic theory of personality development during the 1940s and 1950s, it is understandable that most therapists had a great deal of difficulty in breaking from this model. Most of them were aware of the effect of the family relationships upon a patient. However, they were very resistant toward moving into an active form of therapy that would directly involve the family with the patient. In the early 1950s some of the pioneers in family therapy began to experiment with this method of treatment. As their experiences increased, they soon observed that things happened when patients and families were present that had not been seen during individual psychotherapy. It became obvious that it was impossible to gain the insights into an individual's behavior during a one-to-one relationship that were made possible by observing the individual's behavior in relation to the behavior patterns of his family. One of the earliest pioneers in family therapy was Dr. John Bell.[2] His efforts to involve the family in treatment resulted in observing the phenomenon of resistance used by the family to avoid looking within itself as a causative system, but wanting instead to focus on the identified patient. This initial resistance is frequently encountered by therapists in statements made by the family such as, "He is the patient, why involve us?" or "He has the problem, the rest of us are fine." It is believed that the identified patient serves as a defense for the rest of the family. As long as treatment remains focused on the patient the family avoids looking at itself for pathology.

Another important and basic research study involving the relationship between mental illness and family dynamics was done at the National Institute of Mental Health in Bethesda, Maryland under the direction of Dr. L. Murray Bowen.[3] In this project five families were hospitalized in the institute with the patients and studied closely to observe the interpersonal behavior of families of schizophrenic patients. This study revealed that a problem of faulty communications existed in the families of schizophrenic patients. A double message or double bind type of communication was identified. For example, a parent might profess to the patient that the parent wanted him to become independent, while, at the same time, in various verbal and non-verbal ways, encouraging continuance of the patient's dependency upon the parent. This phenomenon is often observed by family therapists while working with schizophrenic patients and their families.

Another important research group was formed in Palo Alto, California under the direction of the late Dr. Don Jackson. Much of this group's work also focused on the problem of faulty communications within the family of schizophrenic patients. It was theorized that after years of exposure to distorted and double bind type of communications in these families that the children became very confused and automatically accepted distorted communications as normal. Therefore, it was recognized that there was a need during therapy to direct efforts into changing the communication systems within these families.

Other notable studies in family therapy were conducted by Nathan Ackerman, a psychiatrist, and Virginia Satir, a psychiatric social worker.[4,5]

WHAT COMPRISES THE FAMILY?

There are differences of opinion among various therapists concerning who must be involved when we mention family therapy. We generally refer to the nuclear family as comprising the father, mother, and children. The nuclear family would also include any significant relatives living in the same household. Beyond this, we refer to what is called the extended family. The extended family could include significant relatives and friends, such as grandparents, aunts, uncles, very close family friends. It is essential, at least as part of the diagnostic understanding of the family, to try to see the entire nuclear family in the early sessions. Questions are frequently raised about what to do if the family refuses to come. From my viewpoint, whether or not the family cooperates in coming to therapy sessions depends on how convinced the therapist is that it is important to see the entire family. Personally, it is my belief that if the therapist is convinced of the importance of seeing the entire family that he will convey it to the family and they will accept this as the structure for therapy. After the initial diagnostic sessions which may comprise from one to three meetings with a family, it then becomes an individual matter for the therapist to determine how he is going to proceed with the family. My own experience has been to use a great deal of flexibility in this respect. At one time I may meet with the extended family and then set up a subsequent meeting with the parents and children present. In other stages of therapy I may see just the children or the parents.

WHO DOES FAMILY THERAPY?

Family therapy today is being practiced primarily by individuals who have had experience in conducting individual psychotherapy and have come from the professions of psychiatry, psychology, and social work. Most therapists practicing this type of therapy have recognized the importance of moving into the family approach toward psychotherapy. In the United States we are in the early stages of setting up formal training centers for the practice of family therapy. There is a great deal of literature on family therapy. Most therapists have gone into this technique on the basis of their reading and actually trying their own techniques of therapy. Sometimes there are opportunities to learn the technique of family therapy by working as co-therapist with other experienced therapists. In order to do family therapy, however, a person should have a solid base from which to work in terms of a theory of personality development. There should be a definite orientation to one of the basic schools of psychology regarding personality. While family therapy does focus on the present interaction within the family, the therapist does necessarily have to be working within some theoretical concepts of human development and behavior. Opportunities are also becoming available for psychiatric nurses to become involved in family therapy.

USE OF CO-THERAPISTS

Whenever possible, family therapy should be conducted by co-therapists. Because of the complexities of family relationships, it is extremely difficult for one therapist to handle successfully the variety of interactions taking place during family therapy. There are times when the therapists need the mutual support of each other because of the tendency of a family to close ranks against a therapist. During individual therapy the transference and counter-transference problem is more easily dealt with than in family therapy. In family therapy, the problem of counter-transference on the part of the therapist may sometimes become extremely complicated. Therefore, co-therapists are in a position to discuss and interpret the counter-transference problems for each other. Another useful technique that can be used by co-therapists is that of discussion between them concerning their diagnostic impressions and their areas of agreement and disagreement in the presence of the family. The manner in which co-therapists can disagree and work their disagreements through becomes a model for the disturbed family that has been unable to cope with individual expressions and disagreements within the family system.

TECHNIQUES OF FAMILY THERAPY

Many of the techniques of conducting family therapy are so intricate and subtle that the best way for a therapist to learn the techniques is through actual clinical experience under the supervision of another therapist. The family therapist enters into therapy in a very direct and personal way with the family. This is quite different from the non-directive type of individual psychotherapy where the therapist is relatively uninvolved with his patient. With family therapy the therapist becomes very actively involved. Because much of the therapy focuses on actual behavior as it is occurring, the therapist must begin to observe and pick up cues from the interactions as soon as the family starts to enter the room. The family therapist needs to be skilled in dealing with verbal communications as well as the many subtle non-verbal communications that go on within families. The therapist who is perceptive to the non-verbal cues has a very powerful tool with which to move into some of the interactions within the family. The manner in which the family seats themselves will frequently indicate something about the relationships. The following case illustrates how a therapist might move into a non-verbal situation interview. How this developed into expanded areas of interaction within the family of a girl who was in the midst of trying to emancipate herself from the family is shown.

The patient was 18 years old. During the early interviews it appeared that there was a very intense relationship between the patient and her father who seemed to feel very threatened and disturbed by his daughter's efforts toward emancipation. When the family came in for this session the patient sat beside her mother. The father sat at the opposite end of the table with a ten year old sister of the patient who was very well groomed and attractive. During the interview the sister would lean her head on daddy's shoulder and daddy would respond with a great affection. As the interview progressed a great deal of hostility was being expressed between the patient and her father. At this point the therapist commented on the younger sister's warm relationship with her father and asked what the patient had been like at that age. The whole tenor of the patient's relationship with her father seemed to change. The father began to talk very warmly about the patient when she was a little girl. It was apparent that the patient and her father had enjoyed a very close relationship prior to the onset of her adolescence. They then began to communicate more openly and were able to talk about the closeness they had felt for each other. Together they began to explore when the difficulties in the relationship started. From this discussion we moved into establishing that the problems began when the patient became interested in boys. This, of course, opened up the oedipal relationship of the patient and father.

Probably the most important technique used in family therapy is confrontation. Confrontation by the therapist means that the therapist confronts the family in a very direct manner with his observations of their behavior. In utilizing the technique of confrontation the therapist must be aware of his own motives in order to prevent using confrontation in a hostile, attacking manner. A soft benign approach is far more productive. When the therapist observes non-verbal communications occurring in the family he should move in very directly with confrontation. The therapist should learn to observe closely eye contact or lack of eye contact between family members. This can be highly significant in their relationship. The therapist should comment directly on what he observes. Other non-verbal communications can include various types of gesturing, grimacing, and sighing.

Initially, the therapist has to deal with the resistances of the family to looking at the behavior of the entire family. Usually, the early sessions of therapy involve a great deal of discussion about the identified patient and his behavior. During this phase the family will frequently talk directly to the therapist instead of talking to each other. This is something that the therapist needs to interpret to them. In the early sessions family members want to spend a great deal of time discussing past behavior and the effect of outside influences upon the patient. However, it is important for the therapist to remember that we are trying to help the family to begin to look at itself as a system for the causes of the pathological behavior. By having the entire family present the therapist is helped in verifying and reinforcing his impressions. This is a very powerful tool which we do not have in individual psychotherapy.

A technique about which there is some difference of opinion is the history-taking procedure. Satir, one of the early pioneers in family therapy, believes the detailed history is very important. Other family therapists do not see the necessity of getting the family history first. Many times the historical data come to light through observing the present behavior of the family and its development into a presentation of the history by them. The advantage of having the historical data is that it allows the therapist to use more of his own framework associations during therapy.

The use of confrontation concerning the oedipal situation is another family therapy technique. In many families where we are dealing with acting out adolescent adjustment problems we eventually have to utilize the oedipal confrontation. This involves the so called family triangle in which there is usually a very hostile intense relationship between a child and the parent of the opposite sex. The outward behavior that we observe usually involves a tremendous amount of hostility directed towards each other. This is a defense against the underlying strong feelings of affection which they have for each other. The oedipal problem seems to become more intensified in families in which the relationship between the parents is an unstable one. We more or less need to have a realignment take place within the family along the lines of a strengthened husband-wife relationship. Many severe adolescent acting out behavior disorders make a significant improvement when they are confronted with their relationship to the parent of the opposite sex. Preferably, this should take place through some type of visible behavior on the part of the parents with the child present. Frequently, the adolescent becomes less anxious and less vulnerable to acting out behavior when the relationship between the parents is firmly established for him through family therapy. An example of this occurred in a case involving a 16-year-old boy who was seen with his father and mother for family therapy. At first, the boy was behaving in a tyrannical manner towards his mother and attempting to force a divorce between the parents. Underlying this was the oedipal conflict in which he hoped to see the parents divorced and then have mother to himself. The belligerence expressed toward the mother was a defense against his incestuous feelings toward her. The turning point in this case occurred after considerable work with the parents and their relationship. In a very direct manner the father informed the son that this was his wife, that he loved her and that the son was not about to disrupt this marital relationship. Following this confrontation there was a marked improvement in his relationship with his mother.

INDICATIONS OF PROGRESS IN FAMILY THERAPY

During the initial stages of family therapy there exists a very intense relationship between the family members. Initially, little or no humor is observed in their relationships. All of the discussions between them are of an intensity that gives the impression that their very existence is being threatened by each other. One of the signs of progress in family therapy is when we begin to see a lessening of the intensity in the relationships and an appearance of humor. To present a model to the family that problem solving can be done in a less intense manner, the therapist can interject a bit of humor during a therapy session. One of the definite goals of family therapy is to reduce the intensity of the relationships between family members. Another indication of progress is when the family members begin to show some insight into how their behavior is affecting each other. It is difficult to predict when these changes are going to occur. I have had families come to therapy after many sessions of very intense hostility and suddenly begin to talk to each other in a softer, less intense manner. When this stage has been reached the family then seems more comfortable in expressing their viewpoints with each other. A mutual respect seems to be developing among them.

If family therapy is proceeding well it has been my experience to observe the following pattern. Initially, the family begins by focusing on the problems of the patient and blaming outside influences on the individual's difficulties. Gradually, a shift occurs in which they talk less about the identified patient and begin to focus on the interactional behavior of the siblings. The last and most significant stage of family therapy is when the focus starts to shift to the parental relationship. As we begin to explore this relationship the core of the family pathology seems to emerge. At this point the entire family may agree to the parents' continuing in conjoint therapy.

WHAT TYPES OF CASES RESPOND TO FAMILY THERAPY?

There is probably no diagnostic category for which family therapy might not be indicated at certain stages of the treatment program. Although we do not utilize family therapy when the patient is in a severe psychotic depressive state, we do begin to use it when the patient's condition starts to improve. Family therapy appears to be extremely helpful in treating the adjustment problems of children and adolescents. Severe sociopathic character disorders are probably the least likely to be helped. There are differences of opinion among therapists concerning the types of illnesses that are not likely to respond to family therapy. I believe that the technique can be helpful in most cases.

Family therapy, as a technique, is not a panacea and should not be thought of as a replacement for other methods of treatment. It is, however, a very powerful therapeutic method used in conjunction with other psychiatric treatment approaches.

SUGGESTED REFERENCES

Ackerman, N.: The Psychodynamics of Family Life. Basic Books, New York, 1958.

Anderson, D.: Nursing therapy with families. Perspect. Psychiat. Care 7: 21 (Jan.-Feb.), 1969.

Bell, J.: Family Group Therapy. Public Health Monograph #64, U.S. Department of Health, Education, and Welfare, 1961.

Bulbulyan, A.: The psychiatric nurse as family therapist. Perspect. Psychiat. Care 7: 58 (Mar.-Apr.), 1969.

Fagin, C.: Family-Centered Nursing in Community Psychiatry. F. A. Davis Co., Philadelphia, 1970.

Jackson, D. (Ed.): The Etiology of Schizophrenia. Basic Books, New York, 1960.

Jackson, D., and Weakland, J.: Schizophrenic symptoms and family interaction. Archives of General Psychiatry, 1959.

Ostendorf, M.: The public health nurse's role in helping a family to cope with mental health problems. Perspect. Psychiat. Care 5: 208 (Sept.-Oct.), 1967.

Satir, V.: Conjoint Family Therapy. Science and Behavior Books, Palo Alto, Calif., 1964.

Smith, L., and Mills, B.: Intervention techniques and unhealthy family patterns. Perspect. Psychiat. Care 7: 112 (May-June), 1969.

Smoyak, S.: Threat ... a recurring family dynamic. Perspect. Psychiat. Care 7: 267 (May-June), 1969.

Tanner, L.: Family-oriented health care: Is the interdisciplinary health team necessary? Perspect. Psychiat. Care 9: 18 (May-June), 1971.

FOOTNOTES

1. Anderson, D.: Nursing Therapy with Families. Perspect. Psychiat. Care 7: 21 (Jan.-Feb.), 1969.
2. Bell, J.: Family Group Therapy. Public Health Monograph #64, U. S. Department of Health, Education, and Welfare, 1961.
3. Bowen, M.: A family concept of schizophrenia, in Jackson, D. (ed.): The Etiology of Schizophrenia. Basic Books, New York, 1960.
4. Ackerman, N.: The Psychodynamics of Family Life. Basic Books, New York, 1958.
5. Jackson, D., and Weakland, J.: Schizophrenic Symptoms and Family Interaction. Archives of General Psychiatry, 1959.

CHAPTER **29**

Therapy with Tranquilizing and Antidepressant Drugs

Tranquilizing and antidepressant drugs are being used extensively in the treatment of mentally ill patients. Owing to their efficacy, the drugs have largely replaced the physical treatments, such as hydrotherapy, electroshock treatment, and insulin therapy, and the frequency of their use is increasing steadily.

The drugs are not considered cure-alls for mental illness. It is recognized that they help considerably in relieving patients' immediate behavior symptoms (overactivity, underactivity) as well as the distressing feelings of anxiety, fear, insecurity, hostility, depression, worry, fatigue, and the like. This often enables the attending physician to explore with the patient the less obvious, but very important, conflictual emotional aspects associated with the patient's illness.

EFFECTS UPON TREATMENT APPROACHES

Drug therapy has been influential in changing the social structure and organization of hospital wards as well as in reducing the length of illness and hospitalization for many patients. In many instances, patients taking the new drugs are helped to assume more responsibility for their own care and activities in open wards. A considerable number of persons are treated on an outpatient basis in physicians' offices and in hospital and community clinics. In some instances, patients, if treated early enough, are helped sufficiently to enable them to remain at home in the community and engage in their occupations. In other situations, patients may be released earlier from the hospital than was possible formerly, to continue medication at home. Arrangements are made before discharge for the patient to return to the hospital or a community mental-health clinic for observation

361

during the continued treatment period. In some communities, public health nurses visit discharged patients in their homes to observe their progress and reactions to continued medication. Being able to live in the family and community environment is often beneficial for the patient. Contacts with relatives and friends are maintained and these relationships can be emotionally supportive. This is especially true if family members have been instructed by medical personnel concerning their reaction to the patient. All of these newer developments are considered social as well as economic advances in the care and treatment of the mentally ill.

EFFECTS UPON NURSING CARE *interpersonal communication + social skills.*

Tranquilizing and antidepressant drugs have made patients more accessible to nursing personnel, while also making nursing personnel more accessible to patients. The former physical demands of nursing care have been reduced, and nurses have more time to socialize and work with patients. Opportunities for improving nursing care which never before seemed possible are now available. The new drugs highlight the need for nursing personnel to develop competency in interpersonal communication and social skills if patients are to benefit to the fullest degree from therapeutic agents. Nurses should be especially alert to note and report side reactions which may develop following administration of the drugs.

TRANQUILIZING DRUGS

Generally speaking, when effective, tranquilizing drugs produce a state of calm and sense of well-being in patients suffering from emotional and mental disorders. Agitation is reduced, and overactive mentally ill patients become increasingly quieter and more rational in their thinking and behavior as well as more accessible to treatment. Selective tranquilizing medications slow heart action, lower blood pressure, and are effective in relieving a number of somatic conditions which may or may not be accompanied by emotional distress. The clinical behavior state of the patient is more important than diagnostic classification in selecting a tranquilizing drug for treatment.

Dosages

Dosages are adjusted according to the severity of the condition being treated, the route of administration, and the response of the individual patient. The dosage prescribed for emotionally disturbed and mentally ill patients is usually larger than the dosage required for the treatment of somatic conditions and medical disorders, such as nausea, vomiting, hypertension, postoperative pain, and others.

Preparations Available

Tranquilizing drugs are available in various types of preparations. Oral tablets, syrups, concentrates, long-acting Spansules, injectable solutions for intramuscular and intravenous administration, and rectal suppositories are obtainable.

Administration of Injectable Solutions

Intramuscular injections should be given with the patient lying down and remaining so for at least one-half hour after the injection owing to the possibility of hypotensive effects which may cause the patient to feel faint and dizzy. It is good to observe the patient for a period of one hour. The injection site should be massaged to reduce irritating effects which may develop. Extreme care should be taken to avoid accidental injection of the undiluted solution into a vein. These drugs should not be mixed in a syringe with other medications. Solutions should be protected from light because exposure may cause discoloration and alter the potency of the drug.

Side Effects

Some side effects may be mild and transitory. Remedial treatment may or may not be required, dependent upon the reaction and its persistence. During the early period of treatment, when the dosage is being regulated and the patient is becoming adjusted to the medication, side effects may occur and subside within a relatively short period of time. Lassitude and drowsiness, nasal stuffiness or congestion, dizziness, anorexia, headache, nausea, urinary retention, constipation, diarrhea, blurred vision, dilatation or constriction of the pupils, rashes, and other effects should be reported when observed.

More severe side effects occur infrequently but are possible. Their appearance is an indication that the drug should be discontinued or the dosage reduced. Urinalysis, blood studies, renal and liver function tests, other laboratory examinations, and remedial treatment may be required. The appearance of serious side effects should be reported immediately, and the drug should not be continued without a doctor's order. To prevent the development of more serious side effects, most hospitals check the blood pressure of patients taking tranquilizers and antidepressant drugs daily.

Blood studies and urinalysis are also done routinely at periodic intervals to detect blood dyscrasias and blood cell changes.

Agranulocytosis is a rare, but possible and most serious, adverse reaction. Nursing personnel should watch for and report signs of mouth infection, complaints of sore throat, and other symptoms of infection which may be early indications of developing agranulocytosis. Leukocyte and differential blood counts should be done. Significant white blood cell changes are indications to discontinue the drug. Antibiotic therapy is started immediately.

Jaundice is another serious side effect. Urinalysis, to detect the presence of bile, and liver function tests may indicate that the drug should be discontinued.

Extrapyramidal symptoms (Parkinson-like tremors) may indicate that the drug be discontinued, the dosage reduced, and an antiparkinsonian medication be prescribed for the patient.

Significant lowering of blood pressure may warrant discontinuance of the prescribed tranquilizer. If a hypotensive reaction occurs, the patient should be placed in a recumbent position in bed with the head lowered and the legs elevated. The blood pressure should be checked and the physician notified. A stimulant drug (usually Levophed [levarterenol bitartrate] or Neo-Synephrine Hydrochloride [phenylephrine]) may have to be given to raise the patient's blood pressure.

Patients taking phenothiazine derivative tranquilizers should be protected from exposure to the sun, because they may develop photosensitivity, a skin rash which resembles a sunburn.

Contraindications

Owing to their potentiating effects, tranquilizing drugs are contraindicated in patients in comatose states cuased by central nervous system depressants (alcohol, barbiturates, opiates, etc.) and also in patients under the influence of large amounts of barbiturates or narcotics. Adrenalin chloride (epinephrine) should not be given for hypotensive reactions.

Precautions

Patients taking tranquilizing and antidepressant drugs should have their blood pressure checked carefully whenever they are receiving combinations of sedatives or stimulants. Medications should be withheld when there are significant changes in the vital signs.

RESERPINE (SERPASIL)

Reserpine is derived from Rauwolfia, a preparation extracted from the root of the tropical snakeroot plant, Rauwolfia serpentina. For centuries, Rauwolfia had been used in India for the treatment of many afflictions, including hypertension and mental illness. It is often prescribed in general practice to reduce hypertension. Reserpine is not as widely used in the treatment of mentally ill patients as are other tranquilizing drugs which produce less hypotensive effects. The length of time for cumulative effect to take place—about three weeks—is another reason that it is less extensively used than are some other preparations.

Patients taking reserpine usually pass through three consecutive reaction stages, but this is not a constant occurrence. The first stage, characterized by sedation, may start soon after the drug is administered and may last from 2 to 10 days. Patients eat and sleep well and are more receptive towards other persons than they were prior to receiving the drug. Turbulence characterizes the second stage and usually occurs 10 to 14 days following the initial administration of the drug although it may occur earlier. Patients become restless, apprehensive, fearful, and may experience hallunications and express delusional thinking. The third stage, the integrative period, is characterized by the subsiding of turbulence, followed by the appearance of more stable behavior, and is usually reached after two to three weeks of treatment have elapsed.

A daily maintenance oral dose for adults may range from 0.1 mg. for mild anxiety-tension and related disorders to 1.0 mg. for the treatment of more pronounced emotional disorders. In starting therapy for severely agitated, combative patients, reserpine may be administered intramuscularly in order to obtain a rapid sedative effect. A single intramuscular dose may range from 2.5 mg. to 5.0 mg. Oral medication may be started on the same day that the first intramuscular dose is given. When this combined plan is used, a small initial dose is given prior to treatment to test for sensitivity. It may be necessary to repeat the intramuscular injection every day or every other day for several days until the oral maintenance dose required to stabilize the patient's behavior is reached. It is recommended that reserpine be given following meals owing to its irritating effect upon the gastrointestinal tract.

A very few patients taking reserpine have developed moderate to severe depression. Although depression usually disappears when administration of the drug is discontinued, active treatment, including hospitalization for electrotherapy, has been required for some patients. Blood pressure readings should be carefully checked when the drug is prescribed for elderly patients who often have low blood pressure prior to therapy. Readings should also be carefully checked if the drug is being given in combination with other sedative drugs having hypotensive effects.

PHENOTHIAZINE COMPOUNDS

A large number of tranquilizing drugs are derivatives of the phenothiazine compound. The specific action of each phenothiazine drug is said to be related to its individual chemical structure. Manufacturers of these drugs have claimed that the differences in chemical structure have resulted in specific therapeutic effects with improved aspects of tranquilization.

Chlorpromazine (Thorazine)

Chlorpromazine, first used by French physicians to potentiate the effects of surgical anesthesia, is one of the most widely prescribed tranquilizers. Its capacity to alleviate anxiety, tension, and agitation without dulling mental faculties makes Thorazine useful in the treatment of mental and emotional disorders as well as in many different somatic conditions where emotional stress is a complicating or a causative factor.

Oral tablet administration is frequently prescribed. For the treatment of emotional and mental disturbances, the starting adult oral dose may range from 10.0 mg. three or four times a day to 25.0 mg. two or three times a day, dependent upon the severity of the patient's symptoms. After a day or two, the dose may be increased by increments of 20.0 mg. to 50.0 mg. daily at semiweekly intervals until the desired maximum clinical effect is reached. Increments in dosage are given more gradually to debilitated and elderly patients. The maximum clinical dose is usually continued for at least two weeks after which it can usually be reduced to a maintenance level. A daily total dose ranging from 200.0 mg. to 400.0 mg., given in divided doses, is average for achieving a beneficial response. However, some patients have received higher total daily doses. When intramuscular injection is given to control acutely agitated behavior, the starting dose is 25.0 mg. Most patients become quiet and cooperative within 24 to 48 hours following the initial intramuscular injection. Oral medication is then substituted according to an increment regimen.

Nursing personnel who are in frequent contact with Thorazine may develop contact dermatitis. Care should be taken to avoid getting the medication on the hands and clothing. Rubber gloves should be worn when repeatedly handling ampuls, multiple-dose vials, syringes, and especially, oral concentrates. The gloves should be washed well with a good detergent, both before and after removal from the hands. Following removal of the gloves, the hands should be washed with a mild soap or detergent, to remove any possible residue. Contact dermatitis usually subsides when exposure to the drug is avoided. Soothing, protective creams may help to relieve skin discomfort. However, in conditions which fail to subside when avoidance of contact is practiced, a doctor should be consulted.

Promazine (Sparine) *15 - 1500*

Sparine (promazine) is unchlorinated chlorpromazine. It is said to be effective in the management of acutely agitated patients as well as those being treated for acute alcoholism, drug addiction, and acute psychotic states.

Although the oral route of administration is preferred, Sparine may be given intravenously in the management of severely agitated adult patients. When the patient is quieted, Sparine may be given intramuscularly or orally. The oral or intramuscular adult dose may range from 10.0 mg. to 200.0 mg., given at four to six hour intervals, depending upon the patient's response. The initial dose given to an acutely inebriated patient should not exceed 50.0 mg. This precaution prevents a greater potentiation of the depressant effects of alcohol. The patient should be carefully observed and kept in bed following intravenous and intramuscular injections.

Prochlorperazine (Compazine) *15 - 150*

Compazine is said to be rapidly effective in its tranquilizing action for the control of anxiety, agitation, tension, and confusion which may be observed in a number of psychiatric disorders. Patients who have failed to respond to previous therapy may respond favorably to Compazine, becoming calm, accessible, and free from hallucinations. The drug may help them to develop insight into their illnesses.

A usual starting oral tablet dose for adult patients is 5.0 mg. given three to four times a day as prescribed. Some patients may require higher doses.

Triflupromazine (Vesprin) *100 - 150*

Vesprin is said to be a drug having increased tranquilizing effects without increased toxicity, made possible through a modification of the phenothiazine structure. According to the literature, it is helpful in controlling delusions and hallucinations and does not lower the convulsive threshold.

For institutionalized mentally ill patients the total daily oral adult dose may range from 100.0 mg. to 150.0 mg. given in divided doses as prescribed. The dose for geriatric patients is 10.0 mg. given two to three times a day.

Trifluoperazine (Stelazine) _₂_ ³⁰ᵐᵍ

Stelazine is said to be effective in the treatment of withdrawn, hypoactive psychotic patients as well as hyperactive, agitated patients. It is also said to have a marked, beneficial effect on delusions and hallucinations. In the treatment of chronic anxiety, as seen in outpatients, Stelazine can restore drive to normal levels in patients who are either hypoactive or hyperactive.

The usual starting oral adult dose for hospitalized mentally ill patients is 2.0 mg. to 5.0 mg. given twice a day as prescribed. Occasional reactions of drowsiness, dizziness, or stimulation may be observed which are often transitory symptoms. A few patients may experience a transient unpleasant stimulation or jittery feeling characterized by motor restlessness and sometimes insomnia. The dosage of Stelazine should not be increased while these side effects are present. In some instances, it may be necessary to reduce the dose if these symptoms are particularly distressing.

Although the increased mental and physical activity frequently seen with Stelazine therapy in apathetic patients is usually beneficial, it may be an undesirable side effect in patients afflicted with physical illness which necessitates limitation of activity. Patients having angina pectoris should be carefully observed for such unfavorable responses so that any reaction may be reported and use of the drug discontinued. Patients having a history of cardiovascular conditions should be carefully observed for hypotensive reactions.

Fluphenazine Hydrochloride (Prolixin)

It is claimed that Prolixin produces a rapid onset of antihallucinatory and antidelusional effects, followed by sustained and prolonged action. It has also been stated that this drug appears to produce less of a sedative reaction than most of the phenothiazine derivatives.

The starting oral adult dose for anxiety and tension states is usually 1.0 mg. A second or higher dose may be prescribed. Six to eight hours should elapse between the first and second doses.

Thioridazine (Mellaril) 30 – 800

Because it acts directly upon certain areas of the brain with very little "spill-over" into other sections, Mellaril is said to be more specific in its tranquilizing action and therapeutic effectiveness. Its minimal sedative effect makes it possible for patients to resume normal daily activities in the hospital, at work, or at home. Owing to its minimal photosensitivity effects, Mellaril is often prescribed as a drug of choice during the summer. These advantages are said to represent improved tranquilization with a greater margin of safety in general office practice, in psychiatric outpatient clinics, and in hospitalization.

The usual starting oral adult dose for non-psychiatric patients may range from 10.0 mg. three to four times a day to 25.0 mg. three to four times a day. Psychotic patients may require 100.0 mg. three to four times a day as a starting dose.

Perphenazine (Trilafon) *6 – 64 mg / day.*

Trilafon may be used in treating agitated mental and emotional disturbances whether of functional or organic origin. The lowest dosage that will produce the desired effect is prescribed.

For mild anxiety and tension states the usual adult dose, by tablet, is 2.0 mg. or 4.0 mg. given three to four times a day. Adult hospitalized psychiatric patients may require 8.0 mg. to 16.0 mg. administered two to four times a day as a starting dose. An early reduction is made in the dosage.

Patients having a history of convulsive disorders or severe side reactions to other phenothiazine medications should be closely observed for side reactions. A significant, not otherwise explained, rise in body temperature may indicate individual intolerance and necessitate discontinuance of Trilafon.

TRANQUILIZERS DERIVED FROM OTHER COMPOUNDS

Chlordiazepoxide (Librium) *FAT*

Librium is completely unrelated chemically or pharmacologically to any other tranquilizer or antidepressant agent. It is said to be virtually specific for the relief of irrational fears, anxiety, and tension. Librium has also shown an antidepressant effect in some patients.

For mild to moderate anxiety and tension states, the usual adult oral dose is 5.0 mg. or 10.0 mg. given three to four times daily. For the treatment of more severe emotional disturbances, the oral adult dose may be 20.0 mg. or 25.0 mg. given three times a day. Geriatric patients and those afflicted with debilitating illnesses are usually given the smallest effective dose (usually 5.0 mg. given two to four times a day, as prescribed.)

Diazepam (Valium) — *emotional origin*

Valium is said to be especially helpful for patients whose somatic complaints are of emotional origin. The rapid onset of its calming effect (within 15 to 30 minutes) makes it useful in treating patients manifesting agitated behavior with secondary depressive reactions. The sedative effect of Valium is said to be minimal.

The dosage for mild to moderate psychoneurotic tension anxiety states and agitated depressive episodes is 2.0 mg. to 5.0 mg. two or three times daily. For severe psychoneurotic reactions the dosage is 5.0 mg. to 10.0 mg. three or four times a day. Valium is contraindicated in patients having histories of convulsive disorders or glaucoma. It is not of value in the treatment of psychotic patients in lieu of other appropriate therapy.

Chlorprothixene (Taractan)

Taractan also produces a rapid calming effect with a minimal risk of deepening depressive symptoms and is said to be helpful in the treatment of patients manifesting agitation with coexisting depression. When given to newly admitted patients, its rapid effect permits early use of psychotherapy.

The recommended dosage for the adult patient is 10.0 mg. three or four times daily in the treatment of mild to moderate behavior disorders. For treating severe neurotic and psychotic states, the dosage is 25.0 mg. to 50.0 mg. four times daily.

Meprobamate (Miltown) (Equanil) — *muscle relaxant — voluntary*

Meprobamate, also known by the trade names, Miltown and Equanil, is a synthetic muscle relaxant which acts upon voluntary muscles without affecting the muscles of the diaphragm. It is said to be safe in the relief of respiratory muscle spasm encountered in poliomyelitis, cerebral palsy, hemiplegia, and paraplegia. It also produces a tranquilizing effect on the central nervous system. In the treatment of the mentally ill, it is used to reduce psychic tension with accompanying anxiety and fear. Patients taking the drug maintain their alertness as psychotherapy is facilitated. Meprobamate is claimed to calm the individual without producing a clouding of consciousness and a "hangover" following sleep. It is also said that persons taking the drug are able to look at problems without fear. Mostly, it has been prescribed for psychoneurotic and milder emotional disorders, and particularly for patients who are not hospitalized.

Meprobamate differs in its chemical structure as well as its action from other tranquilizing drugs. The initial dose is usually one 400.00 mg. tablet given three or four times daily. For patients requiring less medication than average, or for those whose medication is being reduced, 200.0 mg. may be a satisfactory dosage.

Meprobamate is said to be unusually free of side effects, and those which do occur are usually of a minor nature. Susceptible persons who have taken Meprobamate for long periods of time have been known to develop a dependence upon the drug. When excessive dosage has been continued for weeks or months, the dosage should be reduced gradually because abrupt discontinuance may precipitate withdrawal reactions.

ANTIDEPRESSANT DRUGS — *psychic energizers*

Generally speaking, antidepressant drugs referred to as "psychic energizers" produce in depressed patients a feeling of well-being, increased alertness, a more optimistic outlook, improved appetite, and enjoyment in activities and social relationships with other persons. These drugs are not recommended for the treatment of essentially normal responses to temporary emotionally depressive situations. When they are administered, careful observations should be made of the patient because the possibility of suicidal attempts cannot be overlooked until remission is complete. Significant changes in vital signs should be reported as well as any other reactions which may be indicative of side effects requiring a change in the dosage or discontinuance of the drug.

There are precautions against giving certain antidepressant drugs in combination with any drug which inhibits monoamine oxidase activity. It is recommended that a two-week waiting period elapse between the use of an antidepressant drug which has failed to produce a therapeutic response in the patient and the administration of another drug.

Dosages

Dosages are prescribed and adjusted according to the individual needs and responses of patients. Geriatric and adolescent patients usually cannot tolerate as high a daily dosage as is given to adult patients. Dependent upon the drug given, it may take from several days to a few weeks or longer to achieve and observe a therapeutic reaction in the patient. After a favorable behavior change is observed, the dosage is reduced gradually to a

maintenance dose. Some patients continue to take a prescribed maintenance dose after being discharged from the hospital.

Preparations Available

Antidepressant drugs are available in oral tablets and solutions for
intramuscular injections.

Side Effects *anxiety episodes manic or hypomanic reactions*

Patients may occasionally develop acute anxiety episodes and become
agitated during therapy. It may be necessary to reduce the dosage or
prescribe an additional tranquilizing drug. Hypomanic or manic reactions
may occur occasionally, probably as manifestations of underlying cyclic
disorder. Discontinuance of the drug may be necessary.

Because of their stimulating effect upon body systems and organs,
antidepressant drugs should be prescribed and given only under careful
supervision and observation to patients afflicted with cardiovascular disease. Low dosages are given to these persons as well as to elderly patients
who may fall and suffer bodily injury during therapy.

Mild and transitory side effects may occur during the early period of
treatment when the patient is becoming adjusted to the drug and the
dosage strength is being adjusted. Some of these reactions may require
remedial treatment, dependent upon the appearance and persistence of
symptoms.

Antidepressant drugs may produce any of the less severe as well as the
more severe side reactions observed when tranquilizers are taken by patients (see pp. 363, 364 for description and treatment).

While one would expect the possibility of hypertensive reactions with
stimulating drugs, some antidepressant medications have been known to
produce hypotensive as well as hypertensive reactions in individual patients. The more severe side effects of jaundice, extrapyramidal symptoms,
and agranulocytosis are infrequent, but possible, reactions to anticipate.

Contraindications *liver disease convulsive disorders*

According to the literature, antidepressant drugs are contraindicated
for patients having histories of liver disease and convulsive disorders.

Precautions *V S B P Blood studies - urinalysis - liver function*

Because of the potentiating effects of antidepressant drugs, careful observations of vital signs, especially blood pressure, and other reactions should be made when patients taking these medications are given central nervous system stimulant or depressant drugs or hypotensive medications.

Generally speaking, the nurse giving medications of any kind should make it a rule to observe and report any and all unfavorable reactions in order to be certain that it is safe for the patient to continue taking the medication.

During prolonged therapy with tranquilizing and antidepressant drugs, it is recommended that blood studies, liver function tests, and urinalysis be done routinely at prescribed intervals in order to detect effects upon body systems and organs.

Imipramine (Tofranil) *100 mg no side effects - don't give ō MAO inhibitors*

Tofranil is prescribed for the relief of depression of varying degrees with associate symptoms related to changes in energy drive, eating, sleeping habits, etc.

It is not possible to describe a dosage schedule of Tofranil that will provide optimal results in all patients. Tablets are available in 25.0 mg. and 10.0 mg. sizes. An initial total daily dosage for adult patients of 100.0 mg. given in divided doses, as prescribed by the physician, is recommended. Increments may be required. Therapy for geriatric and adolescent patients may be initiated with a total daily dosage of 30.0 mg. or 40.0 mg. given in divided doses. The single dose prescribed for these patients is usually 10.0 mg. After a therapeutic response is observed, the dosage is gradually reduced to a maintenance dose. Tofranil should not be given in combination with any other drug which inhibits monoamine oxidase activity. It is said to be tolerated well and rarely produces serious side effects.

Phenelzine (Nardil) *MAO inhibitor*

Nardil, an inhibitor of monoamine oxidase activity, is said to be effective in the treatment of depressive states ranging from mild to severe.

For initial therapy the usual adult dose is one 15.0 mg. tablet three times a day. The dosage is maintained until remission of symptoms is achieved. Maximum benefit is usually observed within a period of two to six weeks following initial administration of the drug. The dosage is reduced slowly over several weeks. A maintenance dose, as low as one tablet a day or every other day, dependent upon the individual patient's response, may be continued as long as required.

Tranylcypromine Sulfate (Parnate) MAO I

Parnate is an inhibitor of monoamine oxidase activity said to be beneficial in the treatment of depressive reactions of varying degrees.

The recommended initial dose for adult patients is 10.0 mg. given twice a day, once in the morning and once in the afternoon. This regimen is continued for two to three weeks. If a satisfactory response is not produced, the dose may be increased by 10.0 mg. a day. If the daily dose is increased, 20.0 mg. is given in the morning and 10.0 mg. in the afternoon. As soon as a satisfactory response is achieved, the dosage may be reduced to a maintenance level of 20.0 mg. or 10.0 mg. a day, dependent upon the individual patient's requirements. Parnate should not be given in combination with Tofranil, and it should not be given for at least two weeks after a regimen of treatment with Tofranil.

Amitriptyline Hydrochloride (Elavil)   100-mg - nolan MAO I

Elavil is described as a potent antidepressant agent with a low degree of toxicity. It is not a monoamine oxidase inhibitor. Elavil has a tranquilizing component to its action which is helpful in achieving a therapeutic response in patients manifesting depression with predominant symptoms of anxiety and agitation.

The majority of adult patients will respond favorably to an ititial dose of 25.0 mg. three times a day. If, during treatment of more severely ill patients, it is necessary to increase the dose of Elavil, it is recommended that a 25.0 mg. increment be given with the evening medications. At breakfast and lunch time the patient receives 25.0 mg. At supper time and again at the hour of sleep the patient is given 50.0 mg. The dosage is gradually reduced to the smallest amount necessary to maintain relief from depressive symptoms. Most patients respond well to a maintenance dose of 25.0 mg. given two to four times a day.

SUGGESTED REFERENCES

Ayd, F.: The major tranquilizers. Am. J. Nurs. 65: 70, (April), 1965.
Ayd, F.: The minor tranquilizers. Am. J. Nurs. 65: 89, (May), 1965.
Ayd, F.: The antidepressants. Am. J. Nurs. 65: 78, (June), 1965.
Cohen, S., Ditman, K., et al.: Psychochemotherapy. The Physician's Manual. Western Medical Publications, Los Angeles (Printed for Hoffman-La Roche Inc., Nutley, New Jersey), 1967.
Elavil.* Merck, Sharp & Dohme, Division of Merck & Co., Inc., West Point, Pa.
Let Your Light So Shine.* Roche Laboratories, Division of Hoffmann-LaRoche Inc., Nutley, New Jersey, p. 49.
Miltown—Physicians' Reference Manual.* Wallace Pharmaceuticals, Cranbury, New Jersey.

Nardil.* Warner-Chilcott Laboratories, Morris Plains, New Jersey.

Nurse's Guide to Mellaril Therapy.* Sandoz Pharmaceuticals, Division of Sandoz, Inc., Hanover, New Jersey.

Physicians' Desk Reference, ed. 26. Medical Economics, Inc., Oradell, New Jersey, 1972.

Prolixin.* E. R. Squibb & Sons, New York.

Rodman, M.: Drug therapy today: drugs for managing mood disorders. R.N. 33: 43 (Dec.), 1970.

Rodman, M.: Drug therapy: the major tranquilizers and antidepressants. R. N. 68: 53 (Aug.), 1968.

Shaffer, J.: Allergic reactions to drugs. Am. J. Nurs. 65: 101, (Oct.), 1965.

The Psychiatric Nurse's Guide to Therapy with Thorazine, Compazine, Stelazine, Parnate.* Smith, Kline & French Laboratories, Philadelphia.

Tofranil.* Geigy Pharmaceuticals, Division of Geigy Chemical Corporation, Ardsley, New York.

Trilafon.* Schering Corporation, Bloomfield, New Jersey.

Vesprin.* E.R. Squibb & Sons, New York.

*Pamphlets may be obtained from Product Information Divisions of the pharmaceutical company converned.

For reviewing this chapter, grateful acknowledgement is made to Mr. Ben Feigan, pharmacist.

UNIT 8

Behavior and Nursing Care of Patients

CHAPTER 30

Behavior Reactions
During the Senile Period: Nursing Care

Admissions to psychiatric hospitals of persons afflicted with reactions associated with the senile period have increased, owing to the fact that medical science has made it possible for older people to live longer. The life expectancy of the American population has been extending for a century and a half, and there appears to be no reversal of this trend. Today there are more than 14 million Americans over 65 years of age, and their numbers are growing steadily.

THE SENILE PERIOD

The senile period usually commences at the age of 60 years. Some individuals for some unknown reason, however, do develop pre-senile changes and manifest these developments between the ages of 40 and 60 years of life.

MENTAL HEALTH INFLUENCES

The mental health of the aged is largely influenced by cultural concepts, attitudes, social changes, and the degree of adjustment the individual has demonstrated throughout life toward changing situations and problems. It is generally believed that social, psychiatric factors play a more important etiologic part than do organic changes in the development of senile mental disturbance. Indeed, some investigators believe that an individual who has managed to maintain a good disposition toward change and problems, and who retains some social contacts and interests in the later years of life, rarely develops mental illness during the senile period.

SOCIAL, CULTURAL FACTORS

As people get older, they become less energetic and physically incapable of accomplishing as much as they did previously. Their interests and enthusiasms wane, they become self-centered, and tend to socialize less with other persons. Children in the family usually marry, establish new homes, and transfer with them their interests, enthusiasms, and affection. Deaths of relatives and acquaintances gradually reduce the older person's social contacts. Occupations may necessitate the migration of some family members to distant regions so that they experience little opportunity or occasion to visit with parents.

There is general agreement that the American culture does not provide enough satisfying roles for older people. It is said that our concept of old age is a product of the agricultural and rural society of the nineteenth century, when elderly persons retained their homes, lived with the family as it enlarged, and performed tasks which were available in rural or semirural environments. Actually, many aged persons are living alone today in large cities in small apartments and rooms. There is little opportunity for employment and social contacts. The American concept of the United States as a country of young, vigorous, successful people also affects the aged. This is reflected in motion pictures, popular magazines, and advertisements. A high value is placed upon work so that a person who does not work is thought of as a useless member of society. This value is obvious in the current attitude towards people of wealth, who are encouraged to find something to do in order to be useful. Working is more than a way of earning a livelihood in the United States; it is a way of keeping one's self-respect. The emphasis in American industry upon compulsory retirement at a certain age has resulted in a loss of self-respect in some older individuals. Indeed, many persons between the ages of 45 and 60 years report that it is difficult to obtain employment, owing to their advancing years.

PHYSICAL CHANGES

Many physical changes, considered quite normal, occur during the senile period. Senile persons usually eat less, lose weight, and often have gastric and many other somatic complaints. The individual's skin appears dry and inelastic because of a reduced secretion of lubricants, and may feel cold, owing to poor circulation. The underlying adipose tissue disappears, and the skin assumes a wrinkled look and can be rolled up with the fingers. Brown spots (keratoses) are commonly observed on the skin of senile persons. Visual disturbances, such as farsightedness and cataracts, may develop. Many of these individuals must wear eyeglasses. Deafness is frequently observed and often necessitates the patient's dependence upon a hearing aid. Salivation is reduced, and dryness of the mucous membranes of the mouth results. The teeth may become infected and require repairs or extraction. Many aged persons wear dentures and may manifest difficulties in swallowing and chewing. There may be distortions in the sensations of taste and smell. The hair loses its luster and usually turns gray. Sleep disturbances are common, especially reversed sleep patterns wherein the patient sleeps during the day and awakens in the night manifesting confused, restless, and agitated behavior. Elimination may be affected, resulting in complaints of constipation, retention, or diarrhea. Muscular weakness, incoordination, and sometimes tremors develop which affect the patient's ability to grasp objects, walk steadily, and write legibly. Coexisting sclerosis of the cerebral arteries may produce symptoms of headache, dizziness, and sometimes vascular accidents. Many senile persons neglect their daily hygiene, dress, and personal appearance.

MENTAL CHANGES

Mental changes may commence with periods of transient confusion and a tendency to be absentminded. Formerly familiar duties require a longer time to perform. Aged persons often become resistive to changes, resent new ideas, opinions, and the behavior of members of the younger generation. Oftentimes they are spunky, irritable, and quarrelsome. As time goes on, they manifest more marked symptoms of senile mental disorder, such as impairment of thinking, reasoning, judgment and memory. They do not remember recent events but readily recall remote events and are often referred to as being in their second childhood. These persons may become disoriented as to time, place, and persons. Sometimes they speak of relatives and acquaintances who are dead as if those individuals were alive. It is not unusual for them to misidentify people. Hiding and hoarding of food or articles of little or no value, suspiciousness, hallucinations, and persecutory delusions may be observed.

In the home, their behavior has often been a cause for concern. Some of these persons have wandered about during the night in a confused state, tampered with the time setting of clocks, turned on gas jets, and become excited.

In general hospitals, they frequently react to precipitating factors such as surgery, drugs, infection, and hypoglycemic reactions. Frequently they manifest confused and delirious behavior which is reversible with alleviation of the precipitating cause. Problematical sexual behavior, involving sexual advances and indecencies, is not uncommon.

ETIOLOGY, DYNAMICS

Patients with senile brain disease usually have histories of emotional insecurity, inflexibility, set habits, and poor adjustment to life situations and changes. Any threat or loss, during advancing years, produces feeling influences to which the patient reacts strongly. Many psychiatrists believe that the behavior of senile persons is consistent, to an exaggerated degree, with their normal temperaments and previous personality patterns. Depression, delusions, and agitated behavior reactions constitute a resort to the use of lifelong defense mechanisms in the resolution of conflict.

Reduced social contacts result in feelings of loneliness and rejection and of being unloved, unwanted, and unnecessary; depression is a response to all of these. The economic threat of advancing years and the need to be dependent may be extremely frightening. Loss of a job produces feelings of fear, insecurity, lowered self-esteem, and anxiety. Hiding and hoarding are reactions to threats to security. Irritability, resistance, inflexibility, and aggression are hostile but fearful responses toward feelings of insecurity, lowered self-esteem, and the need to be dependent. Suspiciousness, persecutory delusions, and hallucinations are projections of these individuals' innermost fears and thoughts. Questionable sexual behavior is a compensatory defense mechanism toward a waning, functional capacity.

TREATMENT ENVIRONMENT

Sometimes it is possible to care for the aged who have milder forms of senile mental reactions in the home, where the environment is familiar. Usually these persons are much happier in their homes than in an institution, where routines frequently exist to which the patient must adjust, necessitating a change in well-established, lifelong habits. There are times, however, when it is necessary to hospitalize the patient who requires special medical and nursing care and protection. Patients who may sustain an injury, wander in their confusion, and manifest homicidal or suicidal tendencies are usually not manageable in the home. Physical handicaps such as blindness, deafness, convulsive seizures, and crippling defects of the extremities may also require that the patient be hospitalized in a therapeutic, protective environment.

NURSING CARE

Nursing of the aged is most effective when personnel recognize that the needs of these patients are much like the needs of other people. One must have a genuine liking for older persons and an interest in helping to make them feel accepted, worth while, and approved. It will be necessary to adapt the plan of nursing care to the individual patient. There will be times when it will be difficult to gain the patient's cooperation, particularly if the individual objects to any form of routine which interferes with his former habits. To determine the wisest approach, the nurse will want to be alert to the patient's feelings and needs so that his values may be weighed with those values of immediate concern to the staff and hospital. Quite often, it is possible to satisfy the patient's needs and preserve his dignity with some minor adaptations.

To give good care to geriatric patients, the nurse must be skillful in managing the patient without making it obvious to the patient that he is being managed. Some of the following suggestions may be helpful in caring for these individuals. Sympathy, kindness, and thoughtfulness should be extended without introducing an element of pity. Tolerance and being able to accede to the patient's wishes on occasions and injecting a kind sense of humor can often accomplish much. A sensitivity to the patient's need for physical assistance enables the nurse to know when to give aid without making it necessary for the patient to make a request for it. Consideration for the patient's particular circumstances of being unemployed, possibly impoverished, helpless, and dependent is a desirable nursing quality. Many of these persons have been accustomed to private homes, have claimed ownership to certain possessions and known much more privacy than the ward of a large psychiatric hospital. The nurse who listens to the patient and learns all she can from available records and other sources of information about the person's background and home environment will be able to offer effective emotional support. There are times when it is possible to draw a screen around a patient's bed when giving nursing care. A single room, or the ward dining room, may sometimes be used to allow the patient a quiet, private visit on occasion. These are little considerations for which many underprivileged patients, so to speak, will be extremely grateful. Patience and tact are necessary when the aged person becomes "ornery," unreasonable, and opinionated. Frequently, it is helpful to allow these persons to be heard because they have a need to talk and express their viewpoints, especially when they have underlying doubts and fears. Careful explanations are always helpful in alleviating their fears and anxiety. An optimistic attitude is vitally essential if these patients are to be remotivated and rehabilitated. There exists an unfortunate, contagious attitude of chronicity and hopelessness on the part of some nursing personnel concerning senile patients. Actually, many of these patients can be rehabilitated sufficiently to adjust to their particular infirmities and engage in some social and recreational activities. Many of them are able to take care of their intimate physical needs with a minimum of assistance. The

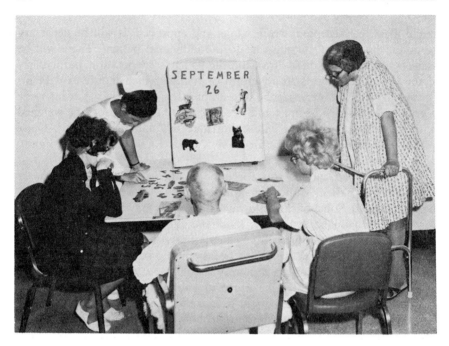

Fig. 1.   Reorienting an elderly group through word picture association aids. (Courtesy of Arkansas State Hospital, Little Rock, Ark.)

idea that it is easier and less time-consuming to do everything for the patient can be equally demoralizing. It is necessary to remember that morale is built not only by what the nurse can do for the patient, but also by what the patient can do for himself and others. Hurry should be avoided because it produces feelings of inadequacy and frustration.

If these patients can get around, either on foot or in wheel chairs, they should be introduced to other ill persons. This is one way of helping them to develop a stimulating outside interest. It is surprising how often some of the more able individuals can, and do, enjoy assisting less able patients. They may help others to get out of bed, dress, and walk to the bathroom and about the ward, and assist with feeding at mealtime.

Visits from family members should be encouraged when these occasions are pleasing to the patient. Many aged patients, however, appear to be forgotten or do not have relatives. These are the lonely patients who enjoy little chats, a visit from the clergy or a hospital volunteer.

Patients who are able to read may be given literature or allowed access to the hospital library. Quite often the librarian or a volunteer will visit the ward to distribute books. Some patients may not read but enjoy looking at colorful magazines.

On special occasions, such as birthdays or holidays, these patients enjoy the recognition and attention attached to a greeting card, a birthday cake, or some small token of remembrance. Oftentimes they can help to plan and participate in parties and social gatherings.

Many elderly patients can and do learn. In fact, some, like the late Grandma Moses, the well-known artist, produced their best works in their later years. They can be stimulated to engage in creating works of art and crafts. Many enjoy drawing, painting, making favors, pasting decals, etc. An occasional word of praise bolsters their morale and sense of achievement. Engaging in these activities is helpful, also, in preventing physical contractures. It keeps patients mentally alert and diverted from preoccupation, feelings of loneliness, and helplessness.

In warm weather these persons can spend considerable time sitting in the open air, provided they are protected from undue exposure to the sun. In cool weather, they must be dressed appropriately to protect them from catching cold.

Good physical care requires that all complaints or symptoms of illness be investigated. Elderly persons may develop conditions which require medical attention. Upper respiratory infection, constipation, and diarrhea are commonly observed. If medication is required, it should be prescribed by a physician. Diarrhea should always be cause to consider the possibility of a fecal impaction which may necessitate an enema or removal of the retained mass. Routine toileting of patients after meals is a recommended habit-training procedure. When nursing personnel are too busy to supervise this practice each time, they can teach some of the more able patients to initiate and carry out the plan. Habit training reduces incontinence, soiling, constipation, and also influences favorable responses in the patient's feelings and the ward environment.

Patients with physical handicaps may require various degrees of assistance, dependent upon the particular patient's infirmity. Blind persons usually enjoy having someone to chat with, or the companionship of an individual who has time to read to them occasionally or walk them around the ward or outside of the building. Patients with crippling defects may need assistance in handling objects, dressing, walking, getting in and out of bed, the bath tub, etc.

It should not be assumed automatically that all aged persons are deaf. Some of them can hear well when the nurse stands directly in front of them and speaks slowly and distinctly so that they can lip read if necessary. Oftentimes, senile patients will indicate verbally, or with gestures, that they wish the nurse to speak louder.

SOCIAL TRENDS

There is a widespread concern about the problems and needs of the aged. Many people feel that geriatric patients should be cared for in special hospitals, other than psychiatric institutions, in which special attention and facilities may be provided for them. Some states have already passed legislation that prevents their admission to mental hospitals. Increasing emphasis is being placed upon caring for these individuals in long-term care facilities and foster homes. Legislation has been enacted to provide them with some economic security through social security and old age assistance programs. A great effort is being made to encourage industry to reappraise their compulsory retirement plans and make some provisions for the employment of older persons. While industry may be inclined sympathetically toward this viewpoint, they have a restraining influence placed upon them when attempting to purchase workmen's compensation insurance plans. The belief that aged persons are more susceptible to disease, injury, and long-term illness prevails.

Many ideas regarding housing for the aged have already been demonstrated and advanced. The geriatric clinic, where these persons may go for health examinations and assistance, have been inaugurated. Recreation centers where both sexes of the older group may meet for social activities, discussions, and planned educational programs have become firmly established in some large metropolitan areas. Housing projects have been constructed which include a certain number of apartments equipped with special living conveniences and facilities for older persons. A building supervisor has the responsibility of visiting the occupants daily. Another plan has been to provide a large, central dining room, in such apartment houses, in which the elderly might dine. In another community, consideration has been given to the suggestion that the local high school cooking classroom be converted into a dining room each evening so that aged persons might have one hot meal served to them during the day. In some communities an ingenious plan has been worked out, by a group of club women, to carry hot meals into the homes of some of these persons. These evidences are encouraging in that they indicate a real effort being made to meet the needs of aged persons.

SUGGESTED REFERENCES

Amburgey, P.: Environmental aids for the aged patient. Am. J. Nurs. 66: 2017 (Sept.), 1966.
Anderson, C.: Instituting change in psychiatric geriatric settings. J. Psychiat. Nurs, 8: 13 (Jul.-Aug.), 1970.
Bozian, M.: Nursing in a geriatric day center. Am. J. Nurs. 64: 93 (April), 1964.
Burnside, I.: Crisis intervention with geriatric hospitalized patients. J. Psychiat. Nurs. 8: 17 (Mar.-Apr.), 1970.

Burnside, I.: Group work among the aged. Nurs. Outlook 17: 68 (June), 1969.

Conti, M.: The lonliness of old age. Nurs. Outlook 18: 28 (Aug.), 1970.

Culbert, P., and Kos, B.: Aging: considerations for health teaching. Nurs. Clin. N. Am. (Dec.), W. B. Saunders Co., Philadelphia, 1971, p. 605.

Dowling, E.: They're giving the aged a new will to live. R.N. 27: 57 (Oct.), 1964.

Goldfarb, A.: Responsibilities to our aged. Am. J. Nurs. 64: 78 (Nov.), 1964.

Hulicka, I.: Fostering self-respect in aged patients. Am. J. Nurs. 64: 84 (March), 1964.

Ouimette, H.: When your elderly patient can't sleep. R.N. 27: 65 (Dec.), 1964.

Peszczynski, M.: Why old people fall. Am. J. Nurs. 65: 86 (May), 1965.

Smith, E.: Nursing services for the aged in housing projects and day centers. Am. J. Nurs. 65: 72 (Dec.), 1965.

Stevens, R.: Treatment of the aged in state hospitals. J. Psychiat. Nurs. 9: 31 (Jan.-Feb.), 1971.

Wolff, K.: Helping elderly patients face the fear of death. Hosp. Commun. Psychiat. 18: 142 (May), 1967.

CHAPTER 31

Drug Addiction Causing
Dependence Behavior: Nursing Care

Drug addiction is characterized chiefly by an overpowering desire or need to continue taking a natural or synthetic drug having habit-forming properties. Repeated consumption of the same dose produces a declining effect (tolerance) which results in a tendency to increase the dose. The addict develops a psychological and sometimes a physical dependence on the effects of the drug. Psychological dependence develops owing to the relief from tension and emotional discomfort which use of the drug effects. Drug addiction is a serious public health problem.

ETIOLOGY, DYNAMICS

Some persons commence the drug habit when they take medication prescribed for the relief of a painful condition. Other individuals become victims of suggestion in seeking the experience of something new and thrilling. It is generally believed that many persons who develop the drug habit have a basic sociopathic-personality character structure. Emotionally, they are immature, unstable individuals with strong dependency needs and underlying feelings of inadequacy and inferiority. Neurotic persons, who frequently have physical complaints and experience much discomfort through anxiety, also become addicted. Drug addiction is often found among residents of large cities and persons who engage in underworld activities. Doctors and nurses, who develop addiction, are probably influenced by easy access to drugs.

Peddlers involved in illegal traffic of narcotics extract exorbitant sums of money from their purchasers. Frequently the addict is involved in financial and legal difficulties. Morally and socially, the person regresses. In order to obtain opiates or the money necessary to procure them, the individual will associate with undesirable persons, commit crimes, and submit to perverse sexual acts.

ADDICTION TO OPIATES

There are individuals who become addicted to opiates and develop a chronic physical and emotional dependence upon them. Morphine and heroin appear to be the drugs of choice; addiction to codeine is rare. Morphine substitutes, which are related in chemical structure to other drugs but produce opiate-like effects, are also favored by addicts. These drugs are Demerol (meperidine hydrochloride) and methadone (Adanon, Dolophine).

Opiates produce feelings of serenity, relief from anxiety, and a generalized pleasant sensation of warmth and relaxation. Primitive needs and motivations, such as hunger, sex, and pain, are reduced. A feeling of sexual gratification is experienced by some addicts.

PHYSICAL AND MENTAL EFFECTS

In the early dependence period, the person resorting to the use of opiates feels exhilarated and even ambitious. His activity performance increases. Gradually the addict comes to rely upon the use of opiates to bolster his self-confidence in difficult problematical situations. As time progresses, the addict's tolerance to dosage increases, and it becomes necessary to increase the amount taken. Eventually, the body commences to react to the depressant effects of opiates. The individual loses his appetite, vim, and vigor. He develops an emaciated appearance, with sunken cheeks and pale, grayish complexion. Physically, his job performance decreases, thus reducing his social productivity. Gradually, the person withdraws from normal social contacts.

Continuance of the habit causes the addict to develop an overwhelming craving and physiological need for opiates to maintain emotional and physical equilibrium. Without the drug, there is grave danger of body shock and a fatal collapse. When the individual is unable to obtain opiates, he becomes moody, irritable, tremulous, unable to relax or sleep, and develops serious physical, debilitating symptoms. Chronic addiction produces impairment of the patient's judgment and intellectual abilities. Deterioration of the person's ethical sense and standards of living occurs. The addict's whole purpose in life appears to revolve around obtainment of the drug.*

SOCIAL CONTROLS

Narcotics are under the legal supervision and control of federal and state governments. Penalties for violations of control measures commenced with the Harrison Narcotic Act of 1914. Legally, these drugs are unobtainable without a physician's written prescription.

The United States Public Health Service maintains federal hospitals at Lexington, Kentucky and Fort Worth, Texas, in which addicts, prisoners, and probationers convicted of federal narcotic law violations receive priority treatment. Voluntary patients may also seek treatment in these hospitals. Female patients may receive treatment only in the Lexington hospital. For information concerning admission to the federal hospitals, one may write to the Surgeon General of the United States Public Health Service.

For many reasons, there is strong opposition to current proposals to legalize the distribution of opiates to addicts in controlled clinics. There is a marked trend toward recognizing drug addiction as an illness and social problem instead of a criminal offense.[1] It is recommended that addicts be treated either privately or in a government hospital. Treatment on an outpatient basis is not recommended.

ADMISSION OF PATIENT TO HOSPITAL

Under ordinary conditions, the patient admitted to a hospital for withdrawal treatment should be received, undressed, and bathed in an area which is removed from the location of his permanent room. Clothing must be carefully searched, including all pockets, linings, and other places of concealment. The physician may order an enema. Women patients may be given a vaginal irrigation when the treatment is prescribed. Addicts have been known to conceal drugs in unusual places, including body orifices. The patient should be dressed in hospital clothing until the end of the withdrawal syndrome in order to prevent his escape and attempts to obtain drugs outside of the hospital. Visitors and mail should be carefully supervised. Nursing personnel should never mail a letter outside of the hospital

---

*Oakland, California, police have been using subcutaneous injections of nalline hydrochloride (N-allylnormorphine) to identify opiate addicts. The drug produces withdrawal symptoms when given to individuals who are taking opiates. This makes it possible to detain the person legally on charges of possession of illicit drugs. Oakland claims that this procedure has reduced its crime rate.

for these patients as they may be attempting to contact someone who will supply the drug through some obscure channel.

When an addict is admitted to a hospital in a state of physical collapse, it is usually impossible for the physician to obtain sufficient history from the patient or relatives to make a diagnosis. There are, however, some telltale signs which may be observed. Addicts usually prefer the intravenous method of injection, owing to its rapid effects. Needle marks and abscess scars may be observed on the skin over the victim's veins. The application of external heat, sedative prescription, and intravenous fluids usually produces immediate therapeutic effects.

WITHDRAWAL OF DRUG

Withdrawal of opiates cannot be commenced safely until the patient's condition improves.

Abrupt withdrawal of the drug from the patient is not considered humane and may even be dangerous[2] in depriving the body too suddenly of something it presently requires. Physiological shock and fatal collapse may be avoided when gradual abstinence treatment is instituted. Treatment is commenced by giving the patient a sedative dose of the same drug to which he is addicted, or a substitute drug. The sedative dose is reduced appropriately each day, or every few days, as indicated by the patient's reaction, until the person is able to go without medication.

Methadone appears to be favored for withdrawal purposes, owing to its relatively long duration of action. It can be given both orally and intramuscularly, as indicated. Withdrawal reaction symptoms are milder when methadone is administered.

WITHDRAWAL REACTIONS

Nursing personnel may expect to observe such withdrawal reactions as anxiety, irritability, tremors, gastric complaints, inability of the patient to relax or sleep, and muscle cramps. These patients sometimes beg for medication, but it will be necessary for the nurse to adhere to the physician's orders while remaining kindly toward the patient, who actually feels most uncomfortable and often frightened. Warm baths may be soothing and relaxing and help to reduce tremors and muscle cramps. However, the patient should be supervised carefully in the bath, which should not be prolonged, owing to the patient's usually poor physical condition.

More painful and serious reactions should be reported immediately, such as excruciating abdominal pains, diarrhea, vomiting and convulsions. Sometimes it is necessary to increase temporarily the amount of sedation being given until the patient's condition improves. Artificial fluids may be required to maintain body fluid balance.

REHABILITATION

It is recommended that persons admitted to institutions for treatment of drug addiction remain for several months in the hospital following the completion of abstinence treatment. The physical and emotional rehabilitation is considered of vital importance. Most authorities do not believe this can be accomplished in less than nine months to one year. Carrying out this proposal, however, often becomes a real problem in a private hospital.

NARCOTICS ANONYMOUS AND SYNANON

Treatment and rehabilitation approaches have been strengthened through Narcotics Anonymous and Synanon. These methods have proved sufficiently beneficial to prompt the establishment of special facilities in some states, notably California and New York where drug addiction is a serious problem. Narcotics Anonymous uses a group therapy approach similar to that used by Alcoholics Anonymous (see p. 406).

Synanon, an organization started by Charles Dederich, uses a group therapy approach that differs from the standard technique. The word Synanon was coined by an early member of the group who was attempting to pronounce simultaneously the words symposium and seminar.

Synanon members live in a large community home having an environment like that of a therapeutic milieu. Physicians, psychologists, nurses, and social workers supervise, counsel, and guide the work done by the ex-addicts who staff the house and actively assist with the program. Ramirez describes progressive steps of treatment utilized with the basic Synanon approach. The first step is to contact the addict in the community and encourage him to enter a medical facility to be withdrawn from the drug. After detoxification, the addict lives in a residential center and participates in group living and therapy. In the third phase, the addict is assigned to work making contacts with addicts in the community and as an aide in the medical treatment center. His response to treatment and work assignments are evaluated before he is certified as rehabilitated. After this, the ex-addict may choose to work with the program as an employee, if he qualifies in competition with others, or to do other work. He is eligible for vocational training, individual treatment and counseling, and educational opportunities sponsored by the program. He also agrees to cooperate with any follow-up procedures which may be required for research purposes. It may take as long as three years for an addict to be certified. The employed ex-addicts are trained to lead group sessions which are held weekly or when specially called to discuss some immediate happening constituting a crisis situation or problem which involves and requires group action. Unlike regular group therapy, the membership of each Synanon meeting is always different. This prevents members from forming emotional ties that would promote mutual agreements between them to prevent the revelation of emotionally painful material at a meeting. The basic Synanon approach is "attack." The participants criticize weaknesses and censor certain behavior. The objective is to help the addict face reality, gain insight, and develop self-awareness and the strength to resist and abandon "the habit." An active social program, including recreational and occupational therapy is maintained. Weekly meetings with family members and visitors are held in the home. Special meetings on topics of interest, led by an outside speaker and followed by group discussion, are held regularly. The success of the treatment plan is attributed largely to the understanding of the ex-addict which is reflected in his work with other addicts. In addition, working with patients undergoing treatment is a reminder to him of what he once was and constitutes a preventive social control.

PROGNOSIS

Although a few patients manage to abstain from drugs for periods of a few to five or six years following withdrawal treatment and rehabilitation, many of these persons tend to relapse into the habit. Most authorities believe that a complete cure is rare. The early reports and follow-up studies of addicts treated in a Synanon home have been encouraging. It is hoped that as more centers are established, there will be a more hopeful outlook toward recovery from drug addiction.

ADDICTION TO COCAINE

Cocaine, derived from the cocoa plant, is a drug to which sociopathic persons become addicted.

The intravenous route of injection is usually preferred, owing to rapid effects of the drug's action. Subcutaneous injection produces abscess and scar formation.

Addiction to cocaine always occurs as a result of association with cocaine addicts, who induce individuals to acquire the habit and assist each other in procurement of the drug and other habit-forming drugs, especially morphine and barbiturates.

Cocaine stimulates the cerebral cortex and produces a state of alertness, exhilaration, and a generalized feeling of ecstasy described by authors as similar to sexual orgasm. Under its immediate effects, the addict becomes active, talkative, gay and witty. When the effects of the drug wear off, the person becomes most irritable, and remains so until another dose is received. Malnutrition and emaciated appearance are observed about the addict, owing to cocaine's depressive effects upon the appetite. There is no evidence to indicate that cocaine addicts develop a tolerance for, and physiological dependence upon, the drug.

Persons addicted to cocaine do not as a rule use it continuously, but instead resort to its use for short debauches. To recapture fleeting sensations of ecstasy following injection, the individual has a compulsive tendency to repeat the injection of cocaine, as frequently as every 15 or 30 minutes, until the supply available is exhausted.

PHYSICAL AND MENTAL REACTIONS

Excessive stimulation of the cerebral cortex and sympathetic nervous system eventually produces extreme anxiety, fear, apprehension, tremors, formication, tachycardia and hypertension. Patients taking large daily doses may have marked psychotic reactions, manifested by visual and auditory hallucinations and delusions. They have been known to commit some of the most serious crimes during such periods, including murder and sexually perverse acts. Socially and morally, they regress to the lowest level. Morphine comes into use when the individual reacts fearfully to the development of severe anxiety and apprehension and attempts to counteract the cocaine effects.

TREATMENT

Emergency treatment of overactivity, apprehension, and anxiety with hallucinations and delusions is effective when one of the rapidly acting barbiturates such as pentobarbital is administered intravenously. Morphine is an effective antidote and is the one preferred by the addict.

PROGNOSIS

The prognosis is poor. It is worse when addiction to both cocaine and morphine is observed. Relapse frequently occurs. Many of these persons die from physical collapse or upper respiratory infections.

BARBITURATE POISONING AND ADDICTION

Acute barbiturate poisoning is frequently superimposed on barbiturate addiction. For that reason and because nurses often see the intoxicated reaction, it is discussed here. Barbiturates taken in excess of amounts prescribed for therapeutic purposes produce physical and emotional changes referred to as acute barbiturate poisoning. Occasionally an individual manifests a sensitive reaction to barbiturates, but most frequently the condition results from a suicidal attempt. Approximately 1500 deaths occur from barbiturate poisoning each year in the United States. It is more common in women than in men, in persons ranging in age from 30 to 50 years than in older or younger persons, and in urban areas than in rural districts. Barbiturate addiction complicates about half of all cases of morphine addiction. Many of these individuals are also addicted to alcohol.

Chronic addiction to barbiturates is always associated with some psychiatric disorder, usually a psychoneurosis or personality disorder. Neuroses associated with anxiety and insomnia are particularly important psychogenic factors. Barbiturates diminish anxiety and ego controls and allow the person to act out a solution for, or satisfy directly, basic primitive drives. The mechanisms underlying an individual's tolerance to, and physical dependence upon, barbiturates is not completely understood. The drugs most commonly used are Nembutal (pentobarbital), Seconal (secobarbital), Amytal (amobarbital), Luminal (phenobarbital), and barbital.

Barbiturate addicts may use these drugs while on a spree of less than 24 hours, or they may resort to them for debauches lasting from a few days to several weeks. Barbiturates may also be taken in large daily doses for months or years.

EFFECTS OF DRUG

Barbiturates produce depressive effects upon the central nervous system. The particular drug, dosage taken, and the lapse of time between ingestion and identification of the reaction influence the physiological reaction. Rapidly acting barbiturates, such as Nembutal and Seconal, produce coma quickly, but recovery is also relatively rapid. Barbital and phenobarbital produce coma slowly, but recovery is also slow. The difference is due in part to variations in the speed of the detoxification of the particular drugs and their storage in fat depots.

TYPES OF REACTIONS

There are four grades or depths of reactions observed, ranging from a mild reaction in which the patient is asleep but can be aroused to answer questions to a comatose condition in which body reflexes are absent and there is respiratory or circulatory depression or both. Although the patient may be comatose, in all except the mildest reaction the body reflexes are intact in the first two grades. Respiration and circulation are seriously depressed in the fourth or deepest grade.[4] Differentiation of these reactions is important in prescribing treatment and influences the prognosis.

Pneumonia is one of the most serious, and sometimes fatal, complications.

DIAGNOSTIC SIGNS

Acute barbiturate poisoning resembles alcoholic intoxication except that the patient's complexion is pale instead of flushed. In addition, there is an absence of alcohol odor about the patient unless the individual has consumed both drugs. A diagnosis can sometimes be established with information furnished by relatives or a conscious patient. When the patient is unable to respond and relatives are absent, an immediate diagnosis may be made by observing the physical signs and the discovery of empty bottles, pills or capsules in the victim's residence. Parts of colored capsules are often found in the patient's mouth or in the gastric contents when a lavage is performed.

TREATMENT

Treatment of barbiturate poisoning depends upon the severity of the patient's reaction. Patients manifesting mild reactions require no special treatment, but should be carefully observed and kept awake by repeated stimulation. Talking to the patient, walking him about, and giving him coffee are all stimulating measures. Selective stimulating drugs, such as caffeine sodium benzoate or amphetamine sulfate, may be prescribed by the physician for patients manifesting moderate reactions. Gastric lavage is performed only if barbiturates have been ingested within a few hours preceding admission of the patient to the hospital. There is always the risk of lavage producing pulmonary aspiration. Therefore, great care must be taken to avoid misplacing the tube into the lung. Hemodialysis may also be used, especially for those patients who have ingested large amounts of long-acting barbiturates.

Treatment of the deepest grade of barbiturate intoxication is an emergency procedure. The patient should be placed in a semiprone position with one hip elevated and the bed raised in the middle. The patient's dentures are removed, and his mouth and pharynx kept free of mucus.

Adequate pulmonary ventilation must be maintained. An airway is inserted and kept open and clean. In the most severe cases an endotracheal tube may be required. Measures are taken to combat circulatory collapse. If the patient is in shock, a plasma expander or a transfusion of whole blood is administered. In severe poisoning, an approved type of automatic positive pressure respirator or an external (Drinker) respirator is used. Artificial respiration may have to be carried on for days.

After recovery from an intoxication reaction, it should be ascertained whether or not the patient is addicted to barbiturates. If so, barbiturate intake is restored until the patient's condition permits the commencement of the withdrawal syndrome.

Barbiturates should not be withdrawn abruptly, owing to the possibility of severe abstinence reactions and a fatal convulsion. Gradual, carefully regulated abstinence is recommended. Dosage is reduced each day or every few days as indicated by the patient's reaction. If the patient becomes extremely anxious, develops insomnia or becomes tremulous during the withdrawal procedure, reduction of the drug should be stopped temporarily until these symptoms subside. Withdrawal should always be carried out in a hospital where it is possible for the medical staff to maintain control of the treatment environment.

A patient admitted under ordinary conditions to a hospital for purposes of treatment of chronic addiction to barbiturates and barbiturate withdrawal should be supervised during the admission procedure and thereafter, as is done with persons addicted to opiates (see p. 390).

REHABILITATION

Attention to the patient's physical needs, diet, rest, exercise and recreation is important during the convalescence stage, following withdrawal of drugs to which persons are addicted. Social psychiatric rehabilitation is of vital importance but often impossible to achieve. Unfortunately, the addict usually returns to the same environment and conditions which were partly responsible for his addiction. Many local social service agencies, too, resist accepting and aiding drug addicts.

PROGNOSIS

The prognosis in mild and moderate barbiturate poison reactions is excellent. It is grave when the reaction is severe, long, and when coma is deep. The prognosis in chronic barbiturate addiction is guarded. Relapse is very common.

MEPERIDINE HYDROCHLORIDE AND METHADONE

Meperidine hydrochloride (Demerol) and methadone (Adanon, Dolophine) are two synthetic drugs given to persons who do not tolerate morphine well. They are also administered to individuals afflicted with chronic conditions associated with mild grades of pain which cannot be controlled by nonaddicting medications. The analgesic effects of these two drugs is somewhat greater than codeine. It is claimed that they produce fewer undesirable reactions. Both meperidine and methadone have a distinct capacity to cause addiction, although tolerance to them is said to develop slowly. Withdrawal symptoms are not as severe as those observed in morphine addiction.

AMPHETAMINE

Amphetamine (Benzedrine) produces a pleasant feeling of well-being and accelerates psychomotor activity. Persons have been known to take this drug indiscriminately in an effort to remain alert and awake for longer than usual periods. The stimulating effect of Benzedrine is, however, followed by fatigue and feelings of depression. Individuals with poorly organized personalities have a tendency to become addicted. Increasing use of the drug produces tolerance and requires larger doses to effect the desired stimulation.

MARIHUANA

Marihuana cigarettes, called "joints," do not produce a biologic dependence. Following inhalation, the individual smoking marihuana feels calm, relaxed, confident, pleasant, and somewhat euphoric. These feelings subside with a few hours of sleep. Owing to the type of social contacts maintained by persons using marihuana, these individuals often become addicted, in due time, to opiates. Use of marihuana has also been known to precipitate a psychotic reaction in individuals with poorly organized personalities. Investigators have pointed out that the use of marihuana does not lead to criminal habits and that alcohol is responsible for more crimes than all of the addicting drugs combined.

HALLUCINOGENIC DRUGS

Self experimentation with the so called psychedelic or "mind expanding" drugs has been a grave medical-social problem during the past several years. Unfortunately, some intellectuals of the collegiate community have appealed to students to use these drugs for the purpose of enlarging their perception, gaining new insights, and releasing their blocked creative powers. Silocybin and Mescaline have been used, but Lysergic acid diethylamide (LSD) has been the most widely used and publicized hallucinogenic drug. The mechanical action of these substances is unknown. Their usefulness in the treatment of mental illness is still in the experimental stage. While some persons using hallucinogenic drugs have reported feeling reactions of rapture, others have experienced fear and simulated or prolonged psychotic episodes. After taking these drugs, an individual may have symptoms of tachycardia, dilation of pupils, chest and abdominal tightness, and nausea, followed by vivid hallucinations, severe anxiety, and delusions. It is true that smoking marihuana, glue sniffing, and LSD "trips" do not produce classical addiction. However, they have been known to produce panic states, uncontrolled aggression, suicidal and homicidal behavior. Some reports also indicate that LSD may do damage to chromosomes. Thus, it is possible that a young person "exploring inner space" may be taking a drug capable of temporarily disorganizing his mental processes and producing long range genetic changes that may affect future generations. These hazardous possibilities are sufficient reason to restrict their availability and use to legitimate scientifically controlled research. When indiscriminately taken for self experimentation, their use is correctly labelled as drug abuse.[5]

SUGGESTED REFERENCES

Beeson, P. B., and McDermott, W.: Cecil-Loeb Textbook of Medicine, ed. 13. W. B. Saunders Co., Philadelphia, 1971, p. 147.

Elliott, H.: Acute barbiturate poisoning. Hosp. Med. 2: 7 (Jan.), 1966.

Fink, M., Freedman, A., et al.: Narcotic antagonists: another approach to addiction therapy. Am. J. Nurs. 71: 1359 (July), 1971.

Freedman, A.: The narcotic addict in the general hospital. Ment. Hosp. 16: 230 (Aug.), 1965.

Freedman, A., and Kaplan, H. (eds.): Comprehensive Textbook of Psychiatry, ed. 1. The Williams & Wilkins Co., Baltimore, 1967, p. 989.

Garb, S.: Narcotic addiction in nurses and doctors. Nurs. Outlook 13: 30 (Nov.), 1965.

Kolb, L.: Noyes' Modern Clinical Psychiatry, ed. 7. W. B. Saunders Co., Philadelphia, 1968, p. 516.

Kromberg, C., and Proctor, J.: Methadone maintenance—evolution of a day program. Am. J. Nurs. 70: 2575 (Dec.), 1970.

Osnos, R.: A community counseling center for addicts. Nurs. Outlook 13: 38 (Nov.), 1965.

Pearson, B.: Methadone maintenance in heroin addiction—the program at Beth Israel Medical Center. Am. J. Nurs. 70: 2571 (Dec.), 1970.

Ramirez, E.: Help for the addict. Am. J. Nurs. 67: 2348 (Nov.), 1967.

Rohde, I.: Panic in the streets. Nurs. Outlook 13: 45 (Nov.), 1965.

Rodewald, R.: Speed kills: the adolescent methedrine addict. Perspect. Psychiat. Care 8: 160 (Jul.-Aug.), 1970.

Rodman, M.: Drug therapy today: drugs used against addiction. R.N. 33: 71 (Oct.), 1970.

Rodman, M., and Smith, D.: Pharmacology and drug therapy in nursing. J. B. Lippincott Co., Philadelphia, 1968, pp. 11, 43.

Taylor, S.: Addicts as patients. Nurs. Outlook 13: 41 (Nov.), 1965.

FOOTNOTES

1. Council on Mental Health: Report on narcotic addiction. J.A.M.A. 165: 1839 (Dec.), 1957.
2. Kolb, L.: Noyes' Modern Clinical Psychiatry, ed. 7. W. B. Saunders Co., Philadelphia, 1968, p. 522.
3. Ramirez, E.: Help for the addict. Am. J. Nurs. 67: 2348 (Nov.), 1967.
4. Beeson, P. B., and McDermott, W.: Cecil-Loeb Textbook of Medicine, ed. 13. W. B. Saunders Co., Philadelphia, 1971, p. 147.
5. Rodman, M., and Smith, D.: Pharmacology and Drug Therapy in Nursing. J. B. Lippincott Co., Philadelphia, 1968, p. 43.

CHAPTER 32

Alcoholism and Its Intoxication Effects upon Behavior: Nursing Care

According to Thompson, an alcoholic is a person who uses alcohol in sufficient amounts to impair his efficiency or to interfere with his occupational, social, or economic adjustment. When a person is unable to avoid the repeated use of intoxicating alcoholic beverages he is considered an alcoholic.[1]

SOCIAL ASPECTS

Alcoholism is a major public health problem. Recognition of alcoholism as an illness, social problem, and social responsibility came in 1944, with the establishment of the National Committee on Alcoholism and the Yale Plan Clinic in New Haven, Connecticut. Some psychiatric hospitals still do not admit alcoholics for treatment. Efforts are being directed toward treating them in special hospitals.

Statistics indicate that five out of six alcoholics are men between 30 and 55 years of age. Thus, the most productive years of these persons' lives are lost to society. Increasing demands and responsibilities during this same period of life are also important factors to consider in the evaluation of alcoholism and its effects.

DRINKING PATTERNS

Some persons are able to take a cocktail or two and stop drinking when they desire. These individuals are thought of as social drinkers who conform and oblige the group in order to be accepted and approved. Another type of social drinker, who is shy and somewhat inhibited in a group, feels at ease, enhanced and more comfortable after a drink or two.

Thus, indulgence facilitates the socialization process. Alcoholics continue to drink after they have tasted the first drink. It is often difficult for the social drinker to understand why other people drink excessively.

ETIOLOGY, DYNAMICS

While many individual factors, including culture, environment, health, psychosexual development and interpersonal relations, appear to contribute to the development of alcoholism, it is generally believed that underlying fear and anxiety, associated with some pressing inner conflict, motivates the alcoholic to drink. These persons usually cannot identify or verbalize their basic conflict with its associated feelings. Alcoholics have poor super-ego control and a low tolerance for stress, strain and frustration. Reactivation of the inner conflict produces unbearable fear and anxiety. Alcohol, being a depressant, aids in relaxing the individual. By its action, however, it also lowers the capacity for use of the repression mechanism, and releases inhibitions, hostility, and primitive drives. Following a drinking episode, the alcoholic develops fear of retaliation, guilt, and anxiety. These feelings are intensified when family members and associates reprimand or reject him because of his behavior. Thus, a vicious circle of behavior is established. Feelings of anxiety and guilt cause the alcoholic to become completely dependent upon alcohol to ease the discomfort of threatening influences. Many persons, who resort to alcohol, drink as if obsessed with a compulsion to do so whenever anxiety arises.

Alcoholics may not be thought of as belonging to a group having a definite type of personality, but they do have some common characteristics of personality. Superficially they are often attractive, charming, warm, friendly, and give the impression of reliability. Beneath this behavior, however, they are immature, unstable, stubborn, often impulsive, unreliable and irresponsible. Goals in life are usually lacking or poorly organized and directed. These persons have poor relationships with others, are very sensitive to personal criticism, react childishly toward authority, and have a tendency to blame other individuals for their own shortcomings and failures. They often represent themselves as abused, misunderstood, and victims of circumstances. Basically, alcoholics have deep inner feelings of inferiority, insecurity, fear of rejection, and anxiety. Feelings of resentment and hostility are harbored during periods of stress and strain until alcohol permits their release. Many of these persons have histories of early-life psychological trauma and are fixed at the oral level of personality development. They have strong dependency needs. Inability to identify with a stable figure is considered a reason for their lack of super-ego control. Many alcoholics have problems in sexual adjustment; some make unsuccessful heterosexual adjustments, some are promiscuous, and others have conscious or unconscious homosexual tendencies. Sexual conflicts may be a cause or result of alcohol indulgence.

MENTAL AND PHYSICAL EFFECTS

When the alcoholic becomes intoxicated, his behavior is obviously in marked contrast to his usual behavior and that of the social drinker, who appears to be stable and well-adjusted. The excessive drinker may suddenly become overly gay, friendly, talkative, impulsive, hostile, profane, and boastful. At times he may be moved to tears and self-pity. Once these persons commence to drink, they may continue to do so for hours and even days, with apparent disregard for family, occupation and financial responsibilities. In the home, they may become abusive and cruel. When confronted with these behavior changes, alcoholics become evasive, facetious, and vague. They are known to gloss over and defend discreditable behavior of other persons, which is interpreted as identification with and defense of their own behavior.

Habitual intoxication produces a reduction in interests, ambition, job efficiency, and impairment of judgment and other intellectual functions. Eventually these persons develop an overwhelming craving for alcohol, and deteriorate mentally. Most of their time is spent in pursuit of a drink or the means to procure it. Social and moral regression takes place. Alcoholics have been known to cheat, lie and steal. As they regress, they become careless and slovenly in personal habits and appearance. They may go for days without food when drinking; thus, their physical health declines and they become emaciated. Many habitual drinkers are transient workers, live in cheap hotels; sleep in alleys, gutters, or on park benches; and live a day-to-day, hand-to-mouth existence. They often resort to begging from others.

TYPES OF ALCOHOLISM

PATHOLOGICAL INTOXICATION

This usually occurs in persons who are emotionally unstable and often possess an epileptic or hysterical temperament. Marked pathological behavior manifested in confusion, disorientation, delusions, illusions, hallucinations, over-activity, or severe depression and suicidal attempts may be observed. These reactions occur suddenly, and may last for a few minutes or hours after such an individual consumes a small amount of alcohol. The reaction is usually followed by a prolonged sleep from which the person awakens with amnesia for the episode.

DELIRIUM TREMENS

Delirium tremens usually develops acutely in the chronic alcoholic following an unusually severe or prolonged period of drinking. This type of reaction is rarely observed in persons under the age of 30 years, or those who have been drinking for less than three or four years. The cause of delirium tremens is unknown, but it is thought to be due to faulty body metabolism or the absorption of toxins from the gastrointestinal tract. This results in edema of the brain and increased spinal fluid pressure. Quite often, these reactions appear to follow an acute injury or infection which may possibly lower the person's resistance to the toxic process. Delirium tremens is characterized by tremors, restlessness, illusions, hallucinations, persecutory delusions, great fear, and anxiety. Patients who are severely ill usually have high temperature elevations, furred tongue, foul breath, and cracked mucous membranes, are dehydrated and may have convulsive seizures. They often pick at the bed clothing, jump at the slightest approach from others, and express fears of bugs, ants, and other insects crawling over them. Their illusions and hallucinations include visions of animals and other strange objects. In their confusion and fear, they often attempt to get out of bed to run from some expected danger. These reactions may last from three to ten days. Convalescence follows a prolonged sleep. Complications of pneumonia and heart failure may terminate in death.

ACUTE HALLUCINOSIS homosexual origins

This is psychogenic in origin and resembles a schizophrenic reaction. Such reactions usually are precipitated by prolonged and excessive drinking. Frequently the persons afflicted have a history of unconscious and unrecognized homosexual tendencies and unsuccessful heterosexual adjustment. Such a reaction is manifested in symptoms of great fear, auditory hallucinations, visual illusions, ideas of reference, and delusions. Voices which they hear accuse them of sexual promiscuity, homosexuality, and perversion. They may respond with expressions of anger, depression, and suicidal attempts. Eventually these persons are usually diagnosed as paranoid schizophrenics.

KORSAKOFF'S PSYCHOSIS

This was first described by the Russian psychiatrist, Sergei Korsakoff. It occurs more frequently in women than in men and in persons who have indulged in chronic drinking for several years. The reaction is caused by degeneration in the cerebrum and peripheral nerves, owing to a dietary and vitamin B deficiency. The distinguishing symptoms of remote and recent memory impairment, confabulation, absent knee jerks, and pain over the nerve trunks may follow an episode of delirium tremens, or may occur independently. The subjects become evasive and jocular in their verbal responses in an attempt to conceal their amnesia. Symptomatic treatment produces only temporary improvement. These individuals do not regain insight, but eventually develop permanent intellectual and esthetic deterioration.

ALCOHOLIC PARANOIA homosexual origins

This is thought to be due to repressed homosexual impulses which give rise to conflicts which the person attempts to resolve with indulgence in alcohol. Thus, a circle of conflict, indulgence, and paranoid delusions continues without interruption. Actually, personality fixation and psychological conditions were favorable for the development of this reaction long before indulgence commenced. During the pre-psychotic period, these individuals are stubborn, suspicious, resentful of discipline, and project blame upon others. Later psychotic symptoms consist chiefly of delusions of jealousy and infidelity, which are motivated by fear and guilt feelings arising from basic homosexual impulses. These individuals tend to socialize with members of the same sex. Continued indulgence may increase their sexual impotence which intensifies their insecurity and incompetence feelings.

TREATMENT OF ALCOHOLISM

Treatment of alcoholism commences with the relief of acute symptoms, such as delirium, overactivity, dehydration, and vitamin deficiency. The immediate treatment objectives are to relax the patient, induce sleep, and restore body fluids and vitamins.

Alcohol may be withdrawn abruptly or gradually from the patient, depending upon the physician's treatment preference. Many doctors prefer the gradual withdrawal procedure, because the physical reactions are reduced in intensity and the danger of collapse is not as great. Patients undergoing withdrawal often become irritable, difficult to manage, plead for alcohol, and may react with physical symptoms of tremors, insomnia, and fear. Critically ill patients in delirium tremens with high temperature elevations require most careful observation, treatment, and care. Complications of circulatory collapse, pneumonia, and meningitis are not uncommon, and fatalities may occur.

Although some physicians still prefer paraldehyde as a sedative, some of the new tranquilizing drugs are being used considerably.

Dependent upon the individual patient's condition, some doctors prescribe a few insulin treatments to utilize carbohydrates, induce sleep and aid in alcohol elimination, through diaphoresis. Fluids are given freely, as well as parenteral injections of vitamin B. Patients must be carefully observed. Convulsions indicate that treatment should be terminated and emergency measures instituted.

Critically ill patients who are near exhaustion are usually given a 5 per cent glucose in saline infusion. Vitamin B and a small dose of insulin are usually added to the infusion. This treatment is ordinarily repeated until the patient improves.

All treatment approaches are usually followed up with daily parenteral injections of vitamin B. Liver extract is frequently prescribed. A high caloric diet with plenty of fluid is given. Later, oral vitamins are administered.

Psychotherapy is considered to be the most essential and helpful of all treatments. An effort is made to help the patient to recognize his innermost conflict and resolve it. No treatment, however, can be successful unless the alcoholic possesses the will to overcome the habit, and strives continuously toward that goal.

REHABILITATION

Psychiatric social rehabilitation is difficult but most important. Unfortunately, these persons are often rejected by other, better-adjusted individuals who could, by accepting the ex-alcoholic, contribute to his social rehabilitation. Thus, the patient is more or less forced back into his old environment and group setting with persons who often constitute an unstable social influence.

ALCOHOLICS ANONYMOUS

Alcoholics Anonymous organizations have been formed all over the United States. This group, founded by two ex-alcoholics, utilizes the principle of group psychotherapy among its members. Meetings are held in their club rooms regularly, and members find companionship and considerable understanding in this environment. Persons join the organization voluntarily and endeavor to abide by its well-known Twelve Steps. The first step consists of an admission, on the individual's part, that he is addicted to alcohol. This is considered the most difficult thing for the alcoholic to do. Later, at open group meetings, many patients willingly discuss their illness and its development. In doing so, they attempt to identify their conflicts and feelings which motivated habitual drinking and describe how they were able to overcome excessive drinking. The alcoholic who is listening is, thereby, encouraged to discover that he is not so different from many others. Indirectly he learns how alcohol has been, and can be, avoided. The organization encourages its members to contact headquarters immediately whenever they feel they may relapse into excessive drinking. When this occurs, a member who has discontinued drinking and is considered capable aids the other member, remaining with him until the overwhelming craving has been conquered. Many patients claim they have received help in overcoming the habit through this organization, and physicians have commended the group's work.

PROGNOSIS

The prognosis is guarded. It is generally believed that the chances for recovery are increased when the condition is treated in its very early stages of development. Many patients relapse into the habit; complete recoveries are rare.

NURSING CARE

When the patient is hospitalized for treatment of acute symptoms he must be kept in a quiet environment, free from exciting influences. Delirious alcoholic patients often manifest a state of physical exhaustion, dehydration, and elevated body temperature. In some instances, physical depletion, delirium, and tremors require immediate treatment constituting emergency care. During this period, usually a few days, careful observation of the patient's physical condition as well as protective nursing measures are essential. These patients may be so restless, confused, and fearful that they may become resistive toward nursing personnel and difficult to protect. They can be prevented from falling out of bed and injuring themselves by placing them in a crib bed. Restraint of any type is undesirable because it may increase their fears, cause them to struggle, and may result in a circulatory collapse.

Well-lit rooms help to reduce the fears and illusory experiences of delirious alcoholic patients. Shadows cast by bright corridor lights upon the walls and ceiling of a dimly lit or darkened room may be stimuli which induce illusions of animals, bugs, or other disturbing objects.

Because these patients are often in poor physical condition and incontinent they need to be kept clean, dry, warm, and protected from drafts and upper respiratory infections. Sudden, abrupt approaches can be very frightening and stimulating. The nurse should always approach quietly and speak gently to these patients. When it is necessary to move or turn them, change their bed linen, or administer medications and treatments the nurse should explain what she is going to do before starting the procedure. When the patient is too weak and tremulous to drink from a cup or feeder the nurse may spoon-feed the fluid into the side of his mouth, allowing it to trickle slowly down into the alimentary tract, reducing the possibility of aspiration.

To understand the alcoholic, it is important to look beyond the symptoms and learn about the person. These patients are in need of physical as well as social rehabilitation. Attention to their rest, diet, personal hygiene, and appearance is important for reasons of health and morale. Once they begin to feel better they usually want to be discharged from the hospital and will express the belief that they do not require further treatment and can manage to abstain from alcohol without supervision. Such reactions are indications of their lack of insight into the emotional aspects of their illness.

During the recovery-rehabilitation period the acceptance of the patient by the nurse is very important because the patient has previously experienced rejection in the home and social environment following drinking episodes. The nurse's acceptance may be the action which encourages the patient to socialize and participate in planned ward activities. Because the alcoholic patient has inferiority feelings and a low self-esteem the nurse's participation in conversation, ward activities, and occasions of some comradeship are supportive approaches.

The nurse should be aware of these patients' tendency to rationalize their behavior and to seek sympathy and special privileges which would set them apart from the patient group. It is well to listen but also to recognize that emotionally it is difficult for them to perceive the reality of their behavior. Many of these patients are attractive and have a magnetic-like influence upon people. It is not unusual for nursing personnel to be won over to their way of thinking to the extent of being overly sympathetic instead of empathetic.

The compulsion to drink is quite strong in the chronic alcoholic patient. The patient may make efforts to smuggle alcohol into the hospital. It is important to be aware that this could happen and to prevent liquor from being brought into the premises. Patients may also leave the hospital with or without permission and return intoxicated. The nurse should receive the patient without commenting about the condition observed. The occurrence should be referred to the physician.

Because many of these persons cannot afford to be absent from employment or to finance prolonged treatment in a hospital, some community mental hygiene clinics have arranged special hours for them to receive continued therapy.

The public health nurse has an important role in the care and rehabilitation of alcoholic patients and their families. It is said that the marital partner is always involved in the psychological processes of the alcoholic. Reciprocal relationships between husband and wife are often seen. As the patient improves, the adjustment of the spouse frequently deteriorates. The spouse is often ambivalent about the patient's recovery as if deriving neurotic satisfaction from being needed—a response which may be on an unconscious level. The inadequacy of the sick partner makes the mate feel needed and more adequate. Conversations of such spouses revolve around having to struggle to keep the family together, being both mother and father to the children, and like topics. Wives of alcoholic patients have also been observed to resent the husband's therapist whom they view as a threat to their control of the patient. The nurse going into such a home environment is challenged to withhold any negative feelings she may recognize in her reactions to such observations.

Nurses can encourage the spouse to join Alanon, the associate group of the Alcoholics Anonymous organization. Members of Alanon endeavor to learn about alcoholism in an effort to understand better the effects of their relationships with the alcoholic patient. In some instances they may be able to get a spouse to receive psychiatric consultation. A censoring marital partner is less likely to influence the alcoholic to abstain from drinking than is a noncensoring one. The nurse who gains the confidence of the family may be able to identify medical, psychological, economic and social problems for which community assistance is available from such agencies as Child Welfare, Public Assistance, Vocational Rehabilitation, Child Guidance, and family services. She is also in a position to interpret the family situation to school teachers who may be attempting to resolve problems of children reared in disturbed home environments of alcoholic patients.

Although many alcoholic patients may never be completely cured, they can improve. A patient who has never been sober for more than a few days or weeks over a period of years may abstain from drinking for six months following hospitalization, treatment, and follow-up care. The patient may drink again at the end of that period, but maintenance of the longer period of sobriety indicates improvement. From the realistic viewpoint it is important for the nurse to anticipate improvement instead of complete cures and to appreciate it as progress for the patient when it does occur.

Attitudes shown toward an alcoholic patient's relapse should be no different than those expressed toward relapses occurring in association with other illnesses. Expressions of kindness and being nonjudgmental, accepting, consistent, and understanding in approach influence favorable relationships which affect the alcoholic patient's response to treatment.

SUGGESTED REFERENCES

Alcoholism, addiction, depression: nurse's story. Nurs. Outlook 13: 48 (Nov.), 1965.
Block, M.: Alcoholism is many illnesses. Nurs. Outlook 13: 35 (Nov.), 1965.
Chafetz, M., Blane, H., and Hill, M.: Children of alcoholics: observations in a child guidance clinic. Ment. Health Digest 4: 35 (Feb.), 1972.
Coulter, B.: Our whole community is helping to fight alcoholism. R.N. 28: 52 (Dec.), 1965.
Fowler, G.: Understanding the patient who uses alcohol to solve his problems. Nurs. Forum 4: 61, 1965.
Gelperin, A., and Gelperin, E.: The inebriate in the emergency room. Ment. Health Digest 2: 33 (Nov.), 1970.
Hoff, E. (ed.): Aspects of Alcoholism. J. B. Lippincott Co., Philadelphia, 1966. (Printed for Hoffman-LaRoche Laboratories, Nutley, New Jersey.)
Johnson, M.: Nurses speak out on alcoholism. Nurs. Forum 4: 16, 1965.
Kimmel, M.: Antabuse in a clinic program. Am. J. Nurs. 7: 1173 (June), 1971.
Kolb, L.: Noyes' Modern Clinical Psychiatry, ed. 7. W. B. Saunders Co., Philadelphia, 1968, p. 193.
Mechanic, D., and Sewell, B.: Community action and alcohol rehabilitation. Ment. Hyg. 49: 288 (April), 1965.
Moore, M.: An account of a nurse's role and functions in an alcoholic treatment program. J. Psychiat. Nurs. 8: 21 (May-June), 1970.
Morton, E.: Nursing care in an alcoholic unit. Nurs. Outlook 14: 45 (Oct.), 1966.
Price, G.: Alcoholism—A family, community, and nursing problem. Am. J. Nurs. 67: 1022 (May), 1967.

FOOTNOTES

1. Thompson, G.: Acute and Chronic Alcoholic Conditions. American Handbook of Psychiatry, Vol. II. Basic Books, Inc., New York, 1959, p. 203.

CHAPTER 33

Behavior of Patients Having Convulsive Disorders: Nursing Care

The chief manifestation of convulsive disorders is a seizure. Seizures vary in type. They are usually characterized by recurrent episodes of changes in the state of consciousness which may or may not be accompanied by convulsive movements or disturbances in feeling or behavior or both. Epilepsy, a term derived from the Greek word meaning to be seized or fall upon, was formerly considered a disease entity. It is now regarded as a symptom complex characterized by occurrences of convulsive seizures. Convulsive seizures may be acquired or idiopathic.

ETIOLOGY

Acquired, symptomatic seizures may be precipitated by head trauma, fever, infection, neoplasms, degenerative brain disease, abrupt abstinence from continuous ingestion of drugs, and neurosurgery. Symptomatic seizures are usually acute reactions which often subside with alleviation of the precipitating cause. Idiopathic epilepsy is the spontaneous occurrence of convulsive seizures which cannot be attributed to any known underlying pathologic state. Some investigators believe that in this type of seizure there is some inherited or constitutional flaw in the brain which causes the nerve cells to discharge explosively.

RESEARCH REPORTED

More than 75 years ago, Doctor John Hughlings Jackson postulated that convulsions were accompanied by an abnormal discharge of energy in the cerebral cortex of the brain. Doctor William Lennox, well-known investigator of epileptic disorders, later applied the term "cerebral dys-

411

rhythmia" to this discharge phenomenon. Jackson's theory was confirmed in 1929 with the development of the electroencephalogram by Doctor Hans Berger of Germany. While the electroencephalogram reveals the presence of cerebral dysrhythmia in the graphic record produced during the course of a patient's examination, it fails to reveal the underlying pathogenesis. Thus, considerable research into the etiologic basis of convulsive disorders is still in progress.

There is a tendency to consider epilepsy as a central nervous system reaction to an injurious stimulus. Convulsive seizures are probably produced by a variety of internal and external stimuli. Some investigators believe that a hereditary predisposition plus a precipitating factor is required for the development of convulsive disorders. The predisposition may remain dormant in the person if the precipitating factor can be avoided.

A most distinctive brain wave pattern observed in the electroencephalogram is associated with the production of convulsive seizures. This same pattern persists during the interval between attacks. It is of interest to know that this typical brain wave pattern may also be observed in the electroencephalograms of persons who have never manifested a convulsive seizure. The pattern has also been observed in a large percentage of records of parents and near relatives of individuals afflicted with epilepsy. The occurrence is eight times greater in both identical twins than in fraternal twins. This evidence has led to the hypothesis that persons who demonstrate cerebral dysrhythmias in their electroencephalograms possess a hereditary predisposition and might develop convulsive seizures in the presence of precipitating factors. The possibility that some parents are carriers of the disorder has been considered. However, heredity is still a controversial issue among researchers.[1]

TYPES OF CONVULSIVE SEIZURES

There are several types of convulsive seizures, but four main types are recognized by most authorities: grand mal, petit mal, psychomotor, and jacksonian.

GRAND MAL

This is known as the major type of epileptic seizure. A large number of patients experience an aura (premonition), usually just previous to the seizure. Feelings of nausea, numbness, tingling sensation, or headache may represent the aura in some persons. Some individuals experience a subjective impression of bright flashing lights. Investigators are of the opinion that the particular aura may indicate the initial site of energy discharge.

Many patients elicit a sharp, piercing cry just previous to the attack. The patient falls to the floor or ground, loses consciousness, and presents a general picture of body rigidity at the start of the seizure. This is called the "tonic phase." The clonic phase follows soon after, and is characterized by generalized muscular twitchings of the entire body and stertorous breathing. The patient usually froths at the mouth, becomes cyanotic, and may be incontinent. Gradually the twitchings cease, and the person becomes relaxed. He usually falls into a deep sleep for several hours following this type of seizure and has an amnesia for the episode. Successive seizures without intervening recovery of consciousness are referred to as "status epilepticus," a condition which is more serious than a single attack and may be fatal if not treated.

The appearance of a grand mal seizure sometimes reveals the real meaning of minor symptoms which may have been obvious but disturbing and puzzling to family members, physicians, and other persons. Local muscle spasms, dreamlike states, mental blocking, and defects of attention may have been observed for lengthy periods, sometimes years.

PETIT MAL

There is an absence of the aura in petit mal seizures which are characterized by a fleeting loss of consciousness lasting from 5 to 30 seconds. These attacks begin and end abruptly. The patient does not fall but suddenly maintains a fixed posture, empty facial expression, stops whatever he is doing at the time, and drops anything he may have in his hands. Slight twitching of the eyelids, eyebrows, and head may be observed. Upon regaining consciousness, most patients are aware that a seizure has occurred, but some individuals may remain unaware. Petit mal seizures occur most frequently in children between the ages of 10 and 18 years. One, two, a few, or a great number of attacks may occur in one day. These seizures may disappear entirely or be replaced by other types. Many children afflicted with petit mal seizures develop grand mal seizures. Grand mal and petit mal attacks may coexist. Studies of petit mal seizures have revealed that they often occur in maladjusted children who harbor conscious or unconscious feelings of parental rejection and insecurity. Frequently these children are antagonistic and rebellious towards their parents.

PSYCHOMOTOR SEIZURES

Seizures that are not grand mal, petit mal, or jacksonian are generally considered to be psychomotor types. In appearance they may range from mild, dreamlike confusional states to more prolonged accentuations of a manifest mood, such as fear, depression, and irritability, to an advanced state known as the epileptic furor. The activities carried on by the person during psychomotor seizures are not recalled later, a reaction that is difficult for observers to understand owing to the impression received that the individual was acting with conscious awareness in spite of the so-called "blacking out" that is often claimed. During the epileptic furor the person may be responding to very vivid, frightening hallucinations, run berserk, and commit hazardous, homicidal, and destructive acts. This type of seizure as well as those in which personality characteristics of mood constitute the seizure are known as epileptic equivalents. Psychomotor seizures are observed more frequently in adults, have a tendency to increase with age, and may occur in combination with grand mal seizures.

JACKSONIAN SEIZURES

These seizures are characterized by a twitching or numbness of an extremity or side of the face, which may increase in severity. The patient does not usually lose consciousness. Neurologists are always interested in knowing the particular part of the body involved in the seizure (left or right side of face or extremity). The affected area may indicate that a focal lesion is present on the opposite side of the brain.

When the focal discharging lesion is in the occipital, parietal, or frontal lobes of the brain, the patient's symptoms are largely neurological. If the focal lesion is located in one or both temporal lobes, the clinical picture is predominantly psychiatric or that of psychomotor seizures. Therefore, it is important for nursing personnel to describe carefully their observations of all convulsive seizures so that the focal site may be identified.[1]

TREATMENT AND NURSING CARE

When the patient has a grand mal attack, he should be permitted to lie where he has fallen. His head should be protected from injury with a pillow or any suitable protective device immediately available. His bodily movements must never be restrained. Clothing about the person's neck and waist should be loosened. A soft gag or roll of bandage may be inserted between the patient's teeth to prevent injury to the tongue. Doctors advise against forcing a gag between the patient's teeth once his jaws are locked. Saliva should be wiped from the patient's mouth to prevent choking. This procedure also permits air to enter the respiratory system more readily. Some physicians administer phenobarbital sodium or Amytal Sodium (sodium amobarbital) intramuscularly following a grand mal seizure, usually to prevent a recurrent seizure.

OBSERVATIONS TO RECORD

The nurse or the person who is with the patient having a seizure should note and record the following:

1. Something about the situation and background in which the seizure occurred.
2. Was there any warning, outcry, or other premonitory sign?
3. Did it occur during the day or night? If at night, was the person asleep?
4. The duration of the convulsion as accurately as possible.
5. The duration of unconsciousness.
6. Was the convulsion generalized or limited? If the latter, to what part of the body?
7. Was there frothing at the mouth?
8. Was there incontinence of urine or feces?
9. What was the color of the face and extremities?
10. Was there perspiration?
11. Were the eyes rotated to one side? If so, which side?
12. Were the pupils of the eyes dilated?

Epileptic patients must be nursed in a quiet, nonstimulating environment. They are very sensitive to their surroundings and associates, and are less apt to develop seizures if they can be kept content and made to feel secure. These persons should be encouraged to carry on with normal activities. Most of them can attend to their immediate personal needs and hygiene.

PREVENTIVE MEDICATIONS, EDUCATION

For grand mal seizures, phenobarbital 0.1 gm. (1-1/2 grains), or Dilantin Sodium (diphenylhydantoin sodium), 0.1 gm. (1-1/2 grains), may be prescribed three times a day for adult patients to prevent subsequent attacks. When Dilantin is prescribed, the patient is frequently given phenobarbital, 0.06 gm. (1 grain), at bedtime. A combined preparation of Dilantin and phenobarbital (Phelantin) is also available. Mesantoin (methylphenylethyl hydantoin), 0.1 gm. (1-1/2 grains), may be prescribed for all types of seizures. Tridione (trimethadione), 0.3 gm. (5 grains), is prescribed for patients who suffer from petit mal attacks. Mysoline (primidone), 0.25 gm., may be prescribed initially for grand mal and psychomotor seizures. More recently some of the tranquilizing drugs, such as Thorazine (chlorpromazine) and Miltown (meprobamate), have been prescribed for the treatment of convulsive disorders. Evaluation of the effects of these drugs as compared with other medications is not complete.

Anticonvulsant drugs, being taken regularly, should not be discontinued abruptly owing to the possibility that the patient may develop status epilepticus.

Patients afflicted with a convulsive disorder should be urged to take prescribed medications faithfully. Authorities believe that this is a most important preventive measure since seizures appear to be more prevalent when this procedure is not practiced.

REHABILITATION

Recently, a great deal of literature has been distributed to lay persons in an attempt to enlist their support in aiding epileptic patients. Families of such patients are instructed in their management and encouraged to keep the home environment free from exciting influences.

Dr. William Lennox believes that two thirds of these persons can be successfully rehabilitated and employed in useful occupations if given an opportunity. He recommends that they be assisted with guidance and counseling for job placement. It is important that they be employed in occupations free from possible hazards. If the person likes his work and is content in his capacity, he can be most successfully rehabilitated.

SUGGESTED REFERENCES

Carozza, V.: Understanding the patient with epilepsy. Nurs. Clin. N. Am. 5: 13 (March), W. B. Saunders Co., Philadelphia, 1970.

Freedman, A., and Kaplan, H. (eds.): Comprehensive Textbook of Psychiatry, ed. 1. The Williams & Wilkins Co., Baltimore, 1967, p. 475.

Hayden, M.: Charting epileptic seizures. J. Psychiat. Nurs. 2: 570 (Nov.-Dec.), 1964.

Kolb, L.: Noyes' Modern Clinical Psychiatry, ed. 7. W. B. Saunders Co., Philadelphia, 1968, p. 259.

Maebius, N.: The nurse as an observer. Am. J. Nurs. 68: 2608 (Dec.), 1968.

Merritt, H.: A Textbook of Neurology. Lea & Febiger, Philadelphia, 1967, p. 753.

Neis, H.: The new look. J. Psychiat. Nurs. 7: 212 (Sept.-Oct.), 1969.

FOOTNOTES

1. Kolb, L.: Noyes' Modern Clinical Psychiatry, ed. 7. W. B. Saunders Co., Philadelphia, 1968, pp. 260, 262.

CHAPTER 34

Moods of Elation and Depression in Affective Behavior: Nursing Care

Affective reactions comprise those psychoses in which ideation and action appear to be characterized chiefly by a dominant affect. Contrasting affective states, elation and depression, might characterize the same patient during different reaction periods.

MANIC-DEPRESSIVE REACTIONS

The manic-depressive reactions or psychoses are characterized by mood swings of elation and depression. During these reactions there is a correlation between the symptoms observed and the particular predominant mood.

TYPES

Manic Type

Manic episodes are manifested in elated behavior and may vary in intensity from hypomania to hypermania. Some investigators believe there has been a decline in the prevalence of manic behavior in our culture.

An overly pleasant, euphoric mood may be the first sign of elated behavior. As the patient's mood increases, the individual may flit or prance about the ward gaily, dance, laugh, sing, and become talkative. Many ideas are expressed. The patient may construe or state plans to write a book, launch a new invention, etc. Much activity is proposed or started, but never completed.

Women patients often express their mood by indulging in heavy applications of cosmetics, striking color and dress schemes, floral and jewel

417

accessories, and flirtatious, coy behavior. The elated man may dress in amusing or abbreviated costumes of clothing, often designed by him from whatever is available in his wardrobe or the ward linen and decorative supply. It is apparent, during these periods of behavior, that manic-type individuals enjoy the attention they attract. To maintain control of the environment they resort to rhyming, punning, and exhibitionistic behavior. When elated behavior is allowed to continue, the patient becomes fatigued and demanding. When his demands are not met, he then becomes irritable, often sarcastic, and sometimes threatening.

During advanced manic phases, one may observe the patient boasting and expressing delusions of grandeur and self-importance. Irritability may be accompanied by delusions of persecution. What appears to be a hallucination is thought to be an attempt by the patient to dramatize a delusion. Elated persons are easily distracted by environmental influences and often express a flight of ideas (fragmentary speech with detectable thought connections). Their ability to retain and remember is usually good, the infrequent exception being during an extreme episode. They often do not eat or sleep well.

Depressed Type   withdrawn brooding

The depressed patient's behavior is in marked contrast to that of the manic. The individual's movements and verbal responses are obviously reduced and retarded. Delusions of guilt and unworthiness, which are often attached to and connected with trivial past incidents, are frequently expressed by the patient. Brooding, self-condemnation, and a hopeless outlook are manifested in the person's behavior. There is a loss of interest in personal appearance, the complexion is pale, and anorexia, weight loss, and insomnia prevail. The individual's attention may be gained when he is not unduly preoccupied. The ability to remember is usually good. Depressive episodes may vary in depth from mild to severe attacks.

Circular Type

This type, sometimes described as cyclic, is characterized by alternations between the manic and depressive moods. The duration of each mood is individualistic. Some patients remain in a particular mood for a few days or less, prior to the shift in affect. Others experience longer episodes of one or another of the dominant moods, prior to the change in affect. The manic mood is usually of shorter duration than the depressed mood. When these mood shifts occur, the observer becomes acutely aware of the marked difference in the patient's appearance, facial expression, and behavior as contrasted with the previous affect. This change is so striking that one has the feeling of observing and talking with an entirely different personality.

Mixed Type

During this type of reaction, the patient demonstrates coexisting manic and depressive moods. Physically, the person is overactive, restless, talkative, and paces about freely. Chain smoking by some patients may be observed. Emotionally the individual is depressed, apprehensive, tense, and fearful. While the patient demonstrates much physical energy, he often fails to attend to, or is unable to organize, his daily hygiene, personal care, and other simple requirements of living.

ETIOLOGY, DYNAMICS

While various theories have been advanced concerning the causes of manic-depressive reactions, none has been definitely accepted. Heredity is considered important by some investigators who have studied the family history of patients and discovered evidence of manic-depressive reactions in living or deceased relatives or both. Other scientists, however, discount the heredity theory by stating that most family histories would reveal some evidence of mental illness.

Some analysts believe that manic-depressive reactions are essentially a failure of the individual to function successfully in preserving internal emotional equilibrium. These disorders are conceived of as the end result of an internal psychological struggle between the patient's unconscious wishes and impulses and moral conscience.

Others view manic-depressive psychosis as an extroverted reaction. The manic phase represents the flight into reality by the patient to escape from his inner conflict into the environment where he is at the mercy of many distracting stimuli. The great activity constitutes a defense to ward off every possible source of danger that might affect him as the individual rushes from one to another as he keeps up a steady stream of activity. In his communications, there are often references to longed for past situations which have been repressed. Under the cloak of hyperactivity and flight of ideas, forbidden thoughts invade the conscious mind in a wish-fulfilling drama. It is not so much the nature of the conflict as it is the way in which the patient deals with it. Depression is the result of failing to deal adequately with the conflict, the defenses have failed and the patient is overwhelmed by his moral self and suffers from accusatory delusions.[1]

The personality structure of these patients has been described as oral in character, greedy, and demanding. They are emotionally immature individuals who can receive, but seldom give. Warm relationships, attention, acceptance, and approval are craved by them. They do not appear to be able to moderate or develop the use of a medium of expression which would ease the emotional discord within them. Instead, they attempt to resolve the internal struggle with the use of the mechanisms of repression and suppression, in efforts to forget and suppress their innermost cravings and conduct. When they become ill, these individuals resort chiefly to overt pathological use of the mechanisms of rationalization, projection, and introjection. The struggle between the individual's unconscious impulses and moral conscience produces feelings of hostility, guilt, and much anxiety. To relieve the internal discomfort of these psychological reactions, these persons project their long-retained feelings of hostility onto persons and objects in the environment, during a manic phase. Their demands, irritability, sarcasm, profanity, exhibitionist behavior, destructiveness and threats are manifestations of the projection of hostility. Persecutory delusions and accusations dispense with their feelings of guilt. During the depressive phase, hostility and guilt are introjected obviously toward the self, in suicidal tendencies, self-condemnation and expressions of the need for punishment. These patients rationalize by connecting their affective behavior to conscious experience instead of to the unconscious, repressed material which threatens to invade conscious awareness.

The observer viewing manic and depressive phases gains the impression of two sharply divergent patterns of behavior. Actually both patterns, while distinctly different in appearance, have one same objective: to gain attention, approval and emotional support. The manic patient can be extremely attractive much of the time. Warm, friendly behavior is a superficial reaching out to others in an attempt to gain acceptance and approval. The depressed patient may gain, through behavior, sympathy, attention, and a warm relationship. Even when the patient appears to be rejecting a relationship with another person, the offering by the other person of this relationship is actually emotionally gratifying to the patient.

The precipitating cause is usually some deep personal, emotionally traumatizing loss.

INCIDENCE

Manic-depressive reactions are rare in childhood. When observed in the young, the disorder is usually noted during preadolescence years. The greatest number of episodes occur between the ages of 18 to 35 years. The illness is also observed during the middle years of life (45 to 55 years). The incidence is greater in women than in men and is exceeded only by schizophrenia.

The patient may experience during his lifetime several periodic episodes of depression only, or the attacks may be only the manic type. Chronic depressive states are common. A considerable number of those who become ill demonstrate the circular type of manic-depressive reaction, in which there is an alternation between elated and depressive mood extremes. Patients have been known to have but one attack during a lifetime of either elation or depression, followed by good adjustment.

PROGNOSIS

The prognosis for the particular episode is considered good. There is, however, a strong tendency for the disorder to reoccur. These patients recognize reality but distort it. The fact that the patient does not demonstrate a complete collapse of his integrative capacities assists him in making a good adjustment between attacks. Some psychiatrists believe that a progressive increase in the time span between attacks increases the possibility of the patient's permanent extramural adjustment. A shortening of the time interval between attacks increases the possibility of the patient becoming permanently hospitalized. If the patient is fortunate enough to have unusually understanding, mature individuals who can accept the person's behavior and give strong emotional support, his chances for recovery are increased.

TREATMENT

Tranquilizing drugs have been helpful during the manic phases in reducing the severity and length of an elated period. In fact, we do not see the severity of episodes as was previously observed prior to drug therapy. In the treatment of depressed types of patients, antidepressant drugs have been helpful. Patients who do not respond well to therapy with drugs may respond favorably to electrotherapy.

It is generally believed that psychotherapy is not particularly effective during the attack period because the patient is difficult to reach at this time. Reassurance of the depressed individual or logical reasoning with the manic type is usually ineffective as these approaches are usually completely ignored by the patient and often result in intensified behavior. Psychotherapy is sometimes used to prevent a reoccurrence of the disorder. Unfortunately, however, many of these patients reject this form of treatment, once they have recovered their emotional equilibrium and gain the assumption that they will be well. An adequate diet, attention to personal hygiene, rest, and social therapeutic activities are essential supportive means, regardless of the chosen treatment.

PREVENTION

Prevention starts in childhood. It is important for a child to learn to give as well as receive and to develop a capacity for withholding gratification. In the parent-child relationship, the aim should be to help the child develop feelings of being lovable and accepted. Occasional disappointments are real experiences in living and also strengthen the child's capacity to adapt and adjust to circumstances.

Psychotherapy following recovery has been known to be helpful in the prevention of recurrent attacks. During treatment, the doctor attempts to explain to the patient that the attacks occur because the patient has failed to discover an acceptable manner of expressing to others directly what he feels and thinks in the majority of instances. The therapist tries to educate the individual to realize that because of the patient's deeply sensitive nature, fear of rejection and disapproval is especially painful and actually motivates the behavior pattern in times of stress and strain. The patient is encouraged to identify signs peculiar to him, from past experiences, of an approaching attack of mania or depression. He is advised to return to the physician for early treatment. Such signs may be feelings keenly sensed by the patient, such as being under pressure, undue, unexplainable anxiety, apprehension, etc., with accompanying feelings of fear.

The attempt is made to enlighten the patient to the fact that matured individuals must give as well as receive in a relationship, and accept the pleasant as well as the unpleasant aspects of human behavior. The patient is encouraged to believe that others can be accepting of debatable and unusual behavior, expressed directly, especially when appropriate ways of doing this are developed. The doctor's role is a difficult one. He is required to be patient, faithful, willing to take abuse and disappointment. He must convince the patient that he is interested in him in spite of the patient's illness and rejection of the physician upon certain occasions. All of this constitutes a learning process, which cannot be successful unless the patient shares in the learning. To convince the patient that his directly expressed behavior can be accepted, the physician permits the patient to act frankly toward him, without withdrawing his approval. The approval is of the patient as an individual, but not particularly an approval of his behavior. Finally, a therapeutic relationship is well on the way when the doctor provides emotional support for the patient as the patient attempts to use newly learned methods of directly expressing ideas and feelings. These same principles of approach may be utilized by the nurse, and other therapists, in the interpersonal situation.

NURSING CARE

Manic-depressive patients are motivated by deep inferiority feelings and fear of rejection. They have a need for acceptance and approval, and are seeking a warmer, more receptive relationship. Unfortunately, they have a tendency to ask this of persons who are usually retiring in nature and who consequently lack the ability to respond affectively to the patient's emotional need for continuous evidence of approval and acceptance. One can understand why they attempt to form such a relationship with this type of individual. It is because the retiring person is not, by his very personality structure, a treatening-feeling influence.

The outward demands of the manic type, as well as the withdrawn, self-condemnatory behavior of the depressive type, frequently reach a point where many relatives and nursing personnel grow weary of attempting to meet the patient's needs. These responses are interpreted by the patient as rejection. Thus, a cycle of rejection followed by increased behavioral symptoms representing, in effect, increased demands for acceptance and approval, becomes obvious. It is, therefore, important for all who nurse these patients to be aware of this fact, and avoid rejection of the individual.

During Manic Phase

In the early manic phase the patient may be overly gay, amusing, and attractive, or he may show signs of irritability and a demanding attitude. These outward manifestations are defense patterns the patient uses to project his uncomfortable feelings of inferiority and fear of rejection onto the environment, in an effort to achieve interpersonal security. One pattern is a superficially pleasant reaching out to persons for emotional support. The other is an open, hostile approach to gain control of the environment and the persons within it. The ability to absorb with understanding and without reproach such behavior as overenthusiasm, talkativeness, gaiety, witty remarks and dramatic actions, as well as criticism, sarcasm, dominance, meddling, profanity, and other overt behavior, is a valuable nursing asset.

Unlike schizophrenic patients, these individuals do not behave in phantasy, but recognize reality while they obviously distort it. Because they are in contact, they are able to reintegrate quite well, following a manic behavior phase. Thus, we may assume that behavior is reversible, and upon that principle allow permissive behavior and freedom of expression within the limits of comfort and safety to the patient and others in the immediate interpersonal situation. Cutting off the manic patient's stream of talk only serves to increase the person's anxiety and need for release of ideation and hostility.

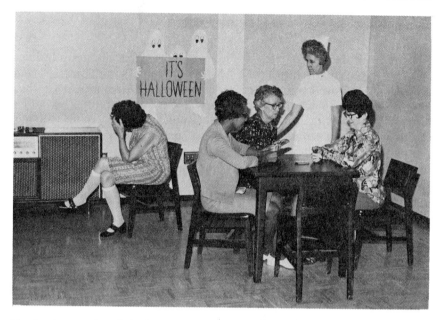

Fig. 1.   A game of cards is therapeutic. (Courtesy of Arkansas State Hospital, Little Rock, Ark.)

It is necessary for nursing personnel to be alert to mounting signs of tension leading to acutely disturbed behavior, so that therapeutic remedial measures may be instituted.

Physical force and vocal methods of reproach are threatening and frightening to the patient. Such approaches frequently produce increased behavior symptoms as well as retaliative, threatening responses from the patient. Meeting the patient's needs with a calm voice and manner and persuading and encouraging him to participate in activities and accept prescribed medical treatment will prove most effective.

The need to remove the patient from a stimulating environment and contact with others by means of seclusion may be eliminated when social activities are utilized therapeutically.

Limitations may be placed skillfully upon the patient's diffuse dispersal of excessive energy. Social diversional activities will help him to utilize constructively his energies. It is important to realize, however, that the patient is easily distracted, provoked and limited in his ability to concentrate and remain at a given activity. Mild exercise in the form of outdoor walks, gardening, putting, ball tossing, and the like, may be very therapeutic. Highly competitive exercise is to be avoided, because these patients respond by attempts to overreach beyond their physical and emotional

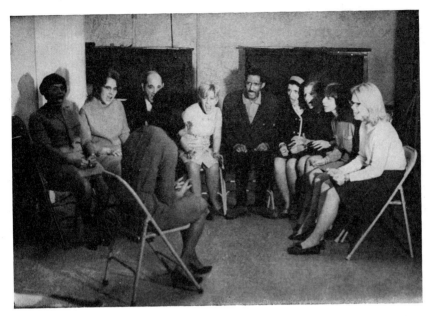

Fig. 2. Speech therapist encourages the expression of emotions. Participants are verbalizing the words "I don't care" which affords the release of hostility. (Courtesy of Essex County Overbrook Hospital, Cedar Grove, N. J.)

endurance. Creativity through occupational therapy provides an opportunity for the patient to design, invent, decorate, and release hostile impulses.

Patients who express a desire to write may be given pencil and paper and allowed to release their deeper feelings in writing. It is not unusual to observe persons so inclined absorbed in penning poetry or voluminous scripts containing evidence of delusions and fragmentary details attached to their deeper anxieties and frustrations. Literary productions provide an excellent channel for release of the patient's feelings.

Simple card games, checkers, jigsaw puzzles, group singing, short circle games and dances may prove enjoyable and not too difficult for the patient's participation.

A well-deserved, tempered compliment may be given to bolster the patient's need for acceptance and approval. It is not advisable to encourage behavior which is ordinarily subject to social restraint, but which may seem entertaining and attractive in the present situation. Encouragement leads to excessiveness of performance by the patient, which is followed by fatigue, irritability, and excitement.

Good hygiene and sufficient rest help to restore the patient's energy and self-esteem. The person feels better physically and emotionally. Attention given to the patient's physical nursing needs will promote rapport in the interpersonal relationship, particularly if the assistance offered to the individual by the nurse is given with obvious sincerity and acceptance. It may be necessary for the nurse to suggest to the patient that he bathe and care for his teeth, hair, and dress when he is highly absorbed in socially unproductive activity.

It is important for the patient to consume adequate nourishment in order to maintain his body fluid balance and prevent dehydration, fever, and subsequent excitement. Delusions, suspicious behavior, and uncooperativeness often accompany highly disturbed behavior. Beverages offered at intervals by the nurse to the patient will reduce an elevated body temperature. The patient will begin to relax, trust others, and cooperate. When the patient is too active to partake of his meals at the regular time, beverages and certain solid foods, such as sandwiches, cookies, and fruit, may be placed directly within the patient's vision and reach. When the patient becomes hungry and stimulated to eat, he will then have these available and maintain his nourishment needs.

During Depressive Phase

In the depressive phase the patient's obvious feelings of despair, lack of spontaneity, pessimism, inactivity, and retardation evoke the attention and sympathy of relatives and nursing personnel. This is emotionally gratifying to the patient, because it is a response to the individual's basic need for acceptance and approval. Outwardly, however, one would not gain the immediate impression that such attention was appreciated by the patient, owing to the fact that the person is usually withdrawn, brooding, and oftentimes uncommunicative.

Feelings of hostility are directed inward by the patient toward the self. The possibility of suicide must be guarded against. Establishing rapport with the individual is the most important suicidal preventive which can be instituted, because it makes the patient feel accepted and worth while. Routine protective measures such as alertness to the patient's whereabouts and actions at all times, careful but indirect and subtle observation, and the removal of hazardous instruments from the patient's environment are also preventive nursing approaches.

Remaining with the patient lends emotional support, even when the patient is inert and uncommunicative. Perseverance in establishing a closer relationship will usually lead to verbalization by the uncommunicative patient of his deeper anxieties and feelings. When hostility and anxiety are expressed openly, the patient will begin to feel relieved and benefit through the nurse-patient relationship.

Some patients who express feelings of guilt and unworthiness may benefit from performing menial tasks, such as cleaning and dusting. Caution should be exercised in the selection of this nursing approach, however, because there are a considerable number of patients who would feel further rejected, inferior, and frustrated. It is necessary to understand the patient's stage of depression, his cultural, educational, and career background in this respect, and to be guided by the doctor's recommendations. In some instances, the patient's self-esteem and morale will be lifted by having him engage in a task which fits in with his previous preparation and experience. To be able to accomplish again, to some degree, what was possible prior to the illness will renew the patient's feelings of hope and confidence.

Conflict between the patient's needs and social restraints may cause ambivalence. The patient is sometimes unable to make decisions, and wavers over small matters. Nursing personnel may give assistance to the patient in making decisions until the individual regains self-confidence. It may be necessary to help the patient to select wearing apparel for the day, decide to attend classes and activities, allow a visitor, and the like. Supervision may be gradually withdrawn as the patient recovers the ability to assume these responsibilities. Depressed patients should never be hurried, because haste arouses feelings of inadequacy and anxiety.

The tension born of brooding, guilt feelings, and anxiety in the patient may cause insomnia. Warm baths followed by a hot beverage, such as milk, before retiring will help the patient to relax, sleep, and restore body energy. Physically and emotionally the patient will begin to feel improved, as time progresses. Early morning awakening is not uncommon in the early depressed phase. During these periods it is advisable to observe the patient carefully, but indirectly. The nurse may sit with the patient and listen to his verbalizations of hopelessness, as he contemplates facing a new day. This simple approach can be very therapeutic.

Attention to the patient's physical nursing needs of bathing, care of hair, teeth, and dress provides a purposeful interpersonal relationship which can be emotionally supportive.

Mild exercise and diversional occupational and social activities are as helpful to the depressed as to the manic patient. All of the activities which are suggested for the patient in the manic phases may be utilized therapeutically for the depressed patient. Stimulating exercise and competitive indoor and outdoor games are to be avoided, because they overtax the patient's physical and emotional endurance and lead to feelings of inadequacy and frustration.

A change of scenery may be introduced with short motor drives. When

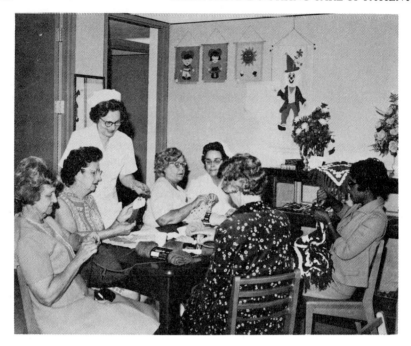

Fig. 3. Creative activity helps to direct patients' interest. (Courtesy of Arkansas State Hospital, Little Rock, Ark.)

the patient is ready for group participation, short table and circle games, as well as social gatherings, musicals, and the like, will be enjoyable and satisfying.

PSYCHOTIC DEPRESSIVE REACTIONS

Psychotic depressive reactions are differentiated from the depressive type of manic-depressive reactions. Patients manifesting psychotic depressive reactions are severely depressed and demonstrate symptoms of gross misinterpretation of reality. Oftentimes they are delusional and hallucinate. There is, however, in their history an absence of repeated depressions or marked cyclothymic swings. A distressing life situation may precipitate the reaction. The approach to and nursing care of these patients is essentially the same as that administered to other depressed patients.

INVOLUTIONAL MELANCHOLIA

Depression, with or without agitation or paranoid ideas, occurring during the menopause, may be diagnosed as an involutional melancholia.

The differential diagnosis is established when there is no evidence of a previous manic-depressive illness in the patient's history. Clinically, the most outstanding symptom is that of depression. Fear of a malignant somatic illness is not uncommon. The patient may brood over past events to a degree that is out of proportion to the life situation. Feelings of guilt and delusions of unworthiness may be expressed. Those patients manifesting agitated depression may pace restlessly about the ward, pick at their clothing, skin, and scalp. Feelings of guilt, apprehension and fear of harm or punishment may be repeatedly communicated. Involutional melancholia is observed more often in women than in men. Women experience the so called "change of life" during their late forties, men experience it during the late fifties. The realization of the approach of the aging process and the end of the child bearing period may be more threatening and disturbing to the personality than the endocrine changes taking place in the body. Many investigators believe that individuals who are characteristically overly meticulous, rigid, inhibited, compulsive, obsessional in temperament, and restricted in their interests are more likely to develop these reactions during the menopause. Of all the depressive syndromes, it is believed that those of middle life present the best prognosis. Relief of the immediate distressing and presenting symptoms may be accomplished with the administration of selected antidepressant and tranquilizing drugs. Hormones may help to restore the endocrine balance and alter mood changes. Psychotherapy is essential treatment for helping these individuals to gain insight into the causes and effects of their illness and dispel abnormal fears of malignant illness. Suicidal precautions may be necessary. Prevention should commence during early life. It is important for people to understand the differences in the physical and emotional development of men and women. Learning to anticipate and accept menopausal changes as a normal life process and extending one's interests beyond the home and family into constructive, mentally diverting activities may be helpful in reducing the incidence of these reactions.

SUGGESTED REFERENCES

Briggs, P., Laperriere, R., et al.: Working outside the home and the occurrence of depression in middle-aged women. Ment. Hyg. 49: 438 (July), 1965.

Crumb, F.: Limited social recovery. Perspect. Psychiat. Care 4: 26 (March–April), 1966.

Crumb, F.: Limited social recovery—further discussion of a depressive behavior pattern. Perspect. Psychiat. Care 4: 32 (May–June), 1966.

Dean, E.: A note on depression. Ment. Hyg. 49: 331 (July), 1965.

Dominick, J.: Nursing care factors in psychotic depressive reactions in elderly patients. Perspect. in Psychiat. Care 6: 28 (Jan.-Feb.), 1968.

Freedman, A., and Kaplan, H. (eds.): Comprehensive Textbook of Psychiatry, ed. 1. The Williams & Wilkins Co., Baltimore, 1967, p. 676.

Isler, C.: What you need to know about depression. R.N. 28: 58, 1965.
Kolb, L.: Noyes' Modern Clinical Psychiatry, ed. 7. W. B. Saunders Co., Philadelphia, 1968, p. 335.
Risley, J.: Nursing intervention in depression. Perspect. Psychiat. Care 5: 65 (Mar.-Apr.), 1967.
Thaler, O.: Grief and depression. Nurs. Forum 5: 8 (Spring), 1966.
Ujhely, G.: Grief and depression—implications for preventive and therapeutic nursing care. Nurs. Forum 5: 23 (Spring), 1966.

FOOTNOTES

1. Pearson, M.: Strecker's Fundamentals of Psychiatry. J. B. Lippincott Co., Philadelphia, 1963, p. 110.

For reviewing this chapter, grateful acknowledgment is made to Doctor Rochus Stiller and Mrs. Selma Taxis, R.N.

CHAPTER 35

Withdrawal from Reality in Schizophrenic Behavior: Nursing Care

There are several types of schizophrenic reactions, each manifesting outwardly symptoms which differentiate one type from another. All types, however, demonstrate a common basic pattern of behavior.

Patients afflicted with schizophrenic reactions are usually of the asthenic body type. Personally, they tend to be introverted, deficient in their affective response ability, self-conscious, retiring, moody, and sensitive.

Generally speaking, schizophrenic reactions are characterized fundamentally by a disharmony between the patient's thinking, feeling, and acting. Thought processes may be disorganized, disturbed, emotion lacking or dissociated in the nature of its peculiar, sometimes bizarre acting out from the content of thought. These persons present failures in adapting to objective reality with its everyday problems, situations and demands and in forming satisfactory relationships with other human beings. Instead of recognizing and adapting to the inevitable frustrations and problems of living, they utilize the mechanism of denial and withdraw from reality. Their retreat is into a world constructed of their fantasies, whims, delusions and hallucinations. Thus, they avoid problems, situations, and social contacts with other individuals. This consistent pattern of failure to perceive and adapt to reality, followed by retreat, becomes so fixed eventually, that the patient's behavior becomes one of concern. Frequently, the patient's abstract ability becomes impaired to the extent that he cannot conceptualize or form logical conclusions. No longer is he inhibited or stimulated by the attitudes of other persons or by the ethical and social codes of society. Instead, through free expression of his repressed cravings and impulses, he acts out in ways which would ordinarily be subjected to social restraint. Hostility, impulsiveness, erotic behavior, primitive regression, and complete dependency are often directly expressed by the schizophrenic patient.

Delusions and hallucinations are accessory symptoms which may also be observed in other psychotic disorders. Oftentimes dreams and hallucinations, seen in a schizophrenic reaction, serve to fulfill denied wishes and to free the patient from intolerable feelings of guilt and anxiety. For instance, the voices the patient hears and attibutes to other individuals are actually outward projections of his own repressed thoughts which he could not bear to accept. Attributing the blame to others serves to protect such a patient against his own, denied impulses.

The term "schizophrenia" (split mind) was coined by Bleuler to describe a lack of integration of the patient's functions. In manic-depressive reactions, the patient's thinking, feeling, and acting are correlated with the predominant mood (elation or depression). In schizophrenic reactions we observe a disharmony, a split. The patient may state that he is being tortured in some grotesque manner, and then proceed to grimace and laugh inappropriately. In manic-depressive reactions, feeling tones change with environmental changes, and the patient is stimulated by external factors. Rarely do schizophrenic patients' feeling tones change with environmental changes. It is well known that these patients are stimulated from within. Nursing personnel may observe this when they enter a ward. The manic patient will approach the nurse. Frequently the nurse finds it necessary to approach the schizophrenic patient if she desires to establish contact.

TYPES OF SCHIZOPHRENIA

SIMPLE TYPE

The onset of a simple reaction is gradual. The subjects are vague, lacking in spontaneity, apathetic, and indifferent to their environments. They may become moody, irritable, lose interest in school, or their occupation, and reduce their associations with other individuals. Under another person's supervision they can perform simple tasks, but they are unable to assume mature responsibilities. Quite often, some member of the family must become responsible for the patient. As the disorder progresses, the patient loses appreciation for esthetic and moral values. He may become an idler, a vagrant, and associate with undesirable persons. Criticism and concern of other individuals makes no impression upon him. This condition may result in deterioration.

HEBEPHRENIC TYPE — *early adolescence*
delusions → cat in straw

Of all the schizophrenic reactions observed, the personality disorganization is the most severe in the hebephrenic type. This disorder has an insidious onset, but becomes full blown usually during early adolescence. These patients' delusions are fragmentary and often bizarre. Somatic delusions are quite common. Patients have been known to insist that one side of the face was wasting away, that the head was shrinking, that the individual was without a stomach and unable to eat, and some women patients have actually clung to the delusion that they harbored an animal, such as a cat, inside of their abdomens. As the disorder progresses, the hebephrenic patient may be observed squatting on the floor in the nude, laughing as if highly amused, wetting, smearing feces, or eating food with his or her fingers as if on an early, infantile level of behavior. Incoherent, unintelligible, babbling speech with neologisms is often heard as the observer pauses to listen to, or attempts to establish contact with, the patient. The patient's emotional expressions are obviously unrelated to reality, and his hallucinations often represent a projection of his repressed impulses or unfulfilled wishes. He becomes highly inaccessible. So absorbed is such a patient in his fantasy that it is frequently difficult to approach him without experiencing an angry, impulsive, threatening reaction.

CATATONIC TYPE

Catatonic reactions are usually acute and precipitated by an emotionally disturbing experience. The disorder occurs most frequently in persons between the ages of 15 and 25 years. The patient may manifest symptoms associated only with catatonic stupor, or at different periods the same patient may demonstrate behavior indicative of either catatonic stupor or excitement. The duration of each phase is individualistic, but the excited phase is usually shorter than the stupor phase. When the patient is in the stuporous phase, one may observe the individual sitting or lying on a bed, standing in a fixed position, or crouched upon the floor for many hours. When lying down, the patient usually keeps his eyes closed. The observer notices that the patient, while standing or sitting, stares downward at the floor. These individuals become immobile, uncommunicative, negativistic, and automatic in their responses to physical suggestion. Catalepsy, which includes the tendency to assume a body rigidity (pathologic limb rigidity) as well as to maintain body postures imposed upon them by others for abnormally long periods of time (waxy flexibility), is commonly observed. The average individual would become most uncomfortable maintaining these postures.

While it is generally known that these catatonic persons are in contact with and aware of their environment and its attending situations, the patient's lack of verbal response to queries has never been completely understood. Levin has expressed the idea that there is a coordination disturbance between thought and speech in the higher cerebral centers which blocks the active verbilization of the patient's thoughts. Levin cites reports of patients who recovered from catatonic stupor phases and gave vivid evidence of their recall of certain situations which occurred during the attacks. These individuals actually believed they had spoken their thoughts.[1] During the stuporous phase they may retain saliva, urine, and feces. Gestures, grinning, and grimacing are also quite common.

Catatonic excitement develops spontaneously, without warning, and at any time of day or night. For instance, a patient who has been mute and unresponsive may suddenly dash into the open ward in an excited manner and in a loud tone of voice threaten, or attempt, to destroy himself or beg others to destroy him. On such occasions, attempts to rush through a window or door have been observed.

PARANOID TYPE

Paranoid reactions occur later than other types, usually between the ages of 30 and 35 years. Suspiciousness and delusions of persecution are the chief characteristics of this type of schizophrenic reaction. These patients are often preoccupied with their unrealistic thinking. Religious behavior such as excessive praying, reading, devotion, and preaching may accompany delusions of omnipotence. Pronouncements of genius or exceptional ability are not uncommon. In the hospital environment these patients are irritable, discontented and unpredictable. When hallucinating they may strike out impulsively at anyone who approaches, since their hallucinations are accusatory. Ideas of reference are frequently expressed by them. One may hear the patient remark that he or she is the object of a remote control influence, that electricity is being sent through the person's body, or that some special radio or newspaper announcement was intended especially for the patient. The paranoid schizophrenic lacks the intense drive for achievement in a career and is likely to give up the environmental struggle and regress further.

CHRONIC UNDIFFERENTIATED TYPE

When any of the schizophrenic reactions appear to be characterized by mixed symptomatology, which may involve symptoms observed in one or several types of reactions, it is impossible to draw clear lines of demarcation which would assist in identifying this aggregate of symptoms as a clearly defined type. The patient may demonstrate such mixtures of symptoms as apathy, ideas of reference, delusions, grimacing, and negativistic behavior, manifested over a long period of time.

ACUTE UNDIFFERENTIATED TYPE

A wide variety of schizophrenic symptoms such as confusion, anxiety, perplexity, ideas of reference, impoverished relationships, and a general turmoil of emotion and fear, sometimes associated with dream states, are observed in this reaction type. These symptoms emerge acutely, and often without obvious precipitating stress or strain to account for them. A careful history, however, usually reveals evidence of early and gradually developmental symptoms.

SCHIZO-AFFECTIVE TYPE

These patients manifest both schizophrenic and manic depressive reactions. They may think and verbalize predominantly like schizophrenics and demonstrate bizarre behavior, while their mood is either pronounced elation or depression. Usually after repeated episodes, they manifest more clearly recognizable schizophrenic features.

CHILDHOOD TYPE

Schizophrenic reactions which occur before the age of puberty (12 years) are categorized in this group.

Childhood reactions have been observed in a great number of children, some as young as two or three years of age. They tend to demonstrate the schizophrenic pattern of withdrawal from reality, autism, fantasy, uncommunicativeness, a lack of interest in other people, and an anxiety which is unrelated to reality. Some of these children may express delusions and hallucinations. They do not relate well to other people but may relate to inanimate objects. They have an obsession for sameness in arrangement of objects, furniture, and the like, in the environment, and they usually resist, either passively or aggressively, the attempts of other persons to change their surroundings or to relate to them.

The attention being focused upon childhood schizophrenia today is probably the basic reason why we have more information about this disorder than was available in the past. Dr. Lauretta Bender, child psychiatrist, suggests in her hypothesis that the condition may begin at birth, explaining that an encephalopathy (dysfunction of the brain) may interfere with the child's normal biological and social personality development. Dr. Leo Kanner, also a well-known child psychiatrist, has had considerable experience with such children. He reports that many of them are the offspring of intellectual parents who spend much of their time following their vocational pursuits and the arts, while remaining frigid and demonstrating little warmth in their family relationships.

RESIDUAL TYPE

Patients with this type of reaction have already demonstrated a definite psychotic schizophrenic reaction, from which they have sufficiently recovered to return to the community and adapt themselves well enough to get along with the members of their local society. At the same time, they do manifest recognizable, residual disturbances of thinking, feeling, and behavior. They appear to be shy, shallow individuals who become easily irritated. This is the type of individual with whom the casual observer may come into contact in the community, and be told by other persons that the individual is somewhat "queer" or "peculiar."

ETIOLOGY, DYNAMICS

Schizophrenia is one of the most baffling mental disorders. Investigators disagree as to its cause and have failed to identify a single positive etiologic factor.

One group of researchers believes that heredity is important. Doctor Franz Kallmann, who did much research with identical twins, reported that if one twin developed schizophrenia, the expectancy rate for it to occur in the other twin was 85.8 per cent. Contrasted with this was a 14 per cent expectancy rate in twins born of two separate cells. The incidence rate of the disorder among siblings in general is the same as that obtaining in fraternal twins, and this fact lends credence to the theory of a hereditary basis.[2,3] The validity of this evidence has been disputed by investigators who claim that the statistics fail to include facts concerned with the individuals' life situations and family relationships.

Another group of doctors believe that schizophrenia is caused by disturbances in the person's metabolism, endocrine balance, and body chemistry.

Anthropologists suggest that the illness is probably due to a combination of genetic, cultural, environmental, social, and psychological factors.

The late Adolph Meyer believed that schizophrenic reactions developed as the result of an individual's persistent faulty reaction to his environment. He believed that the individual made increasing use of poor, ineffective mechanisms of adaptation instead of effective ones. The result of this behavior was considered to be a disorganized personality with final withdrawal from reality. The patient's behavior represented an attempt to reconstruct his personality and maintain emotional equilibrium.

While none of the theories postulated has been abandoned, and research into the causes of schizophrenic reactions continues, the present trend is to relate this illness to the psychodynamics of personality development. Much stress is being placed upon the influence of early interpersonal relationships.

Studies of the schizophrenic process indicate that it begins very early in life and is the result of relationships, attitudes, and experiences of childhood. Attitudes are acquired through the processes of identification and introjection. The attitudes of parents toward children, and the experiences to which children are exposed, are reflected in the child's concept of himself and others, his future relationships, and the defense mechanisms which he develops.

A child must experience feelings of security with an adult in his early relationships before he can gain sufficient trust and confidence in others to form additional relationships. Children who have failed to experience warmth and affection in their family relationships feel rejected and insecure. They cannot give in return to others what they themselves have failed to experience. These children conceive of themselves as being unwanted and unloved. The contemplation of relating to others becomes fearful anticipation. Withdrawal protects the child from further, painful rejection.

Parents have emotional needs, too, and there are some parents who have a need to have their children openly demonstrate affection and feel dependent upon them. A shy child may be rejected by a parent who is acutely sensitive to this lack of emotional warmth in the child's relationships with others. The parent unconsciously withdraws from the child, thus reinforcing the child's pattern of moving away from reality. A similar process may be observed among children who experience sibling rivalry. Another child in the family may be more outgoing in temperament, or possess some ability which satisfies a long-desired, unachieved ambition of the parent. Through the child's demonstration of ability, the parent receives emotional gratification in a vicarious manner. Goals may be set for the child by parents which are inconsistent with goals desired by the child.

The overprotected child is the offspring of an anxious mother who prevents her child from experiencing normal situations which may require the acceptance by the child of disappointment, failure, the making of decisions, adaptation, and self-protection. It may be that such children are not allowed to walk to school alone or with other children, to engage in competitive games, to pet animals, etc. These youngsters consequently conceive of themselves as helpless and unable to cope with the outside world.

Much evidence appears in patients' histories concerning separations due to homes broken through divorce, illness, or death. It is believed that these factors may cause the person to be poorly prepared to adjust to real life experiences and responsibilities with a matured, confident approach.

INCIDENCE

About 23 per cent of all patients admitted for the first time to state hospitals are categorized as having schizophrenic reactions. The greatest number of these patients became ill during the ages of 15 to 25 years. Few persons develop the illness after the age of 50 years. It has been estimated that more than 50 per cent of all mentally ill persons are victims of schizophrenic reactions. In most instances the onset of the disorder is gradual.

In terms of social losses, schizophrenic reactions extract a stupendous toll from society, both financially and productively. Not only are many of these persons unable to provide for their own needs, but they are individuals who will not marry, form family units, or assume a career in which they might contribute or create something of beneficial use to society.

PROGNOSIS *early treatment; worse later in life*

It is generally believed that the chances for recovery are increased when the disorder is identified and treated in its earliest stage. The expectancy for recovery is reduced with each year of continued illness. Of the number of patients who do improve, about 80 per cent are discharged during the first year of hospitalization. There is a tendency for the illness to progress, but not always is there permanent disorganization of the personality. Schizophrenic patients have responded sufficiently well to intelligence tests to indicate that intellectual deterioration does not always occur in these patients. In some subjects, the illness does progress continuously. In other individuals, the episodes occur at intervals. The longer the interval between attacks, the better the prognosis. The recovery possibilities are strengthened if the patient still possesses some affective capacity to respond. The amount of individualized personal care given to patients bears an important relationship to the recovery of the person. Patients afflicted with acute reactions present a more favorable prognosis, particularly if these persons succeed in forming satisfactory, sustaining types of relationships. It has been suggested that the higher mortality rate observed in public hospitals is directly related to the pessimistic attitude of the staff. The prognosis is less favorable when the reaction occurs in later life.

TREATMENT

The schizophrenic patient is difficult to treat, owing to the individual's denial of and withdrawal from reality. In denying reality he moves away from the real, underlying conflicts which he has failed to resolve, and about which he does not communicate freely. In addition, he maintains strong negative attitudes, frequently becomes suspicious, and resists, actively or passively, persons who attempt to form a therapeutic relationship with him. Loss of the ability to affect a satisfactory communicative feeling toward others, in a relationship, often prevents such a patient from making a positive transference toward the therapist.

Some success has been experienced by analysts who have spent several months, or a few years, in their attempts to be accepted by the patient. With the deeply regressed individual, the therapist usually approaches the patient only briefly each day, in an effort to get the person simply to recognize the analyst as a part of his existence and to expect the therapist consistently to return. Once the patient is able to accept the analyst, these visits may be lengthened. The therapist does not probe deeply into the patient's unconscious or attempt to make verbal interpretations to the patient of obvious, repressed material. Instead he focuses upon listening to the patient, lending emotional support and discussing the person's methods of defensive behavior. The objectives during these sessions is to get the patient to perceive reality and recognize attitudes of understanding, acceptance, confidence, and kindness so that he will develop trust and confidence in himself and others.

Selective tranquilizing drugs have largely replaced insulin therapy and electrotherapy in treating schizophrenic patients. Some of these medications have antihallucinatory properties which are helpful in treating patients who hallucinate. As a rule, insulin therapy and electrotherapy are used when the patient does not respond to drug therapy. Best results have been obtained with insulin therapy when the patient was treated during the first six months of the illness.

Some doctors believe that prolonged, intensive electric convulsive treatment (about 20 treatments in a series) is just as effective as insulin therapy. It has been suggested that this method of treatment probably disrupts the process of psychotic organization which is in progress at the time of treatment.

Spontaneous remissions have occurred in some instances. While the therapeutic agent has not been established, it is believed that these patients made contact with some person, possibly a member of the nursing staff who persevered in giving individualized attention, succeeded in communicating with the patient, and thus established a beneficial interpersonal relationship.

Several investigators believe that the recovery rate is influenced positively when the patient can receive individualized attention.

PREVENTION

It is believed that the prevention of schizophrenic reactions is dependent upon educating parents, parent substitutes, teachers, and all persons who come into contact with the young child, since the reaction toward a schizophrenic individual may be influenced by the misunderstandings which exist.

Changing attitudes which will modify behavior are dependent upon having experiences which influence desirable feeling reactions. Thus, it is important for children to experience security feelings in family relationships.

Education involves helping parents and other individuals to realize the importance of making children feel accepted and loved, as well as to consider the intense feelings of abandonment and rejection which may develop in children who are the victims of broken homes.

Children need to be socialized as early as possible in order to experience the realities of living, of giving and receiving, of learning to consider feelings of others, and to enjoy the companionship of other human beings. They should be encouraged to be good losers in the face of defeat, being cognizant of the fact that everybody admires a good loser. Reality has its failures as well as its successes, and success is often built upon the experience of failure. Therefore, it is well to stimulate a child to face failure with the determination to try, try again until he experiences the joy of victory. Self-achievement strengthens the child's feelings of confidence in himself, thus enabling him to accomplish and to face the later frustrations of life.

Schoolteachers are being urged to play a role in the prevention of mental disorders. There is a strong trend toward educating this group to recognize early patterns of withdrawal in children and to appreciate the fact that such children have unresolved conflicts. Many schools have well-formulated plans to refer such children to psychiatrists or child guidance clinics, so that preventive steps may be taken to inhibit the progress of a schizophrenic process.

NURSING CARE

The meaning of the social distance maintained by the schizophrenic patient has become increasingly understood as a sensitive, interpersonal pattern of isolation, motivated by the patient's fears of rejection, repressed hostility, and a lack of faith and confidence in himself and other people. Ambivalent feelings of love and hate toward parents, siblings, and close associates are often observed in schizophrenic patients. These contrasting, conflicting feeling tones are acutely sensed and feared by the patient,

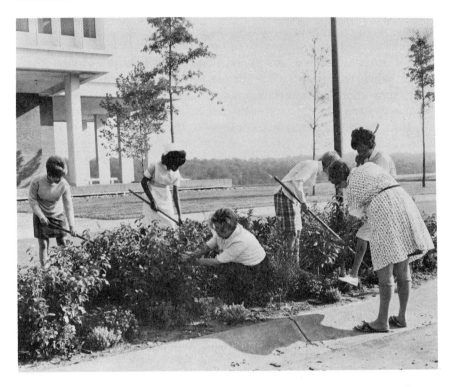

Fig. 1. Nursing students lead a "green thumb" gardening brigade. (Courtesy of Arkansas State Hospital, Little, Ark.)

causing intense anxiety and guilt reactions. Therefore, what the patient says and does is largely a reflection of these feelings. Through their behavior, these individuals are unconsciously defending themselves and attempting to communicate something to nursing personnel. Withdrawal is a defense mechanism against rejection, a reaction which the patient has grown to expect automatically in all relationships. Separation from other persons is also a protective, restraining measure against the potential destructiveness of the patient's hostile impulses toward other persons.

Many of these patients are intellectually and creatively endowed. Restoring them to health brings its rewards. Nursing personnel play the most influential role in the patient's recovery. Whether or not the patient identifies with positive attitudes of acceptance, warmth, sincerity, security, confidence, and love will depend very much upon the attitudes of nursing members. Behavior is modifiable and can be changed for the better, dependent upon the attitudes reflected in the nursing care given to the patient.

Successful recoveries can be achieved only when nursing personnel appreciate why the patient behaves as he does, maintain an optimistic, hopeful attitude toward recovery, and proceed on the premise that schizophrenic patients are not absolutely inhospitable toward overtures from others. When nurses appreciate the fear beneath the patient's social distance, they endeavor to establish contact with the patient and to lend emotional support.

Because these patients lack trust and confidence in other persons, they have a need to test reality many times before they become receptive. To test, they use the trial-and-error method. A nurse who is attempting to establish a relationship with such patients will find it most difficult to persevere in this respect, unless she realizes immediately that the patient may use negative methods to test her sincerity and interest. The patient may seemingly ignore the nurse's presence, move away, or tell the nurse to leave. Nurses attempting to approach these patients may be scorned or rebuked with sarcastic remarks, threats, or impulsive physical outbursts. A very sensitive nurse may react with obvious feelings of discomfort, embarrassment, hostility, or anxiety and develop a tendency to avoid the patient. Avoidance will reinforce the patient's expectations of rejection and the withdrawal pattern. When the patient is allowed opportunity for continuous preoccupation and isolation, he comes to gain satisfaction in his unreal world and prefers it to reality. One of the major requisites for good psychiatric nursing is possession, on the part of the nurse, of the ability to anticipate and accept the patient's testing and negative responses.

Many schizophrenic patients say one thing while meaning another. Basically they are lonely people who, while wanting attention and companionship, have never learned positive methods of achieving these. Instead they often unconsciously provoke rejection, and feel inwardly depressed afterwards, but simply do not know how to resolve the disharmony between their feelings and actions. A nurse who really wants to help a patient must be willing to subjugate her own sensitive nature. She must return again and again, attempting different avenues of approach, until the patient demonstrates recognition of her presence and interest.

It is obvious, then, that the first step in the nurse's plan of care is to persevere in breaking through the patient's defenses, attempting to decrease them with each contact, and increase movement of the patient toward reality. Most schizophrenic patients sustain some measure of contact with reality. Patients who have experienced remissions have divulged the information that their failure to respond to others, during an attack, was due to their frightening delusions or to threatening auditory hallucinations.

Reality is not stereotyped; it is, instead, ever changing. The perception of reality by an individual is dependent upon stimulation. Through nursing

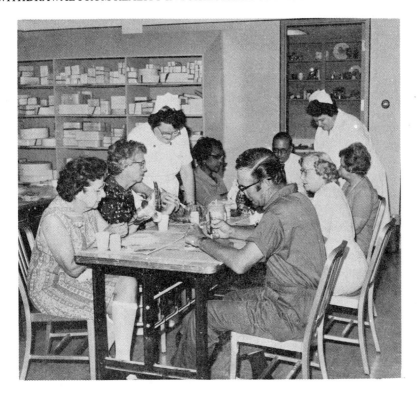

Fig. 2.   Instruction in a variety of crafts. (Courtesy of Arkansas State Hospital, Little Rock, Ark.)

care, the patient's special senses, intellect, and esthetic response may be stimulated. Simple, primary activities directed toward the achievement of simple goals should precede movement toward more complex activities and goals.

Giving the deeply regressed patient intimate physical nursing care may be the only possible avenue of approach toward establishing a successful interpersonal relationship. Feeding the patient, bathing with warm water, the touch of clean linen, the pleasant smell of bath soap, powder, colognes, and lotion may all stimulate the patient's special senses. Special attention to the patient's coiffure (if a woman patient), to fingernails and selection of wearing apparel reflects attitudes of acceptance, interest and sincerity. The individual's esthetic response can be stimulated and attitudes modified. When this type of care becomes a daily approach, the nurse may gradually encourage the patient to participate actively, thus working toward the goal set for the patient to assume responsibility for personal physical care. Patients who are unable to participate actively, or to socialize with others, may be stimulated through music which is played within their hearing range.

When initiating activities which will stimulate the patient, it is well to remember that, because these persons suffer from a severe compulsion to maintain negative attitudes, it will be difficult for the patient to cooperate. Negative attitudes are one of the basic manifestations of a schizophrenic reaction. Acceptance by the nurse of this concept requires serious respect, if one is to hope for a successful recovery of the patient. Getting the individual to relinquish the defense mechanism of negativism requires understanding, time and patience.

Oftentimes there is a tendency to let immobile patients sit or lie in the same room or area of the ward. They should not be left in the same environment, for they require a change. Taking patients out of doors provides an opportunity for them to respond to the radiance of sunshine, fresh air, garden arrangements, the fragrance of flowers, the singing of birds, and other aspects of reality within their sensual range. A picnic or an automobile drive will introduce diverse elements of reality. Whenever possible, these patients should be allowed to attend movies, dances, and other recreational activities taking place in different areas of the hospital. Outwardly they may not appear to be greatly impressed, but this change and introduction of a variety of experiences allow for an increase in movement and stimulation of their special senses and esthetic responses.

In the beginning, the patient may not be ready to socialize with others. Gradually, the nurse should work toward and encourage group association. The patient should feel secure in sustaining the nurse's relationship, but this should not be allowed to become a crutch.

Patients may be introduced to many simple table and circle games which can be enjoyed, dependent upon the season of the year and weather conditions, in the ward living room or out of doors. Crafts and hobbies such as weaving, pasting decals, brush and palette painting, finger painting, drawing, coloring, making holiday favors and decorations, tearing and braiding cloth strips for mats and rugs, and making shell jewelry are simple activities which may be enjoyed. Checkers, dominoes, monopoly, and card games may be played. Tossing quoits, playing handball, and taking short walks outdoors may also appeal to the patient. Many of these patients enjoy television programs and thumbing through colorful magazines. Later they may learn to knit, crochet, tat, and accomplish more complex activities which stimulate intellectual and creative functions. Many patients come to enjoy choosing colors and patterns, as well as the creation of new designs.

Patients who succeed in mildly competitive games, socializing, and accomplishing the goal of a creative project respond well to rewards, which should be given immediately. Perhaps a genuine compliment or a somewhat more complex activity may be suggested as a reward. These approaches reinforce the patient's confidence in his own ability.

Schizophrenic patients frequently become tense, apprehensive, and defensive toward attempts to engage them in verbal communication. They do not like to discuss their feelings and, with a protective barrage of incoherent chatter, will ignore all queries. Probing, therefore, should be avoided.

The language of schizophrenic patients, being symbolic of deeper underlying conflicts, is often unintelligible. One must listen carefully for cues which will guide the observer toward appropriate responses. A word repeated many times, or some topic woven into their apparently jumbled conversation, often appears to be associated with anxiety-producing motivation. For instance, a patient kept weaving into his obvious verbigeration the mention of biology and plant life. The observant nurse remarked, "You seem to know a great deal about biology." To this the patient responded in the affirmative. He then proceeded to discuss at length his ability in this area. Surrounding his communication, however, was obvious conflict concerning the acceptance by others of this concept of his ability. It was obvious that his efforts in this direction had failed. This traumatizing situation, to which he was not able to adapt, was probably the precipitating factor in his illness. Listening to the patient often leads to better understanding by the nurse as well as relaxation and feelings of trust in the patient. Later on, the patient may verbalize his deeper, underlying conflicts.

Word-construction games such as anagrams, Scrabble, and Skip Across are excellent approaches when one is attempting to encourage the patient to communicate. There is a simple little word game which any nurse may construct on ordinary, letter-size paper. The nurse draws several blocks. In the left-hand margin blocks, she prints the letters of a simple word. Or she may ask one of the patients to suggest a word for that area. In each block across the top of the page, the nurse places a topic heading. Patients and nurse take turns in filling in the remaining blocks with their verbal suggestions of words which correlate with the topic and letter indicated. This game is intellectually stimulating and mildly competitive.

Another approach toward encouraging the patient to communicate is to pick out something which appears to be of value to him, such as a known interest, hobby, or ability. Mention it, and quite often the patient will respond.

Psychological trauma is damaging to the patient. When a patient makes an overture, nursing personnel should recognize this immediately as a sustained emotional capacity and desire, on his part, to remain in contact. Unfortunately, in large and busy hospitals, patients who have at-

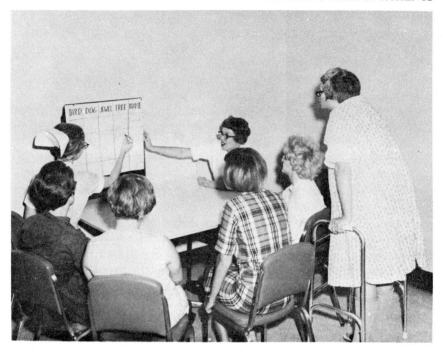

Fig. 3.   Encouraging verbalization through a simple word game involving recognition and recall abilities. (Courtesy of Arkansas State Hospital, Little Rock, Ark.)

tempted to establish a relationship through simple gestures have been rebuked. When a negative response is given by the nurse in this type of situation, it leads to withdrawal and progression of the psychotic organization.

Schizophrenic patients need a demonstration of consistent acceptance, interest, and encouragement. Each new success in the interpersonal situation reduces the patient's anxiety and guilt, and will heighten his self-esteem. Dereistic gratification then becomes less necessary and attractive. Reality is easier to face and accept.

CARE OF CHILDREN

Schizophrenic children have never fully established or have lost partially or completely the ability to test reality. Some of them are unable to differentiate their own bodies from those of other persons. Frequently they avoid looking directly at individuals and show no emotional response to the comings and goings of persons while they are engaged in their preoccupations. There is a marked disinterest in play and external events. Much of their time is spent wandering about the ward, secluding themselves in closets, far-off corners or remote places which are lacking in opportunities for human contact. Body rocking, skin picking, and head banging are common manifestations of behavior. They may remain mute or respond only briefly. Their speech is often fragmentary or filled with neologisms. Some of these children speak of themselves in the third person, thereby demonstrating a lack of the self-concept.

The schizophrenic child may hallucinate, giggle, grimace, or sometimes hum in a monotonous tone of voice. When approached during periods of preoccupation he may react with temper tantrums, panic, attack or withdrawal. It is very difficult to interrupt these acts of behavior to bathe, feed, dress, or put the patient to bed.

Some investigators believe that schizophrenic children should be removed from the mother who is either sick or unable to provide a normal warm, mothering type of relationship. It is also suggested that they be cared for in a special ward because they do not respond well in an environment provided for other sick children. They need special attention and a program geared to their own rate of response. When mixed in with other children and expected to participate in the same activity program, they tend to develop temper tantrums, panic states, or to withdraw.

Nursing care should be given by personnel who are assigned consistently to the ward. Changes in the nursing staff create feelings of insecurity and anxiety reactions. It takes months for personnel who give consistent care to establish a relationship which may lead to a small response from such children.

The nurse may communicate her liking for the child and her interest in him through physical avenues of approach, such as leisurely feeding, bathing, and dressing the child. While giving physical care the nurse can help the child to identify his own body and its parts, differentiating it from hers and those of others. At the same time the nurse is offering a protective closeness. Sometimes a child will cuddle closely to the nurse and then suddenly commence to bite or pinch her as if harboring fear or ambivalent feelings. As the nurse talks to the child she can make clear use of the pronouns "I" and "you," which will help the child to develop a concept of himself as a separate being.

A play area inside the ward and outdoors provides opportunity to divert the child's self-interest. Nurses may teach the child the use of certain toys, such as riding a two-wheeler and participating in the occasion. Learning new skills can be a source of pleasure and a means of strengthening the child's self-confidence. The child is more apt to turn to the adult who does not overwhelm him with affection, or the incentive to achieve for praise.

When the nurse succeeds in breaking through a child's autistic barrier, she needs special support and consultation from the therapist to enable her to provide the remedial mothering relationship needed by the child to influence the development of his self-concept and ability. There is real need for the team approach in the care of schizophrenic children.

At the appropriate time during therapy these children may be taken for walks about the hospital grounds, to the park, or to other places of interest. They may ride in an automobile or on a bus. Such activities provide opportunities for a change in environment and reality experiences which bring them into contact with other human beings. These occasions should be short experiences which do not fatigue the child or produce anxiety. Reaching this point of activity requires many months for most schizophrenic children to accomplish. Some may respond favorably to care, others may regress and never recover.

SUGGESTED REFERENCES

Alexander, L.: The austic child. R.N. 28: 59 (Nov.), 1965.

Arbuckle, J., and Cohen, M.: Rehabilitation nursing in a state mental hospital. Nurs. Outlook 14: 61 (Oct.), 1966.

Carl, M.: Establishing a relationship with a schizophrenic patient. Perspect. Psychiat. Care 1: 20 (March-April), 1963.

Earle, A., Lynn, F., et al.: The role of the psychiatric nurse in the rehabilitation of the schizophrenic patient. J. Psychiat. Nurs. 8: 16 (Jan.-Feb.), 1970.

Freedman, A., and Kaplan, H. (eds.): Comprehensive Textbook of Psychiatry, ed. 1. The Williams & Wilkins Co., Baltimore, 1967, p. 593.

Goodman, L., and LaBelle, M.: The schizophrenic mother. Nurs. Outlook 11: 753 (Oct.), 1963.

Hartman, C.: Psychotic mothers and their babies. Nurs. Outlook 16: 32 (Dec.), 1968.

Juzwiak, M.: The search for the causes of schizophrenia. R.N. 30: 44, 1967.

Kolb, L.: Noyes' Modern Clinical Psychiatry, ed. 7. W. B. Saunders Co., Philadelphia, 1968, p. 355.

Moore, J.: The dynamics of schizophrenia. Perspect. Psychiat. Care 4: 10, 1966.

Moser, D.: Communicating with a schizophrenic patient. Perspect. Psychiat. Care 8: 36 (Jan.-Feb.), 1970.

Phinney, R.: The student of nursing and the schizophrenic patient. Am. J. Nurs. 70: 790 (April), 1970.

Post, J.: Cyclic staff responses to chronic schizophrenic patients. Perspect. Psychiat. Care 2: 13 (May-June), 1964.

Probst, M.: Helping the schizophrenic patient enlarge his perceptual field. Perspect. Psychiat. Care 5: 236 (Sept.-Oct.), 1967.

They said we caused our son's autism. R.N. 28: 54 (Nov.), 1965.

Wildman, L.: Reducing the schizophrenic patient's resistance to involvement. Perspect. Psychiat. Care 3: 26 (May-June), 1965.

FOOTNOTES

1. Levin, M.: Motor hallucination: some motor aspects of mentation. Am. J. Psychiat. 113: 1020, 1957.
2. Kallmann, F.: The genetic theory of schizophrenia. Am. J. Psychiat. 103: 307, 1946.
3. Ewalt, J., and Farnsworth, O.: Textbook of Psychiatry. McGraw-Hill Book Co., New York, 1963, p. 208.

For reviewing this chapter, grateful acknowledgment is made to Doctor Rochus Stiller, Mrs. Selma Taxis, R.N., Mrs. Vivian S. Bryan, R.N., Mrs. Mabel Robinson, R.N., and Miss Florence E. Newell, R.N.

CHAPTER 36

The Persecution Complex in Paranoid Behavior: Nursing Care

The constellation of symptoms observed in the behavior of some persons constitutes a persecution complex. The outstanding characteristics of behavior in the constellation are exaggerated suspicion, delusions of persecution, and pathological use of the defense mechanism projection. In medical literature, these disturbances in behavior are known as paranoid reactions of which there are two distinct types, paranoia and paranoid states.

PARANOIA

The type of psychiatric disorder known as paranoia is rarely seen in the psychiatric hospital. It is believed, however, that there is a greater incidence of it among the general population. The majority of persons afflicted with paranoia are hospitalized only when they are discovered to have committed a violent act or seem about to commit one. Bonner said, because of the low incidence of commitment, we still have a very inadequate conception of this psychosis. Our knowledge of the etiological features, in particular, is limited; and our diagnoses are characterized by doubt and uncertainty. Clinical psychologists are seldom willing to diagnose a case as paranoia, even when all symptoms incontrovertibly indicate it.[1] This is not difficult to understand. Psychiatrists are well aware that these patients frequently involve the therapist in their intricate delusional systems and often resort to legal action. Furthermore, such patients have been known to harbor emotionally dangerous impulses.

Paranoia appears to follow a fundamental pattern of behavior. Persons so afflicted are indignant and suspicious in manner, and nurture a logic-tight delusional system. Superficially they appear to be normal, socially

449

acceptable, and in good contact with their environments. Frequently they are highly intellectual and extremely capable. Some have been considered geniuses. Judgment is impaired only in relation to the individual's unchanging delusional system. The true paranoiac has delusions which are firmly fixed. The delusional system is so well organized and stable at its level that it serves as the defense without affecting deterioration of the intellectual capacity of the psyche. In spite of overwhelming evidence against the validity of their beliefs they do not change them. Instead of developing the apathy, withdrawal, and regression observed in the paranoid schizophrenic, the paranoiac never gives up the struggle. Such individuals go from one situation to another, maintaining the strength of their delusions. With renewed vigor, they subsequently involve still other people in their expanding delusional systems. They do not hallucinate, as do schizophrenic patients of the paranoid type.

PERSONALITY CHARACTERISTICS

A study of the personalities of paranoiacs reveals them to be perfectionistic, jealous, aggressive, and ambitious in their drive for success. They are basically hypersensitive to criticism and control in the discharge of their duties, and to minor slights and humiliations. They appear to falsify their perceptions and judgment in relation to the attitudes of persons in their environment, whom they mistrust and incorporate into their delusional systems. Turning against persons close to them is commonly observed. They have histories of failure after failure in their career relationships. Repeated failures, followed by feelings of frustration, cause them to become hostile and increasingly aggressive and suspicious. They express delusions of persecution and sometimes accessory ones, such as delusions of importance, wealth, and infidelity. Their delusions represent an attempt to make an adjustment, but they fail because of their pathological content and ideation.

ETIOLOGY, DYNAMICS

The literature concerned with paranoia does not support an organic or hereditary theory. There appears to be wide agreement that the illness is related to the psychodynamics of personality development. Some investigators believe that the paranoid reactions may be occasioned by structural conditions of the cerebral cortex, but life histories of these persons also demonstrate basic personality developmental defects.

Studies of the cultural aspects of the patient's history reveal, more often than not, an authoritarian family pattern where harshness, rigidity, suppression of assertion of the child's personality, and frequently cruel treatment are observed. Parents often demonstrate psychotic trends. They have dominated, controlled, and humiliated the patient from early childhood into adulthood. The child feels threatened, but recognizing his inability to cope with the situation, becomes submissive yet filled with a hatred which often leads him to visualize symbolically the violent reactions he feels toward this parental relationship. Feelings of hatred and aggression in the child are repressed or inhibited. Thus, the individual grows to adulthood unable to assert himself, and always feeling suspicious, mistrusting, and misconceiving of the attitudes of those concerned in his interpersonal relationships.

As a consequence of his early affective frustrations and parental domination and cruelty, the person tends to withdraw from normal social contacts. These patients do have suppressed and repressed wishes for affection and closeness which, unconsciously, carry them again and again into situations where they might find satisfactory relationships if only they could trust people. However, no one can ever really get close to them. They tend to be evasive, superficial in their responses, and rigidly unyielding toward others. They have grown to anticipate disappointment, failure, and deceitfulness from others, who they fear will try to use them to gain for themselves some personal advantage. Beneath this behavior, these patients crave attention, affection, and recognition; but since they cannot trust others, they increase their distance (physically and emotionally) from those other people, in order to protect themselves from feelings of insecurity.

Sigmund Freud believed that the paranoid disorders were due to repressed homosexual impulses, but modern psychiatrists, while accepting Freud's theory of a repressed homosexual drive directed toward sexual gratification as one motive, are interested in what appear to be two other drive components. These additional motivating impulses are considered to be power and dependency motivations, directed toward gratification of the need for self-esteem and the need to be dependent. Power and dependency instinctual urges are discussed as pseudohomosexual, as in reality their goals are not directed toward the gratification of a sexual impulse.[2]

We see the need for power in the person who, when placed in authority or invested with some power, becomes overly conscientious about minor details, fault-finding, and difficult and stubborn to the point of exasperation, causing a decline in group morale. Sometimes these individuals manage to gain the leadership of a group, but eventually they become a destructive force in the maintenance of discipline and morale to such an extent that society as a whole becomes the victim, until their lead for power is seized.

The person with a dependency need often has a history of forming a close relationship with an older person of the same sex and becomes frustrated when that person divides or transfers attention to another individual of the same sex, thus failing to provide the emotional support which would meet the person's dependency needs.

Robertson[3] describes four stages of development observed in the progression of paranoia. These are: (1) normal, (2) difficult, (3) paranoid, (4) true paranoia. It is interesting to read Robertson's description where he observes the progression in a typical patient who gave evidence of high intellectual and vocational ability at an early age, then became overly perfectionistic, conscientious, and difficult in the discharge of his duties. He became paranoid when, because of these socially undesirable personal features, he was bypassed for promotion. The final stage erupted with the person expanding his delusions to include society at large. This description can be equated with the newspaper accounts of a person described as being afflicted with paranoia, who terrorized a large metropolitan city with the placement of bombs in public places. Investigation revealed that this had been going on for several years, that lives had been lost or endangered, and several persons injured. When apprehended, the defendant gave evidence of an expansive delusional system which had started with feelings directed first against his employers for having failed to meet his dependency needs during a severe chronic illness. The expansive delusions are obvious in his attacks upon society at large.

Persecutory delusions are defense mechanisms which explain the patients' failures, while absolving them of blame for inability to adjust and to succeed. Persecutory delusions may also be projections of their intense feelings of hatred and violence toward others involved in their delusional systems.

Delusions of infidelity are considered to be a defense against repressed homosexual impulses, or pseudohomosexual impulses which activate feelings of guilt. The person projects the feelings of guilt and fear attached to these delusions upon the spouse. Such an individual may adopt a suspicious attitude toward the mate, make sarcastic remarks of an accusatory nature, and try to humiliate him or her before others. Observers say that these incidents appear to occur following experiences which spend or reduce the heterosexual drive. The homosexual impulse or conflicts emerge following heterosexual experiences and personally traumatizing failures, activating feelings of guilt and fear.[4,5]

Delusions of importance are compensatory mechanisms utilized in attempts to raise the feelings of self-esteem, which are woefully weak.

PARANOID STATES

The paranoid state is characterized by delusions which lack the logic and systematization observed in paranoia. Instead, the delusions are transitory. It also differs from the schizophrenic paranoid type disorder, in that the patient does not manifest the bizarre deterioration observed in schizophrenia. Paranoid states are usually acute reactions of relatively short duration, although there are instances in which the condition appears to become persistent and chronic. When these persons are hospitalized they are confused, demonstrate a loss of memory, and hallucinate. They will express ideas of reference by insisting that others are talking about them, or that they are being controlled by mental telepathy. Their persecutory delusions usually are related to plots by others against them, being followed by the police, and the like. They appear extremely frightened and may sometimes be tremulous.

ETIOLOGY, DYNAMICS

Paranoid states have been observed in aliens who, through circumstances (e.g., prisoners of war), experience changes leading to a dissociation of their environment, former contacts, and the native language.[6] The stress and strain of war, a strange environment with new associates, and inability to communicate effectively appear to activate feelings of fear, ideas of reference, and mistrust. They become aggressive, hostile, suspicious, and filled with persecutory delusions.

Paranoid states may be observed during a manic or depressive phase of an illness or as an accompaniment of alcoholism or drug addiction; they have been known also to occur in association with the delirium following a brain injury. There are investigators who believe these states may be observed in every psychosis and neurosis. Paranoid states have also been demonstrated following the administration of certain drugs, such as amphetamine (Benzedrine) and its derivatives.[7] Investigators believe that there is a strong possibility of these causative physical agents producing an alteration of cerebral physiology and functions. In addition, it is also possible that the pre-psychotic personality adjustment of the individual is the dynamic contributing factor.

INCIDENCE

Paranoia is a rarely observed condition. The onset of the disorder is insidious, and it is progressive in nature. It is usually recognized relatively late in life, generally between the ages of 35 and 55. The average age computed by Bonner is 45.6 years.

Paranoid states are observed more often. Investigators believe that they may be manifested in practically all of the neuroses and psychoses.

PROGNOSIS

Patients afflicted with paranoia do not believe they are ill and thus lack insight. The prognosis is considered poor. Many authorities stress the incurability of the disorder.

Features of the paranoid states disappear as the acute stage of the precipitating disorder subsides. Those who become ill, owing to the strangeness and conditions of an environmental change, do improve when they are removed from the personally threatening experience and replaced in their former familiar surroundings. The discontinuance of drugs which appear to activate a paranoid reaction results in reversal of personality changes in due time.

TREATMENT OF PARANOIA

Paranoia is difficult to treat, in view of the patient's lack of insight and his tendency to involve the therapist in his delusional system. Modern psychiatrists believe that individual psychotherapy should be attempted, as instances have been demonstrated where some patients did at least gain a measure of insight into their conditions which enabled them to function, to a certain degree, on a socially acceptable level.

Sulzberger believes that the best atmosphere for treatment is a mild, positive transference. If the transference reaches a certain point and approaches love in its intensity, the patient is immediately tempted to turn these positive feelings into hate. Vague and evasive remarks cause the patient to experience feelings of panic. Statements made by the therapist should be true, necessary, and agreeable, owing to the patient's suspiciousness and fear of criticism. Once rapport has been established which is not overly friendly, it may be possible for the therapist occasionally and openly to criticize the patient carefully, provided this criticism is free of rancor. Sulzberger believes that this approach is tolerated better than allusions or sarcasm. Thus, the situation becomes less emotionally charged and is viewed somewhat more objectively. The approach recommended would appear to imply that the therapist recognize and discuss the patient's ability to do good work in his respective capacity and then subtly comment on how the patient's opinions of other persons' attitudes and feelings unfortunately affect the maximum achievement which the patient could, no doubt, make in view of his obvious ability. A skillful therapist may make use of these principles.

TREATMENT OF PARANOID STATES

The paranoid states usually subside with the alleviation of the acute phase of the precipitating disorder or situation. Supportive psychotherapy and replacement of displaced persons, such as the reference to prisoners of war previously given, are helpful by transferring these persons to their former environment and providing the emotional support and feelings of security they need. The renewal of contacts with family, relatives, and former associates, together with the ability to understand the language and engage in communications, are the obvious therapeutic factors. The paranoid states resulting from the cumulative effects of drugs such as amphetamine and its derivatives, alcoholism, etc., subside in due time following the withdrawal of the apparently toxic agent.

PREVENTION

Unfortunately psychological tests now in use are not satisfactory in screening persons with paranoid reactions. It is to be hoped that better technics will be developed. Legal measures related to the control of the prescription of certain drugs which produce toxic cumulative effects resulting in paranoid states are helpful.

Feelings of trust are developed in children who have experienced trusting relationships with their own parents and in the immediate family circle. These feelings are engendered both directly and indirectly. Parents who contradict each other in the presence of their children may transfer to the offspring undesirable attitudes of mistrust, thus adversely affecting future adult relationships. The child who listens to parents expressing persecutory feelings about the neighbors and others within the community with whom they are in relationship indirectly conceives of other people as being untrustworthy and unreliable.

It has been recommended that the elements of paranoiac behavior be taught as part of a school subject. This envisions an attempt to enlighten people to recognize the moment an individual manifests paranoiac behavior. In this way, it is believed, society at large would be protected from the likelihood of being duped into becoming involved with persons who for reasons of their own attempt to exploit paranoid attitudes at the expense of racial, religious, or national minorities.[9]

Bonner[1] believes that the authoritarian controlled family pattern is perpetuated from generation to generation. He believes that persons who are victims of this authoritarian parental control learn it and, unconsciously, practice it with their own families. Thus, perhaps we may conclude from this observation that the process of acculturation will be a means in reducing this parental control pattern in the years to come. Perhaps the fast-developing means of travel, particularly by air, which has caused experts to predict "one world," in the future will create a more flexible family relationship in the average home, replacing the rigidly controlled environment with a more democratic philosophy of family rule.

NURSING CARE

Authoritarian approaches and regimental procedures reactivate feelings of being controlled, humiliated, and threatened, thus reinforcing the patient's desire to resist control and retaliate. A flexible approach, within the limits of safety and protection to the patient and others, allowing the individual more freedom of movement and choice of activity, will do more to gain the patient's cooperation.

The nurse, while making an effort to maintain a kindly attitude, should avoid being overly friendly toward the patient. Otherwise, the patient may involve her in his delusional system.

When the patient becomes aggressive, hostile, and possibly sarcastic, it is well to recognize this behavior as resulting from reactivated feelings associated with past experiences retained in the unconscious mind. The patient actually fears the impulse to hurt other people and fears subsequent rejection by nursing personnel, which he believes will follow a demonstration of such behavior. That is why it is important for nurses to remain consistent in their approach to these patients at all times. It is necessary to refrain from obviously avoiding the patient or showing evidence of personal emotional distress. A consistent, yet altruistic approach will reduce considerably the patient's anxiety and instill a small measure of trust toward others.

Nurses should avoid low or whispered conversation in the patient's presence as this may cause the individual to gain ideas of reference. Direct, or indirect but obvious, probing of the patient during conversation should be avoided. Questions or requests from the patient should not be evaded but should be answered sincerely. Feelings of suspicion grow out of both probing and an evasive manner on the nurse's part.

Since repeated failures are believed to cause feelings of anxiety and frustration, these patients need to experience success in activities as well as in their interpersonal relationships. This means that an attitude of acceptance toward the patient, continued over a long period of time and accompanied by encouraging approaches during activities, and later vocational rehabilitation, are vital in strengthening the patient's needed trust in others.

Never argue with these patients or ridicule their delusions. Neither should delusions be reinforced with an attitude of acceptance of them by the nurse. It is best to respond somewhat as follows: "Was that how it happened?" or, "For what reason would someone want to hurt you?" This approach raises microscopic doubts of the validity of the patient's interpretations and may, possibly, cause the patient to go over his ideas later with a more objective viewpoint.

Physical complaints should be reported and approached by the nurse according to the doctor's suggestions. Quite often these complaints concern the patient's genital zone and are thought to be related to basic homosexual motivations and fears.

Persons afflicted with paranoid states, which are more acute at the onset, are very frightened and in need of reassurance. It is helpful to reorient them to their environment in a calm, soothing voice and manner. It is well to assure them in every way that there is nothing to fear. If the patient cannot understand or speak the language, an interpreter may be very helpful in giving the necessary assurance.

SUGGESTED REFERENCES

Freedman, A., and Kaplan, H. (eds.): Comprehensive Textbook of Psychiatry. Williams & Wilkins Co., Baltimore, 1967, p. 665.

Grant, V.: Paranoid dynamics: a case study. Am. J. Psychiat. 11: 143 (Aug.), 1956.

King, F.: Aliens' paranoid reaction. J. Ment. Sci. 97: 589 (July), 1951.

Klein, H., and Horwitz, W.: Psychosexual factors in the paranoid phenomena. Am. J. Psychiat. 105: 697 (Mar.), 1949.

Kolb, L.: Noyes' Modern Clinical Psychiatry, ed. 7. W. B. Saunders Co., Philadelphia, 1968, p. 401.

Maddison, D., Day, P., and Leabeater, B.: Psychiatric Nursing, ed. 2. E. & S. Livingstone Ltd., London, 1968, p. 229.

Ovesey, L.: Pseudohomosexuality, the paranoid mechanism and paranoia. Psychiatry 18: 163 (Feb.), 1955.

Pearson, M.: Strecker's Fundamentals of Psychiatry. J. B. Lippincott Co., Philadelphia, 1963, p. 141.

Revitch, E.: The problem of conjugal paranoia. Dis. Nerv. Sys. 15: 271 (Sept.), 1954.

Robertson, J.: Development of a true paranoia. Dis. Nerv. Sys. 15: 88 (Mar.), 1954.

Stankiewicz, B.: Guides to nursing intervention in the projective patterns of suspicious patients. Perspect. Psychiat. Care 2: 39 (Jan.-Feb.), 1961.

Sulzberger, C.: Psychoanalytic treatment of the paranoid personality. Am. J. Psychother. 9: 430 (July), 1955.

FOOTNOTES

1. Bonner, Hubert: The problem of diagnosis in paranoaic disorder. Am. J. Psychiat. 107: 677 (Mar.), 1951.
2. Ovesey, L.: Pseudohomosexuality, the paranoid mechanism and paranoia. Psychiatry 18: 163 (Feb.), 1955.
3. Robertson, J.: Development of a true paranoia. Dis. Nerv. Sys. 15: 88 (Mar.), 1954.
4. Revitch, E.: The problem of conjugal paranoia. Dis. Nerv. Sys. 15: 271 (Sept.), 1954.
5. Klein, H., and Horwitz, W.: Psychosexual factors in the paranoid phenomena. Am. J. Psychiat. 105: 697 (Mar.), 1949.
6. King, F.: Aliens' paranoid reaction. J. Ment. Sc. 97: 589, 1951.

7. Chapman, A.: Paranoid psychoses associated with amphetamine usage. Am. J. Psychiat. 111: 43 (July), 1954.
8. Sulzberger, C.: Psychoanalytic treatment of the paranoid personality. Am. J. Psychother. 9: 430 (July), 1955.
9. Rosen, H., and Kiene, H.: Early reversible paranoiac reactions. J. Nerv. Ment. Dis. 109: 319 (April), 1949.

For reviewing this chapter, grateful acknowledgment is made to Doctor George Green, Mrs. Selma Taxis, R.N., Mrs. Vivian S. Bryan, R.N., and Miss Florence E. Newell, R.N.

CHAPTER **37**

Behavior Symbolizing Mental Conflict in the Psychoneuroses: Nursing Care

The chief characteristic of the psychoneuroses is anxiety which may be directly felt and expressed or which may be unconsciously and automatically controlled by the use of various psychological defense mechanisms. The anxiety engendered by some deeper, unconscious, unrecognized conflict is displaced into observable symptoms, situations, or objects which bear a symbolic relationship to the unconscious forces. The mechanisms of displacement and symbolism are utilized in this process.

Patients manifesting symptoms of a psychoneurosis do not grossly distort or falsify external reality. In psychotic disorders the patient often distorts, denies reality, and attempts to substitute something else for it through the use of more pathological behavior.

Frequently, the chief symptom observed in a psychoneurosis provides a clue to the person's underlying conflict. The understanding of a psychoneurosis, however, depends upon the observer's ability to recognize the purpose that the patient's symptom is designed unconsciously to serve.

The specific reaction manifested by the individual represents a defense against an unconscious, anxiety-producing situation which the person is unable to manage by other means. The attempts to prevent or alleviate anxiety result in the various types of reactions observed. Usually the reaction observed will be discovered to be allied to the defense mechanisms the individual has used throughout his life to resolve conflicting life situations.

Although the reaction types are classified according to the predominant defense mechanism employed by the person, it is rare to observe a pure reaction type. There may be evidence of mixed reactions in which one or more of the chief defense mechanisms of other reaction types may be observed.

REACTION TYPES

ANXIETY REACTIONS

In these reactions the anxiety is free-floating and unattached to specific situations and objects, as is observed in phobic, dissociative, and depressive reactions.

If the anxiety is not too distressing, the individual may manage to control it through the expression of certain personality traits. Such persons are chronically tense, worried, timid, apprehensive, indecisive, easily embarrassed, sensitive to the opinions of others, and fearful of making mistakes. These individuals are usually scrupulous, overconscientious, ambitious, and attempt to adhere to self-imposed standards of living.

When the anxiety is more painful, the patient may release it unconsciously through symptoms of weeping, depression, irritability, restlessness, insomnia, paralyzing indecision and outbursts of aggression. Feelings of inadequacy and inferiority, sometimes accompanied by paranoid attitudes, may be apparent. Somatic complaints of fatigue, inability to concentrate, a tight band-like sensation around the head, and a quivering feeling in the abdomen may be made. These patients sometimes express fears of some serious physical disease or mental illness.

Patients manifesting chronic anxiety reactions are sometimes subject to additional, acute, terrifying, panic-like states. These attacks may last from a few moments to an hour. Physical complaints of palpitation, precordial discomfort, nausea, diarrhea, urinary frequency, dyspnea, choking, and suffocating feelings may accompany these episodes. Profuse perspiration, flushed face, rapid pulse and dilated eye pupils are often observed at such times. These patients may complain of feeling dizzy, weak or faint, and express fears of impending death. They often appeal beseechingly for help and want someone to remain with them but are too self-engrossed to engage in conversation.

Anxiety reactions are a response to any life situation which threatens the patient's self-requirements or security. Frustrated ambitions, vocational problems, and difficulties in adjusting to sexual and marital life are often discovered to be the core of anxiety reactions. The many taboos and restrictions of our culture inhibit the expression of some innermost desires, strivings, hostility, and aggression. Social demands require that these impulses be repressed. When an overwhelming, threatening situation cannot be resolved, the patient obtains relief from anxiety through the diffuse displacement of it. The particular traits or symptoms observed bear a symbolic relationship to the underlying conflict and the need it creates.

DISSOCIATIVE REACTIONS

These reactions may be considered as a psychic escape from the memory of painful, affective experiences, or a life devoid of emotional satisfaction. There is a dissociation between the conscious and unconscious aspects or functions of the personality, owing to overwhelming anxiety. The patient's defense mechanisms temporarily govern consciousness, memory, and the total personality. During these reactions there is little or no participation of the conscious personality.

Dissociative reactions sometimes resemble psychotic behavior, especially schizophrenic reactions. The onset of the dissociative reaction is usually more sudden than the schizophrenic reaction and is often preceded by more conscious or felt anxiety. Dissociative reactions have been known to occur following catastrophic situations, such as earthquakes, fire, and military engagements.

Twilight States

Twilight states, involving a clouding of consciousness, are psychogenic, delirious episodes which are preceded by marked emotional experiences. These dream-like episodes are accompanied by confusion, dramatic posturing, activities, and voluminous speech which often appears meaningless and unintelligible to the listener. Closer observation of the patient's talk, however, reveals references to highly impressionable, affective experiences. Occasionally these patients weave rather fantastic tales into the episodes.

Twilight states often represent the dreamlike realization of an unfulfilled wish or the dramatic reliving in phantasy of a stimulating emotional experience. The reality of the outside world is excluded from consciousness temporarily and falsified in accordance with deeply seated motives and unfulfilled wishes. Fantastic tales represent an effort to put romance and adventure into a life which has not experienced emotional satisfaction.

Amnesias

One of the commonest dissociative reactions stimulated by anxiety is amnesia, which is to be differentiated from mere forgetting. Amnesia is an active process of blotting out of conscious awareness certain emotional experiences which produce anxiety. Stupor or twilight states may precede the development of amnesia. These earlier states then become selective and restricted to the particular affective experience which provoked anxiety.

Terrifying experiences, serious difficulties in interpersonal relationships, or past behavior resulting in feelings of shame, guilt, and other strong feeling tones may suspend temporarily the person's ability to recall into consciousness certain factual data connected with the obliterated period. Most dissociative amnesias are of brief duration. They may erase from awareness long periods of time involving the entire previous life of the person. Or, earlier life experiences may be recalled while the amnesia is restricted to events immediately preceeding the development of the dissociative reaction.

Fugues

Dissociative fugues are motivated by unconscious forces which compel the individual to withdraw automatically from highly charged emotional situations. They have been known to occur during a publicized investigation of some serious crime or following military engagements. The person conjures fantastic, related self-involvement.

During the fugue the individual may leave his permanent environment and take a long journey, indulging in fantasy acts which are in conflict with his censoring superego. The purpose of the fugue is to permit the performance of these acts.

To protect the ego, the person often employs the mechanism of depersonalization by forgetting his name and past history. Some individuals manifesting fugues use the mechanism of identification by assuming a false name and identifying themselves with the persons whose names they assume. Dissociating one's true identity is a defense which allows the person to detach himself from, and escape, guilt feelings associated with an illegal or socially unacceptable situation, thus allaying anxiety. A complete amnesia may follow termination of the episode until the memory of it is restored by hypnosis, narcotherapy or other psychic means which reveal the personal, emotional factors which evoked the use of an escape mechanism.

CONVERSION REACTIONS

Conversion reactions, often called conversion hysteria, are the physical expressions of emotional conflict on a symbolic level. Some anxiety-producing situation results unconsciously in the appearance of a functional body symptom associated with the organs of special sense or movement. The mental mechanisms of displacement and conversion are utilized in this reaction.

Some of the common conversion reactions observed are manifested in symptoms of hysterical deafness, blindness, anesthesias, paralysis, tics, tremors, choreiform or clonic movements, contractures, and aphonia. The patient's interest and complaints are focused upon the physical disability, while the emotional factors are obscured from conscious awareness. An examination of the patient fails to reveal a responsible organic basis for the production of the symptom.

Conversion reactions are to be differentiated from malingering, which is the production of a physical symptom on a deliberate, conscious level to achieve a definite objective.

The primary, unconscious purpose of the conversion reaction is to provide relief from the distressing anxiety produced by the emotional situation responsible for the occurence of the physical symptom. A secondary gain is often achieved which allows the patient to control the environment through attention, sympathy getting, and frightening others into submission. Suicidal gestures without real intent may be made to obtain a secondary gain.

The physical symptom observed is symbolic of the underlying conflict which produced the disability to prevent or relieve anxiety and meet some need created by the conflict. The more distressing the conflict, the greater the impulsive strivings, resultant anxiety, and focus upon the physical disability.

Conversion reactions are seen most often in adolescents and young adults. Rarely are they observed during or after the middle years of life when more permanent and adjustive mechanisms of defense have been established by the individual.

A study of the life history of patients manifesting conversion reactions usually reveals them to be narcissistic, emotionally immature, dependent, often childish and dramatic in their behavior and addicted to the habitual use of escape mechanisms. They evade responsibility, desire immediate gratification of their wishes, but depend upon others to achieve their desires for them. Oftentimes they are viewed as basically hostile and aggressive individuals.

The psychosexual development of these persons is usually discovered to be arrested at an earlier level of emotional growth. Many of these patients demonstrate a mixture of sexual desire and aversion, manifesting erotic thinking contrasted with prudish behavior and rejection of situations and ideas related to sex. These individuals react readily to suggestive stimuli. Their defense mechanisms are sometimes patterned after those they have observed to be used successfully by others in similar conflictive situations. Or sometimes, they manifest symptoms which they have heard or read about.

Conversion reactions observed in women are said to have a sexual conflict core. The problems of these patients often arise from such difficulties as unsuccessful love affairs, jealousy, frigidity, undesired marriage, fear of pregnancy, or poor marital adjustment. The basis of conversion reactions observed in men appears to be related to situations which threaten their self-esteem, economic success or self-preservation. Such individuals are often discovered to have strong emotional attachments to their mothers and frequently are unable to emancipate themselves from maternal bonds.

PHOBIC REACTIONS

Phobic reactions are manifested in marked, abnormal fear responses to external objects and situations. The degree of fear expressed by the patient is obviously unusual and out of proportion to the attending circumstances.

There are many types of phobias, some of them having names derived from the Greek language. These include a fear of dirt or germs (mysophobia), heights (acrophobia), animals (zoophobia), and closed places (claustrophobia).

Persons who fear dirt or germs may wear gloves, touch certain objects considered to be contaminating with paper tissues, or open doors with their elbows. Individuals who fear heights cannot ascend to higher levels, such as rooftops, towers, and hills. A fear of closed places may be manifested in a closed room, elevator, subway, pullman berth, or automobile. Fear of animals may cause the person to avoid visits to the zoo, having pets in the house or anywhere in their presence.

Patients manifesting phobic reactions become extremely fearful and sometimes panicky when confronted with the possibility of being exposed to or coming into physical contact with the feared object or situation. They will go to the most unusual extremes to avoid exposure. Oftentimes the mere prospect of encountering the feared object or situation may cause them to become panicky, perspire, feel dizzy, faint, or experience heart palpitation or nausea.

Phobic reactions are a defense against anxiety which arises from some deeper, unconscious source. Usually, an analysis reveals a situation which can be traced back to some earlier or childhood experience which activated fear and threats to security. The feared object or situation is symbolic of the deeper, underlying traumatic experience. For instance, a woman, who feared closed places and exhibited panic when exposed to them, had been locked in a dark closet as a child when being punished for misbehavior.

There is no clear-cut list of phobic interpretations or an identical object-fear relationship to the unconscious producing force. Some examples of their meaning as gained through experience are as follows: Acrophobia may symbolize a fear of suicide. Mysophobia may symbolize a fear of moral contamination. Zoophobia may symbolize fear of the father.

OBSESSIVE-COMPULSIVE REACTIONS

Obsessive-compulsive reactions are characterized by the persistent recurrence of unwanted, distressing thoughts and the compulsion to perform repetitive acts or rituals which are often recognized by the patient as unnecessary and unreasonable.

Obsessive thoughts may be intolerable to the patient's conscious mind, owing to their antisocial, sacrilegious, or forbidden nature. They are often referred to as obsessive-ruminative states. Persistence of an obsessive idea may produce fear of having committed, or the danger of possibly performing some homicidal, blasphemous, or socially unacceptable act. Such thoughts may arise from repressed, hostile, aggressive, or erotic impulses which threaten to invade conscious acceptance. Continued emergence of obsessive thoughts arouses feelings of fear, guilt, and anxiety. To allay or bind the associated anxiety, the patient attempts to further protect himself by utilizing the mechanism of undoing in the performance of repetitive acts or rituals which channel psychic energy into physical activity. Repetitive stereotyped activities symbolize unconscious experience and provide a defense against anxiety. In addition, these acts may symbolize atonement, penance or self-punishment. Patients manifesting obsessive-compulsive reactions often displace their anxiety through phobias which are expressed in combination with repetitive or ritualized activities.

Compulsive activities may consist of repetitive hand washing which may symbolize the need for cleansing owing to recurring vulgar, obscene thoughts, erotic cravings, or from some past, often trivial event interpreted by the patient as sin. Hand washing may symbolize fear and guilt over masturbation.

Repetitive counting and rechecking of routine duties may symbolize some past mistake, a fear of making mistakes or of failure, and the need for perfection.

Compulsive touching of certain objects may symbolize experiences which created a need to incorporate the protection and security afforded by supernatural forces. Or, it may symbolize the projection of evil influences thought to be retained through past experience, or the need for magical power or intervention.

As repressed, forbidden impulses threaten to invade conscious acceptance, the need for repetitive or ritualized behavior increases. More symptoms are construed to prevent their emergence.

If the patient is prevented from carrying out compulsive activities, anxiety increases greatly. It is said that if the unconscious causes giving rise to the production of obsessive-compulsive reactions can be ascertained, analyzed, and desensitized through psychotherapy, the patient will automatically relinquish the symptom once the need for it is eliminated. In many instances, however, the core of the difficulty is so deeply imbedded in the unconscious that it is impossible to bring it into conscious awareness.

Many of these individuals are so compulsive that their actions seriously interfere with their comfort and efficient performance of their occupations. They are often forced to retire and seek treatment.

Persons who manifest obsessive-compulsive reactions are said to possess compulsive personality traits, are meticulous, rigid, perfectionistic, and overconscientious. Their behavior is considered to be an exaggeration of the personality pattern.

DEPRESSIVE REACTIONS

The term "depressive reaction" is synonymous with reactive depression. Depressive reactions are characterized by social withdrawal, reduced activity, "blue mood," self-depreciatory behavior, and verbal expressions of guilt. They are to be differentiated from psychotic types of depressive reactions in which there may be obvious mood swings, delusions, severe psychomotor retardation, suicidal ruminations, intractable insomnia, agitation, etc.

These reactions, usually precipitated by a current situation, symbolize some loss to the patient. The loss of a loved relative or friend or some highly prized opportunity may precede the development of depressive reactions. Hostile, aggressive impulses producing ambivalent feelings toward the loss can no longer be excluded from consciousness by the mechanism of repression. The degree of the reaction observed may vary and is dependent upon the intensity of ambivalent feelings held toward the loss and the realistic circumstances surrounding it. Because of the love feeling component, hostility cannot be vented freely; therefore, the patient turns hostile impulses back against the self. The incorporation of these feelings results in self-depreciatory behavior which is symbolic of guilt giving rise to the need for atonement and punishment.

ETIOLOGY, DYNAMICS

A thorough study of the psycho-neurotic patient's life history usually reveals evidence of periodic or constant maladjustment of varying degree which has existed since early life. Overwhelming stress and strain in the immediate environment, which strains the ability to adjust, usually precipitates the development of a psychoneurotic disorder. The anxiety felt and perceived by the conscious portion of the personality is produced by a threat from within the personality.

The psychosexual life with its many taboos and social restrictions is not the only causative factor. Any fundamental impulse or desire which cannot be expressed owing to a too severe and exacting super-ego may be stimulated by an external situation which creates anxiety and mobilizes the defenses of the personality. Personal losses, dissatisfactions, disappointments, irritating relationships, fear of new responsibilities, failures, the changes associated with the involutional period and other situations may stimulate supercharged, repressed emotions, such as aggression, hostility, and resentment. Sometimes there is an absence of influential external factors. Anxiety may be produced by internal, unconscious forces.

The significant origin of the psychoneuroses lies in the less obvious, conflicting attitudes of the individual and relations with key childhood figures. A traumatic childhood experience may be an important source of the difficulty but more important are the effects of the whole constellation of experiences and relationships.

INCIDENCE

There is a high incidence of psychoneurotic disorders. Many persons afflicted with these reactions are seen by general practitioners. Social scientists have reported studies in which the greatest incidence was observed in the higher income bracket of society. The majority of these disorders are manifested between late adolescence and the age of 35 years. This is the period of life when individuals are confronted with adult adjustments and responsibilities. It is the time for satisfying social, economic, and sexual strivings. Frustrations may lead to conflict, anxiety, and tensions which can be met by some individuals only through neurotic manifestations. Women are said to demonstrate psychoneurotic disorders more frequently than men, perhaps owing to the requirements of more rigid repression of basic, biological needs and instincts required of them.

PROGNOSIS

Early detection and treatment of a developing psychoneurotic pattern of defense influence greatly the chances for recovery. Unfortunately, many of these persons come to the attention of psychiatrists at a time in life when the reaction pattern is so well established that it is difficult and often impossible to help them change.

The type of reaction manifested also influences the prognosis. Obsessive-compulsive reactions rarely yield to treatment.

Some investigators report that a psychoneurosis often develops into a psychosis. This does not mean that a psychosis is superimposed upon a psychoneurotic disorder; it develops as an additional affliction. Indeed, at a certain point in its development, it is often difficult for the physician to distinguish between a psychoneurotic reaction and schizophrenic reaction.

The degree of flexibility in the patient's personality and the ability to face reality and gain insight into the unconscious causes of the reaction through therapy influence the individual's capacity to learn other, more satisfying and relieving mechanisms of adjustment.

TREATMENT

When the initial physical examination fails to reveal an organic basis for the reaction, it is generally agreed that no further examinations should be conducted. Repeated physical examinations tend to emphasize organic causes, produce more anxiety, and make it difficult to assess psychic causes and to institute proper therapy. The diagnosis is made on discovery of psychogenic etiologic factors.

The most important aspect of treatment involves a study of the patient's personality, an analysis of the present, precipitating causes, and a reconstruction of the life sequences of psychic experiences which have influenced personality development and structure with its established mechanisms of defense.

Psychotherapy is the preferred treatment, but deep analysis may be necessary in some instances. Hypnosis is sometimes combined with these procedures.

After gaining a positive rapport in the treatment situation, the therapist encourages the patient to talk freely about himself and his life experiences. This provides for the ventilation of charged emotions which paves the way toward the development in the patient of a more rational, objective view of attending and past situations. It is not unusual for the physician to discover that the patient will avoid discussing or make only superficial references to some of the more distressing life experiences.

The doctor never infers doubt of the patient's physical complaints but avoids demonstrating serious concern of them. Constant reassurance is considered undesirable because it stimulates new symptoms and greater fear. At the appropriate time during therapy, the therapist commences to explain the unconscious causes of the reaction and their relationship to the patient's symptoms and anxiety. Desensitization of emotional experiences is utilized. Later, persuasion and suggestion are used to reeducate the patient toward adapting better and more effective mechanisms of adjustment.

Some investigators believe that giving medical prescriptions and advising the patient to rest more should be avoided because they tend to convey the impression of physical causes. Others believe that when anxiety is very great, tranquilizing drugs or electrotherapy, used in combination with psychotherapy, relax the individual and make the patient more accessible to treatment.

PREVENTION

It is said that maladjusted individuals create a maladjusted society. Prevention starts in the home where personality traits and patterns of defense may be acquired.

A parent who reacts to ordinary situations with emotional overtones, anxiety, temperamental outbursts, and physical symptoms may unknowingly provide a negative learning experience for children.

Reacting with acute concern toward the usual childhood diseases or calling attention to the appearance of every slight physical symptom in the growing child may teach an individual early in life to manifest neurotic illness to get attention, avoid responsibilities, and control the environment.

Punishment, which should communicate a message, may produce instead feelings of threat and hostility. Harsh psychic punishment or physical hurt are poor methods of discipline because the instinctive reaction of human beings to psychic or physical hurt is to focus aggression on its primary source. Some minor deprivation which carries significant meaning that can be recognized is more effective because it focuses attention upon the reasons for social disapproval instead of confining it to the offense.

Insistence upon meticulous habits in early life may erupt into compulsive patterns. One wonders seriously about the effects of some methods of school discipline. Forcing a child to write over and over on paper or the blackboard the intention not to commit again some act of misbehavior may be emotionally damaging. The question may well be asked: Does this contribute to the development of hostile aggression and compulsive behavior?

The need for security feelings is often dependent upon the setting of limitations. An adult must be able to discriminate between behavior which can be tolerated, although not necessarily approved, and behavior which requires intervention and control measures.

There is an early, powerful urge to be grown up and independent in every child. A youngster's attempt to do something independently, which is obviously physically burdensome, should not evoke reprimands or laughter. For instance, a child who wants to carry a heavy suitcase might be given some article instead to carry which satisfies the need for doing independently.

Youth should be given the opportunity to make decisions and assume responsibility for them. This also implies responsibility for adults who must necessarily control their anxieties at such times.

Civic organizations and schools have recognized the value of developing social interest and responsibility in teenagers by allowing them to take over the mayor's office and other key positions in local government for a day. Student government groups are known to be more punitive in their judgments than is adult jurisdiction.

Individuals should be encouraged to develop a human interest in, and consideration for, other people to avoid the development of narcissistic personality traits. Participation in the activities of many charitable and civic institutions provides an excellent opportunity to develop a desirable social consciousness.

Sex instruction should commence in the home. Individuals who obtain sex information from outside sources often associate it with immorality and guilt. Parents who satisfy their own neurotic needs by keeping a child emotionally attached and dependent upon them may contribute to the arrest of the person's psycho-sexual growth. Problems in heterosexual and marital adjustment have been known to arise from these sources.

A person who has been encouraged to face and solve problems is prepared better to assume later life responsibilities. One who has learned how to accept defeat is able to handle the inevitable disappointments in life.

It is considered beneficial to encourage persons to make the effort to accept an opportune challenge with whatever capabilities and resources they possess. This increases the capacity to assume responsibility.

The fatigue threshold varies in individuals. Some persons play or work so hard that fatigue fails to register until a situation develops which provokes fear, aggressive outbursts, and other neurotic reactions. To be able to view a situation rationally an individual needs to develop during early life healthful patterns of sleeping, eating, and recreation.

Detection of early neurotic personality traits is largely dependent upon good community mental hygiene educational programs which acquaint individuals with these manifestations.

NURSING CARE

Because persons with psychoneuroses are in good contact with reality, it may be difficult for the nurse to conceive of the patient as ill. To be of therapeutic assistance, the nurse needs to develop acceptance of the fact that the patient is experiencing real discomfort and that fear is as distressing as physical pain. The alleviation of this emotion often results in relief from discomfort.

The nurse's attitude is of paramount importance. If she can be genuinely accepting of the patient and consider the symptoms as indications of an illness, she will be fortified against demonstrating attitudes of doubt and avoidance which serve to intensify the individual's symptoms and anxiety.

The best care can be given when the nurse is acquainted with the patient's life experiences and the immediate precipitating causes of the disorder. It is possible to acquire this information through reading the history and in team or individual conferences with the psychiatrist and other staff members. In a large hospital there may be little time available to get this information. Oftentimes the staff is not organized for the team approach. If the nurse has a good understanding of the psychoneuroses and the forces which motivate behavior, she can combine this knowledge with her observations and follow general principles of care.

It is necessary to recognize that the patient has a need for the symptom. If the need can be met indirectly through nursing approaches, tensions and anxiety can be reduced. For instance, the need for attention can be met sometimes by allowing the patient to verbalize or to assist with planning of social, recreational activities. The need for increased self-esteem and confidence may be met through recognition of, and praise for, some artistic creation produced in occupational therapy. Many of these patients are intellectual and well versed in some field of endeavor. Recognizing the person's desire to talk about his experiences or demonstrate an acquired ability, often meets one's need for recognition and self-esteem. It is not unusual to discover accomplished individuals in patient groups. Some are more talented, creative, and informed than others, but even those with an average interest or ability may be striving to be recognized and appreciated. Some of the most successful persons fear failure and have a neurotic need to be strengthened through the emotional support of other individuals.

There are times when the nurse finds it helpful to seek the guidance of the physician. For instance, it may be necessary to know whether symptoms, such as hysterical seizures, should be only subtly or more closely observed in order to provide a better description of their occurrences and the attending circumstances. Or, the patient may complain of nausea or epigastric symptoms. Physical accompaniments which require medical treatment do develop sometimes during an illness.

Some patients become so engrossed in their physical discomfort that they may seek the nurse's opinion concerning the need for medical treatment. This sometimes happens when a new treatment has been widely publicized. Oftentimes, the patient has discussed the matter previously with the doctor. In such instances, it is wise for the nurse to reaffirm her confidence in the physician's judgment and suggest that the patient seek his advice.

Patients who complain of fatigue and wish to avoid participation in social, recreational activities may be encouraged, but never forced, into activity. Frequently, such persons are seeking just a bit of persuasion which meets the need for acceptance and attention. The doctor may wish a permissive attitude to prevail, especially if he is attempting to help the patient develop confidence and make decisions. At other times, the physician may advise the patient to participate and inform the nurse of this approach so that she will observe the individual's reaction to suggestion. Such observations may provide an index of the doctor-patient relationship and the response to psychotherapeutic techniques.

Anxiety may increase following psychotherapy sessions, especially if the therapist has commenced to explain unconscious forces to the patient. It is helpful to listen and observe the individual's reaction, but the nurse should refrain from suggesting that the patient forget about it. Commenting that the interpretation made by the doctor is of interest and worthy of consideration, in view of his experience and ability to help the person, is more apt to help the individual to adopt an objective viewpoint.

Patients who manifest phobias should never be forced into coming in contact with the feared object or situation. At the appropriate time during psychotherapy, when the patient's fear is considerably mitigated through understanding of unconscious forces, the physician may suggest that the patient try to approach the object or situation. Usually someone, perhaps the nurse, accompanies the patient during the attempt. Timidity, fear, and anxiety may be expressed by the patient. It is helpful to encourage the patient, but never wise to propel the individual into contact.

Compulsive behavior should never be ridiculed or forbidden. The patient's immediate need and relief from anxiety can only be met by allowing and providing for the performance of these activities.

When narcotherapy or hypnosis are utilized, the doctor may request the nurse to observe and record carefully the patient's behavior and conversation following these treatments.

Poorly established eating and sleeping patterns may be obvious in psychoneurotic patients. Some persons may call attention to anorexia and eat sparingly. Long-established patterns do not disappear quickly through attention or admonitions. Focusing attention upon a habit usually increases it. Omitting snacks and nourishment between meals may help to stimulate the appetite. As therapy progresses and the patient engages in diversional daily activities, anorexia may subside.

Some latitude may be extended towards patients who insist they cannot retire and sleep well if they adhere to the usual hour of retirement. A privilege may be given which provides limitations and is well within a healthful range of rest.

SUGGESTED REFERENCES

Freedman, A., and Kaplan, H. (eds.): Comprehensive Textbook of Psychiatry. Williams & Wilkins Co., Baltimore, 1967, pp. 857, 1387.
Kolb, L.: Noyes' Modern Clinical Psychiatry, ed. 7. W. B. Saunders Co., Philadelphia, 1968, pp. 324, 458.
Maddison, D., Day, P., and Leabeater, B.: Psychiatric Nursing. E. & S. Livingstone Ltd., London, 1968, p. 162.
Ujhely, G.: The patients whose symptoms are psychoneurotic, in The Nurse and Her Problem Patients. Springer Co., New York, 1963, p. 104.

For reviewing this chapter, grateful acknowledgment is made to Doctor Rigoberto Rodriguez.

CHAPTER 38

Asocial and Antisocial Behavior in Personality Disorders: Nursing Care

Personality disorders are characterized by pathological asocial and antisocial behavior traits and the perception of minimal anxiety by the individual. The degree of anxiety and sense of distress observed in the psychotic, psychoneurotic, and psychosomatic disorders is not observed in personality disorders. In most instances a personality disorder is manifested by a life-long pattern of action or behavior which the individual makes use of to secure adjustment. The personality disorders are divided into three main groups: personality pattern disturbance, personality trait disturbance, and sociopathic personality disturbance.

PERSONALITY PATTERN DISTURBANCES

There is a fixed, life-long, seemingly inherent pattern of behavior in persons with personality pattern disturbances which rarely, if ever, can be altered in its inherent structure. Prolonged therapy may improve a patient's functioning but basic change is seldom accomplished. The constitutional features in some of these individuals obviously resemble to a lesser degree the personality characteristics observed in some of the major psychoses and psychoneuroses. Owing to the depth of the psychopathology which exists, it is frequently impossible for these persons to maneuver under conditions of stress except into an actual psychosis.

INADEQUATE PERSONALITY

These persons fail in their emotional, economic, occupational, and social adjustments. Upon examination they are neither grossly physically nor mentally deficient. They demonstrate an inability to adapt, are inept,

474

exercise poor judgment, lack physical and emotional stamina, and are socially incompatible. Such individuals lack the ability to persevere and achieve even when reward or success is in sight. They are satisfied with the pleasure of the moment and cannot wait for gratification of needs. Their sense of responsibility to themselves and society is defective.

SCHIZOID PERSONALITY

Schizoid persons avoid close relations with others, are unable to express directly hostility or ordinary aggressive feelings, and manifest autistic thinking. These qualities result early in coldness, aloofness, emotional detachment, fearfulness, avoidance of competition, and daydreams revolving around the need for omnipotence. As children, schizoid personalities are usually shy, quiet, obedient, sensitive, and retiring. At puberty, they frequently become more withdrawn, manifesting the aggregate of personality traits known as introversion. They are described as seclusive, unsociable, and often eccentric.

CYCLOTHYMIC PERSONALITY

Personally, these individuals are warm, friendly, generous, and enthusiastic for competition in their adjustment to life situations. Observers view their behavior as a superficial, emotional reaching out to the environment. Some of these persons may demonstrate alternating moods of elation and sadness. Occasionally they may be either persistently euphoric or depressed, without falsification or distortion of reality.

PARANOID PERSONALITY

These persons manifest many traits of the schizoid personality, coupled with an exquisite sensitivity in interpersonal relations. They have a conspicuous tendency to utilize the mechanism of projection which is expressed in suspiciousness, misinterpretation of events, extreme jealousy, envy, and stubbornness. Under stress they may develop a paranoid reaction.

PERSONALITY TRAIT DISTURBANCES

Persons afflicted with these disturbances are unable to maintain their emotional equilibrium and independence under minor or major stress owing to disturbances in emotional development. Some of these persons manifest personality pattern disturbances which are related to fixation and exaggeration of certain character and behavior patterns. Others demonstrate disturbances which are a regressive reaction due to environmental or endopsychic stress. In these disturbances, anxiety and other neurotic-like reactions are relatively insignificant. The basic personality maldevelopment is the crucial distinguishing factor. The individual may or may not be physically immature.

EMOTIONALLY UNSTABLE PERSONALITY

When confronted by minor stress, these individuals react with an excitability which is ineffective. Between their emotional outbursts they are usually friendly, happy and likeable. Owing to poorly controlled hostility, guilt, and anxiety, their relationships with other people are continuously fraught with fluctuating emotional attitudes. One never knows whether they are friend or foe.

When they become excited they may shout, threaten, or even become destructive and assaultive. Sometimes their excitability is exhibited in scenes of futile despair. Or, they may become sulky, irritable, obstinate, and deliberately make themselves inaccessible to others. Suicidal gestures may be made in a situation regarded as intolerable. They often exhibit jealousy and quarrel with members of the opposite sex. Their hostile, threatening reactions are considered to be poorly disguised attempts to cover up an inherent weakness, as well as evidence of an immature personality.

PASSIVE-AGGRESSIVE PERSONALITY

These personality trait disturbances are of three reaction types which may occur interchangeably in the same person. Oftentimes there is a superimposed anxiety reaction which is typically psychoneurotic.

Passive-Dependent Type

Helplessness, indecisiveness, and a tendency to cling to others as a dependent child to a supporting parent are typical of these trait disturbances. There is a frank expression of an absence of mature self-confidence and self-reliance. An unconscious, underlying hostility is disguised in passivity, timidity, fear, and withdrawal from situations which are likely to arouse hostility.

Passive-Aggressive Type

Passive-aggressive traits, such as pouting, stubbornness, procrastination, inefficiency, and passive obstructionism, are utilized in these disturbances. The behavior is obviously immature and designed to thwart, make other persons uncomfortable, gain attention, or control the situation.

Aggressive Type

A persistent, immature reaction to frustration with irritability, temper tantrums, pathological resentment, and destructive behavior is manifested in this type of reaction. Individuals demonstrating this type of behavior have strong dependency needs.

COMPULSIVE PERSONALITY

Compulsive personality trait disturbances are characterized by chronic, excessive, or obsessive concern with adherence to standards of conscience or of conformity. Persons manifesting these traits are rigid, meticulous, perfectionistic, stubborn, hard workers, and lack the normal capacity to relax. They may be overinhibited and overconscientious. Usually they lack self-confidence and are unable to make decisions. Under pressure they are unable to produce well owing to their compulsive, routinized manner of behavior which is necessary. Being unable to perform according to the pattern developed makes them most uncomfortable and often irritable.

A certain degree of compulsiveness may be within normal range for some persons who achieve through their behavior a strengthening of character and ability. The origin of these traits lies in childhood factors which contribute to such character formation. Frequently these individuals have been driven, forced to conform, and received approval only when they met set standards and demonstrated perfection for others.

Compulsive traits protect the individual against the expression of aggression, hostility, and feelings of guilt. Sometimes these persons develop an obsessive-compulsive psychoneurotic disorder as a result of unbearable stress.

SOCIOPATHIC PERSONALITY DISTURBANCES

Persons manifesting sociopathic personality disturbances demonstrate repeated, recurrent maladjustment to the social environment. Their behavior may be differentiated from the more obvious anxiety and psychoneurotic disorders and the frank expression of regressive behavior often associated with psychotic disorders. Sociopathic features of behavior appear to be built into the individual's entire personality character structure, resulting in patterns of acting out their unconsious impulses and conflicts.

The defect of the sociopath is not intellectual. Instead, he is lacking in moral sensibilities, emotional control and the inhibitions of the will. These persons do not possess the normal concern for, and ability to adopt, social values and codes which would help them to adjust to society. Their emotional immaturity is reflected in impulsive, immediate responses to basic primitive instincts which appear to dominate and drive them compulsively toward a gratification which is insatiable. Their behavior gives the impression of continuously seeking an emotional outlet without regard for rational, acceptable conduct, or the feelings and interests of other persons. Frustration impels them toward social acts which connote irresponsible behavior, poor judgment, undependability and unreliability.

When the sociopath is confronted about behavior acts which are unacceptable to society, there is an obvious lack of real concern and an insensibility to the social effects and impact created thereby.

Many of these persons have difficulties in their interpersonal relations which eventually cause them to lose the respect and friendship of acquaintances. Others, but not all of them, become involved in situations which culminate in serious legal problems.

Most sociopaths are intellectually well endowed. In spite of this, many are unable to remain in an opportune, vocational capacity owing to their marked instability, unreliability, poor judgment, immaturity and irrational conduct of matters. They live for pleasure and gratification, attempting to derive these regardless of society's demands and the heartaches which their behavior often brings to relatives and friends.

Failure in interpersonal relations and vocations and punishment for illegal acts do not effect changes in their behavior patterns. These persons are so deficient in emotional control and normal feeling responses that they are insensible to consequences, and fail to profit from experience or punishment.

Typically, the sociopath is affectionless, narcissistic, selfish, ungrateful, exhibitionistic, egocentric, and demanding. Such individuals lack a critical awareness of their motives, foresight, and discriminative, reflective judgment.

Sociopathic behavior may be manifested in various reaction patterns, but a lack of social consciousness is its distinguishing characteristic.

ANTISOCIAL REACTION

Antisocial sociopaths are frequently callous and hedonistic and demonstrate marked emotional immaturity coupled with irresponsibility and poor judgment.

Quite frequently, these individuals make good first impressions upon others, winning their confidence and favor easily. Superficially, they are charming, attractive in appearance, well spoken, and fine mannered. There is a magnetic attraction about them and their charming convincing approach, which is never rewarding to others but more likely to result in emotional distress for persons who take easily and seriously to them and their ways. They are experts in building up another's confidence and trust in them and just as adept in letting the person down. They lie, cheat, and steal even when there is no particular advantage to be gained.

These are the types of individuals who accept social invitations, failing to appear when the occasion arrives, especially if something more pleasurable and gratifying is made accessible at the same time. On other occasions they flatter and entice people into loaning them money or advancing credit, and then fail to repay their obligations. They spend their money on pleasure and neglect to pay their bills.

Marriage is a loose binding contract for them. They are often unfaithful and engage easily in extramarital affairs. Remorse and a promise to remain faithful are only temporary because they have no special feeling for others. Divorce is common among them and a number of them marry more than once, as if always seeking the rainbow and never being able to grasp it.

These persons do not profit from experience or punishment. Many of them manage to remain free of legal complications and have never been hospitalized. They exist, most likely, in every community. Because they lack a critical awareness of their behavior, they do not seek help until some situation focuses attention upon them and their need for psychiatric help.

DYSSOCIAL REACTIONS

Persons manifesting dyssocial reactions disregard the usual social codes and often come into conflict with them as the result of having lived all of their lives in an abnormal, immoral environment. Within the social groups of these individuals their behavior is considered normal. They often adopt crime as another person adopts a career. A number of these persons are considered professional criminals. The dyssocial sociopaths are often so convincing that they easily swindle others, forge checks, and impersonate celebrities and important people. When confronted with their fantastic lies, these individuals readily manufacture new ones to explain the original ones. They are lacking in moral responsibility and rationalize their criminal acts to their self-satisfaction. These individuals cannot understand the viewpoint held by the normal citizen toward their behavior, possessing as they do an almost paranoid attitude toward organized society. They may be capable of strong loyalties to certain individuals, groups, or codes, particularly if their own welfare is involved. Loyalty demonstrations by them are often motivated by a group conviction that a pal should not squeal on a buddy, regardless of the crime or its effects upon society.

Morally, the dyssocial sociopath is often indiscreetly loose in intimate, sexual relationships. A number of them are professional prostitutes. Helping these persons is a real problem because so often they are committed to penal institutions where the procedures and environment are not conducive to treatment results.

SEXUAL DEVIATION

Deviant sexual behavior is considered a surface symptom of a more profound personality disorder. Persons whose sexual impulses are directed toward a normal heterosexual relationship, but who engage in sexual perversions owing to imposed segregation from members of the opposite sex, are not considered sexual deviates.

Very little is known about the causes of sociopathic sexual behavior deviations, although some postulations have been offered to try to explain their motivation. There is considerable agreement that persons manifesting sexual deviations have been arrested in their psychosexual development at some earlier level of emotional growth. The sex impulse has failed to mature for various reasons or has undergone a deviation in the course of its normal development. The defect is not in the physical development of the sex organs but in the psychosexual sphere. Normal psychic aspects of sex are not harmoniously integrated into the total personality. Sexual impulses are gratified through some deviant type of behavior.

Homosexuality

Homosexuality is a sexual attraction or relationship between members of the same sex. Oftentimes these persons manifest physical characteristics of body, voice, walk, dress and mannerisms associated with the opposite sex. Some investigators attribute this disorder to failure of the person to identify with the parent of the same sex. Heredity has also been mentioned but received less attention. Other authorities point out that parents desirous of a child of a particular sex tend to dress and treat the child as a member of the opposite sex. Seduction of the child at an early age by a member of the same sex, resulting in a continued relationship, is also thought to be a possible contributing factor to the development of homosexuality.

Transvestism

This trait is often observed in homosexuals who derive sexual pleasure and gratification from dressing or masquerading in the clothing of the opposite sex.

Voyeurism

This form of sexual deviation is usually observed in men and may consist of a compulsive interest in watching or looking at members of the opposite sex (peeping Tom) or in exposing the genitals (exhibitionism). These acts are accompanied by sexual stimulation and gratification. It is thought that such individuals are the sons of domineering, aggressive, pampering mothers who shower the child with affection. The fathers are weak and ineffective in stimulating male identification and normal sexual development. Being unable to gratify a developmental, incestuous desire for the mother, the boy unconsciously builds compulsive defenses to overcome forbidden wishes.

Pedophilia

Pedophilia is a pathological sexual interest in children, often observed in men who are weak and impotent persons. Some investigators believe that the individual's behavior toward the child is motivated by an unconscious, unfulfilled childhood wish to have the mother behave in the same way toward the person. Other authorities believe pedophilia may be motivated by fears and doubts concerning one's sexual ability which cause the individual to expect rejection and failure in adult, heterosexual attempts.

Fetishism

Fetishism, a perversion observed in men, provides sexual stimulation and gratification through the obtainment of some material object or article, such as a lock of a women's hair or an undergarment. The fetishist is not able to love a real person but instead attaches great value to the article, which, when once obtained, relieves psychic and sexual tensions. Many psychiatrists point out that the behavior of the fetishist symbolizes a genital conflict. Possessing the article may serve to deny the anatomical difference between the sexes owing to the fear generated in early life with the discovery of this fact.

Sexual Sadism

Sexual sadism is not only socially unacceptable but may result in serious crimes of rape, mutilation, and murder which cause society great concern. Some psychiatrists in attempting to explain this behavior postulate that perhaps the normal, aggressive, destructive instincts associated with early personality development fail to subside or get channeled through the process of sublimation. Instead, these instincts continue into adolescence, becoming associated with the sex impulse as it emerges. Each instinct reinforces the other, resulting in sexual sadism.

ADDICTION

Addiction to alcohol and drugs may serve as escapes from overwhelming conflict and frustration. It is well known that many persons who resort to the habitual use of alcohol and drugs have an underlying personality disorder (see Chaps. 31 and 32).

ETIOLOGY, DYNAMICS

The etiology of personality disorders is unknown. Investigators have postulated theories which are considered to be only speculative but worthy of consideration. Further research is still being conducted into the causes of these disturbances.

Most authorities stress the importance of the psychodynamics of personality development and the life experiences which interfere with maturation and the development of a socialized superego. There is strong evidence that internal psychic pressures created by unconscious impulses and conflicts as well as environmental factors contribute to the development of personality disorders.

Many investigators believe there is a constitutional predisposition in the sociopath which is reinforced by the social environment. In considering heredity it has been observed that there are families in which only one sibling manifested sociopathic behavior. Researchers suggest that such evidence leads to the hypothesis that individuals may be exposed to different types of social relationships and experiences in the same family environment. It has been suggested that owing to a parent's illness, separation, or tendency to demonstrate cold feeling tones toward the child the socio-path may fail to experience a primary, warm affectionate, close, sustaining relationship with a mothering figure. Consequently, normal humanistic qualities fail to develop upon a reciprocal basis and are not integrated into the personality structure. This supposedly accounts for the person's insensibility to concern, affection, and loyalty towards other individuals.

The particular experiences which influence identification, attitudes, and feelings are of utmost importance. The social environment of the home and neighborhood with the character of its residents, prevailing values, standards, codes, and material possessions or deprivations may influence attitudes, feelings, the process of identification, and the reinforcement of a sociopathic personality disturbance.

Brain injury or disease may precipitate the emergence of a more severe, underlying personality disorder.

PROGNOSIS

By the time these persons reach treatment, the character structure is so well ingrained that it rarely yields to constructive change. Prolonged therapy occasionally produces only an improvement in functioning. The drive or motivation behind the expression of sociopathic personality disturbances is so intense and forceful that immediate urges take precedence over rational considerations. The lack of insight which these persons possess concerning their behavior often causes them to become antagonistic and to refuse to confide in the therapist. If the individual does make an effort to change, the immediate need for expression usually impels the continuance of the behavior pattern.

TREATMENT

Treatment commences with a study of the individual's personality development through projective psychological techniques which may reveal significant information concerning personality structure, underlying psychopathology, and the areas of major conflict. Psychotherapy which provides for free association and suggestion approaches is considered the choice treatment. Sometimes it is necessary and possible to modify environmental factors or remove the patient from them. During therapy the patient may be able to relate past conflicts associated with present asocial or antisocial patterns of behavior and gain enough insight to result in the adaptation of more flexible, socially acceptable patterns of behavior.

PREVENTION

In view of the lack of specific etiologic data concerning personality disorders, it is difficult to formulate definite preventive measures. Enough is known, however, about the process of personality development and the factors which influence it to suggest that well-organized programs of mental hygiene could acquaint society with the importance of establishing healthy relationships with children which influence their feelings and attitudes towards other human beings.

Teaching all persons who come into contact with children to recognize existing asocial or antisocial patterns of behavior may result in early detection of abnormal reactions to social pressures and conflicts. Whether or not the process of adaptation can be changed is largely dependent upon available, competent psychiatric consultation and treatment.

Prevention is also dependent upon the cooperation of parents and civic authorities who may be helpful in creating constructive change in the social environment, particularly the influences which interfere with maturation and the development of a social conscience. Respect for human beings and society grows out of experiences which are conducive to satisfactions and the recognition by individual members that certain limitations are essential for the preservation of social ideals and values leading to personal happiness.

NURSING CARE

Many of these persons do not believe they are ill or in need of treatment. Oftentimes they project this idea upon the nursing staff and other patients. Some of them look so well physically and conduct themselves so rationally upon first meeting that an inexperienced nurse may overidentify with their feelings and question their hospitalization. If the nurse reads the patient's history, she will usually discover in it considerable evidence of the patient's pattern of reacting which has not been demonstrated in her presence. As she understands more about the illness and gets better acquainted with the patient, she usually discovers more tangible evidence of the reaction pattern in the individual's response to various developments.

Unless there is a well-planned schedule of daily activities, many of these persons tend to sit around and procrastinate about activity. Oftentimes they shift aimlessly without purposeful direction. The nurse should always convey the impression that active participation in social activites is expected.

So many of these individuals are self-centered, self-seeking and sensitive that it is well for the nurse to try to divide her time among all patients in order to avoid having some of them develop the feeling that favoritism is being extended to certain persons.

Special problems may arise which require that the nurse seek the guidance for her approach from the psychiatrist. It may be very important to know exactly how to handle such problems as a dependent attitude, sulking, irritability, deliberate inaccessibility, or the request for special privileges. Some persons may do well in a more dependent or permissive relationship. Others may need to develop self-reliance or the ability to adhere to limitations.

Persons manifesting sociopathic disturbances often create challenging, problematical situations. They may incite other patients to hostile relationships with the staff or to become involved in instigating a break with regulations. Usually, the sociopath manages to remain free of the acute developmental situation. There may be times when it is necessary to recommend the removal of these persons to another location in order to separate them from persons whom they appear to dominate and lead.

The sociopath may express chagrin at his hospitalization, treating it with subtle sarcasm and hostile feelings towards other persons. Often these individuals attempt to win the nurses's sympathy by projecting blame upon others and rationalizing and minimizing their behavior. Unless the nurse is aware of these inherent tendencies in them, she may be influenced to overidentify with their situation. It is well to listen, but also important to retain an objective viewpoint.

It is not unusual for sociopathic persons to prevail upon the nurse for special privileges, the granting of which may not be at all consistent with the aims of therapy.

A nurse who has an unmet need for attention and affection may become easily attracted to the charm and magnetic qualities of sociopathic patients. Nurses have been known to shower undue attention upon these patients and become emotionally involved in their problems. The nurse who recognizes the development of such an attachment should make every attempt to identify the source of her feelings. Talking it over with an experienced doctor or nurse may be extremely helpful for her and in providing the proper relationship with the patient.

SUGGESTED REFERENCES

Cleckley, H.: American Handbook of Psychiatry. Basic Books, Inc., New York, 1959, p. 567.
Cleckley, H.: The Mask of Sanity. C. V. Mosby Co., St. Louis, 1955.
Freedman, A., and Kaplan, H. (eds.): Comprehensive Textbook of Psychiatry. Williams & Wilkins Co., Baltimore, 1967, pp. 575, 937.

Friedman, P.: Sexual deviations, in American Handbook of Psychiatry, vol. I. Basic Books, Inc., New York, 1959, p. 589.

Group for Advancement of Psychiatry: Psychiatrically Deviated Sex Offenders. Report No. 9. Topeka, Kansas, Group for Advancement of Psychiatry.

Kinsey, N.: Homosexual panic: clinical manifestations and the nurse's function. J. Psychiat. Nurs. 2: 73 (Jan.), 1964.

Kolb, L.: Noyes' Modern Clinical Psychiatry, ed. 7. W. B. Saunders Co., Philadelphia, 1968, pp. 325, 501, 510.

Nagler, S.: Fetishism: a review and a case study. Psychiat. Quart. 31: 713 (Oct.), 1957.

The passive-dependent personality (editorial). Psychiat. Bull., Medical Arts Pub. Foundation, University of Texas, Fall, 1957, p. 78.

The schizoid personality (editorial). Psychiat. Bull., Medical Arts Pub. Foundation, University of Texas, Winter, 1957-1958, p. 2.

The sociopathic personality (editorial). Psychiat. Bull., Medical Arts Pub. Foundation, University of Texas, Spring, 1957, p. 32.

For reviewing this chapter, grateful acknowledgment is made to Doctor Edwin Lawson and Mrs. Vivian S. Bryan, R.N.

CHAPTER **39**

Transient Behavior Reactions to Situational Stress: Nursing Care

Transient situational behavior reactions appear to be acute, temporary symptom responses demonstrated by the patient toward emotionally distressing, depriving, or fearful situations. The symptoms observed in these reactions are the immediate means used by the patient to adjust to the overwhelming situation. If the person possesses good adaptive capacity, the symptoms usually recede when the stress of the situation diminishes.

TYPES OF REACTIONS

Gross Stress Reaction

These reactions follow exposure to severe physical demands or extreme emotional stress, such as in combat or civilian catastrophes (earthquakes, fires, explosions, etc.).

Adult Situational Reaction

These reactions occur when the individual encounters difficult situations or newly experienced environmental factors. They may be manifested in anxiety, alcoholism, asthenia, poor efficiency, low morale, unconventional behavior, etc.

Adjustment Reaction of Infancy

In the absence of organic disease, psychogenic reactions may grow out of the infant's interaction with key persons in the environment or the lack of such persons. They may be manifested in apathy, undue excitability, feeding and sleeping difficulties, etc.

Adjustment Reaction of Childhood

The following types of reactions may be responses to some immediate situation or internal emotional conflict:

1. Habit Disturbances: Nail-biting, thumb-sucking, enuresis, masturbation, tantrums, etc.

2. Conduct Disturbances: Truancy, stealing, destructiveness, cruelty, sexual offenses, use of alcohol, etc.

3. Neurotic Traits: Tics, spasms, somnambulism, stammering, overactivity, phobias, etc.

Adjustment Reaction of Adolescence

These reactions are expressions of emancipatory strivings and vacillations and may resemble any of the personality or psychoneurotic disorders.

Adjustment Reaction of Late Life

These reactions are expressions of problems of physiological, situational, and environmental readjustment which may occur with menopausal changes, occupational retirement, and separation from family members through death or other life situations.

ETIOLOGY, DYNAMICS

The precipitating causes of transient behavior disturbances are the special, developmental situations which produce environmental stress. The unique reactions manifested by the individual in response to the precipitating factors are influenced by the life experiences which have contributed to the patient's personality development and methods of reacting to stress. Cultural and family concepts and attitudes may be reflected in the occurrence of these disturbances. Cultural patterns of rearing infants and children, and attitudes expressed towards the menopausal and senile changes appear to bear some relationship to the individual's self concept and attitudes towards changes and environmental demands.

INCIDENCE

These reactions are commonly observed by general practitioners and nurses employed in schools, industry and visiting nurse associations. A number of individuals demonstrating these disturbances are also observed in community mental hygiene clinics as well as inpatient and outpatient psychiatric services of general hospitals.

PROGNOSIS

Many of these patients react favorably to the elimination of the precipitating causes. The ability of the person to develop more effective methods of adapting to stress also influences the prognosis.

TREATMENT

Treatment revolves around the identification of special stress-producing situations and attempting to help the patient, when possible, to develop some insight into the reasons for the reaction. Desensitization may be helpful in certain instances, particularly those reactions which are a response to fear. Medications may be prescribed temporarily to relieve the discomfort of anxiety. It may also be necessary to help the patient develop better health habits related to rest, diet, and recreation. Social rehabilitation may be necessary for some individuals, especially persons experiencing adolescent, menopausal and senile changes. Family members may play an important part in treatment. Quite often the family attitude towards the needs of children, adolescents, and aging persons may be changed to effect better relationships with the patient which helps to meet the individual's emotional needs.

PREVENTION

Prevention is dependent upon community mental hygiene programs which assist in enlightening persons to the common life experiences which may produce emotional reactions and teaching them how to recognize and meet these situations effectively and to help others to adapt to them. Individuals may be made acquainted with the community resources which can be of assistance in providing competent evaluation and psychiatric help.

NURSING CARE

The reactions of infants are often related to the mother's or mother substitute's manner of caring for the child or her pronounced feeling of inadequacy and fear regarding the ability to give proper care to the infant. Nurses who listen to the problems and feelings experienced by such mothers can often provide them with emotional support by explaining the need for a close, affectionate relationship between the mother and child.

Nurses can also strengthen the self-confidence of mothers by teaching them the proper methods of giving physical care to the infant.

Doctor Smiley Blanton cites one of the most vivid, startling accounts of the effects of lack of maternal affection in his book *Love or Perish*. Ninety-seven infants reared in a highly understaffed foundling home in South America responded to lack of affection and attention with vacant expressions, crying, inability to sleep, and loss of appetite and weight. When picked up and fondled by the attending doctor, these infants screamed and became panicky. Twenty-seven of the children died during the first year of life. Seven more perished the second year. This account points up the need for nurses in institutions to give loving care to infants. It emphasizes that attention to physical needs must be supplemented with fondling and affection.[1]

The disturbances of older children may indicate some problem within the home or school environment which produces anxiety and tension and interferes with meeting the child's underlying needs for acceptance, affection, recognition, and security. Home problems may be very intricate and frequently involve parent-child relationships, relationships between parents, or difficulties with other relatives, such as grandparents. Some parents attempt unconsciously to resolve their own conflicts through demands made upon the child or in their unique method of handling a situation. Attending circumstances require careful investigation.

School nurses may visit the child's home and share their observations with school authorities and members of the teaching staff. Sometimes it is necessary to arrange for special physical and psychiatric examinations in order to evaluate children's special problems. Psychiatric consultation and assistance may be required.

Parents may be brought into conferences in an effort to resolve difficulties which contribute to tension-producing reactions in children. Joint plans may be worked out between the medical and teaching staff, dependent upon the situation, to change or initiate some procedure or approach which may be helpful in relieving a current problem in the classroom or school environment.

Community organizations interested in children's and aged persons' problems have provided recreational centers and programs which help to socially rehabilitate these individuals and meet their emotional needs.

Families may welcome the opportunity to talk over certain problems with the visiting nurse. Sometimes emotional problems are detected in family members during home visits which can be referred to the family physician. Nurses may also assist in making arrangements for referral of a patient to a community mental health service.

Industrial nurses often give emotional support to employees by listening to their complaints and occupational or personal problems. Sometimes a change in job or department is recommended by the nurse. Dependent upon the particular situation, the person may be referred to the plant or family physician or a local mental health service.

Nurses caring for patients in the hospital environment can frequently provide emotional support which is therapeutic. Patients are often benefitted when they are able to verbalize their problems and feelings to the nurse. They may also be encouraged to participate in the many social, recreational activites conducted in the hospital setting which help to divert their interests and reduce anxiety.

NOTE: For additional information regarding the roles of visiting, industrial and school nurses see Chapter 9, The Extending Community Nursing Role.

SUGGESTED REFERENCES

Ashford, M.: Home care of the mentally ill patient. Am. J. Nurs. 57: 206 (Feb.), 1957.
Liebman, S.: Management of Emotional Problems in Medical Practice. J. B. Lippincott Co., Philadelphia, 1956.
Liebman, S.: Understanding Your Patient. J. B. Lippincott Co., Philadelphia, 1957.
Manfreda, E.: The school nurse and the exceptional child. Catholic Nurse 6: 40 (Mar.), 1958.
Vonachen, H., and Mason, M.: The employees mental health. Am. J. Nurs. 57: 753 (June), 1957.

FOOTNOTES

1. Blanton, S.: Love or Perish. Simon & Schuster, New York, 1955, p. 39.

CHAPTER 40

Emotions Affecting Body Organs and Behavior in Psychosomatic Disorders: Nursing Care

These illnesses are commonly referred to as the psychosomatic disorders, the name being derived from the two Greek words *psyche* and *soma*. In differentiating psychosomatic disorders from the psychoneuroses, the distinction may be observed in the afflicted person's defense against anxiety which underlies both illnesses. The defense against anxiety in the psychoneuroses is on a symbolic level, the chief symptom being symbolic of an underlying emotional conflict in the absence of demonstrable organic defect. In the psychosomatic disorders the defense is on a physiologic level, the affect being expressed through the body viscera. Persistent psychosomatic reactions may produce structural organic changes leading to the development of chronic disease.

The general ideas concerning psychosomatic medicine have been known for more than 2,000 years, but have received more attention during the past quarter century. In one of his dialogues, Plato, the Greek philosopher, said, "This is the reason why the cure of many diseases is unknown to the physicians of Hellas, because they are ignorant of the whole which ought to be studied also, for the part can never be made well unless the whole is well—this is the great error of our day in the treatment of human bodies, that the physicians separate the soul from the body." These words indicate that Plato was attempting to convey that the intimate relationship between mind and body must be recognized and that the mind should be considered capable of producing organic disease.

It is said that the family physician of the past was unconsciously an expert in treating psychosomatic disorders. Knowing the life history and the family environment of most of his patients enabled him to recognize that some physical illnesses were of emotional origin and required psychologic support treatment.

TYPES OF PSYCHOSOMATIC REACTIONS

Psychosomatic reactions, having related emotional causes which are often unrecognized by the patient, may be associated with any of the body systems. Some of the more commonly observed reactions are as follows:

Skin Reactions

Neurodermatoses, pruritus, atopic dermatitis, hyperhydrosis.

Musculoskeletal Reactions

Muscle cramps, backache, tension headaches, psychic rheumatism.

Respiratory Reactions

Bronchial spasm, hyperventilation syndromes, asthma, hay fever, sighing respirations, hiccoughs.

Gastrointestinal Reactions

Peptic ulcer-like reactions, chronic gastritis, ulcerative or mucous colitis, constipation, diarrhea, hyperacidity, pylorospasm, heartburn, irritable colon, anorexia nervosa.

Cardiovascular Reactions

Paroxysmal tachycardia, extrasystoles, palpitation, vascular spasms, migraine.

Genitourinary Reactions

Dysmenorrhea, dysuria, frequency.

Endocrine Reactions

Hyperthyroidism.

Nervous System Reactions

General fatigue, exhaustion states, certain types of convulsive seizures.

ETIOLOGY, DYNAMICS

Generally speaking, emotions may be regarded as the cause of some physical dysfunctions and distress. Conversely, organic physical illness may provoke the expression of emotions which often aggravate and complicate greatly these somatic disabilities. When the underlying emotional conflict is not treated, the affected organ may be damaged.

There are differences of opinion among investigators as to the chief etiologic factors which produce psychosomatic disorders. Some authorities stress the importance of environmental and interpersonal causes. Others place emphasis upon the particular emotions expressed and their ability to affect specific body tissues or organs. For instance, hostility is said to affect particularly the heart action. Chronic repressed aggression affects vascular system changes. There are also investigators who believe that individuals inherit or acquire systemic weaknesses. Thus, they conclude that the organ which reacts excessively to emotional developments is determined by inherited weaknesses instead of psychologic factors. For instance, a person with a weak heart would be a victim of hostile feeling reactions. An individual with a weak gastrointestinal system might develop ulcer-like conditions owing to suppression of anger, feelings of humiliation, guilt, or resentment.

Some of the emotions which may be experienced by an individual in response to social, environmental or interpersonal situations as well as physical disease may be fear, hostility, resentment, depression, guilt, frustration, and panic states. Anxiety is greatly perceived.

The mental mechanism utilized in the defense process may be repression or suppression of unpleasant emotional experiences. Introjection may be expressed in the patient's interpretations of illness as punishment. Projection may be manifested in blaming other individuals for taking advantage of the person through overwork or contributing in some manner to the wear and tear upon his reservoir of strength. Conversion is often utilized when the patient concentrates exclusively upon the physical symptoms and is unable to recognize related emotional causes.

Patients afflicted with psychosomatic disorders often have underlying needs for dependency, attention, love, success, recognition, and security. When these needs cannot be met, the person clings unconsciously to his physical disability as a substitute means of achieving satisfaction. While most of these individuals truly desire relief from physical symptoms, the disability may be used as a crutch when emotional needs are not gratified. During World War II it was observed that soldiers who developed gastritis, ulcers, and hypertension in the service recovered almost simultaneously with their return to civil life. In other instances, persons have been known to avoid the assumption of responsibility by clinging unconsciously to their physical disabilities. Loving care, attention, and reassurance by family and friends often gratify the patient's need for dependency and security.

INCIDENCE

The incidence of psychosomatic disorders is said to be high in highly industrialized countries, such as the United States, and where rivalry and competition exist. A considerable number of these disorders are thought to be unrecognized. It is estimated that about one million persons die yearly from disorders which are essentially emotional in origin. The high incidence of psychosomatic disorders has created a serious social and financial problem. At one time it was thought that the process of aging was responsible for chronic, debilitating illnesses. However, studies have revealed that many of the patients with chronic diseases are under 45 years of age.

PROGNOSIS

The chances for recovery are influenced when early detection of psychosomatic disorders and skillful psychotherapeutic approaches are made to help the patient recognize and resolve underlying emotional conflicts.

TREATMENT

Authorities believe that when an organic basis for the patient's complaint cannot be found, the patient should never be told there is nothing wrong with him because the emotional causes are actually a disability. Telling the patient there is nothing wrong serves to intensify the physical symptoms and increase anxiety with resulting aggravating effects upon the involved organ. Organic defects which may be discovered should be treated whenever necessary but not emphasized. Repeated laboratory tests and examinations tend to strengthen the patient's concept of physical causes and may produce fear of an incurable disease.

Getting the patient to talk is the most important part of treatment. The sooner the patient can be encouraged to discuss his personal life, the sooner will emotional causes be brought to the surface and detected. Adults frequently experience distressing problems in the home, on the job, and in the community. Family relationships, religious conflicts, sexual problems, and difficulties associated with the choice of associates and vocations are frequent causes of psychologic reactions.

A skilled psychiatrist is capable of determining the appropriate time during therapy to discuss with the patient his emotional involvements and their effects upon his health. Good rapport between the therapist and patient encourages the individual to talk about his personal problems sufficiently to decrease the power of emotion behind them. This enables the person to become more objective and accepting of the psychic components of an illness. Patients can be helped to recognize that when tensions are not released through some channel the body will do so through organ language. Treatment then revolves around teaching the patient more effective ways of reacting to the life situation which has influenced the development of the disorder.

PREVENTION

Early recognition and treatment of children's emotional problems is an important preventive measure. Through the assistance offered in child guidance clinics and community mental hygiene programs, adults can be taught to recognize emotional conflicts and to appreciate the emotional needs of the growing child. They can also be taught how to influence healthy mental attitudes in children which affect personality development and the ability to react properly to life situations. Concomitant learning outcomes of these preventive approaches also assist adults to adjust in society.

NURSING CARE

The nurse's understanding of these disorders and her attitude toward the patient's symptoms is important in the treatment and recovery process.

The patient's discomfort is very real and often frightening to him. When medical treatment is prescribed in the standing orders the nurse should administer it without hesitation. The physician is able to determine best when medical treatment should be discontinued. Making light of the patient's symptoms and procrastinating about giving prescribed treatment intensify the individual's reaction.

It is not unusual for persons afflicted with psychosomatic disorders to awaken in the middle of the night with complaints of physical distress accompanied by outward expressions of depression, fear and much anxiety. A palpitating heart, sensation of choking, difficult breathing and other prominent symptoms may be extremely frightening to patients. A calm, confident approach on the nurse's part as she remains with the patient to listen to his complaints and fears is reassuring and helps to alleviate anxiety.

When patients are unable to verbalize freely their complaints to the medical staff, they tend to project them upon other patients who often become distressed and feel emotionally burdened.

These individuals should not be pushed beyond comfortable limits or allowed to remain preoccupied and inactive for long periods. They should be encouraged and assisted to make use of their intellectual and physical capacities to the best of their abilities. A well-planned but not overwhelming schedule of social, recreational activities throughout the day and early evening hours provides an outlet for the release of tensions and diversion of mental preoccupation over physical disability.

SUGGESTED REFERENCES

Freedman, A., and Kaplan, H. (eds.): Comprehensive Textbook of Psychiatry. Williams & Wilkins Co., Baltimore, 1967, pp. 1049, 1123.

Kolb, L.: Noyes' Modern Clinical Psychiatry, ed. 7. W. B. Saunders Co., Philadelphia, 1968, pp. 324, 413.

Liebman, S.: Management of Emotional Problems in Medical Practice. J. B. Lippincott Co., Philadelphia, 1956, p. 33.

Liebman, S.: Understanding Your Patient. J. B. Lippincott, Philadelphia, 1957, p. 24.

Maddison, D., Day, P., and Leabeater, B.: Psychiatric Nursing, ed. 2. E. & S. Livingstone Ltd., London, 1968, p. 302.

O'Hara, F., and Reith, H.: Psychosomatic Disorders, in Psychology and the Nurse. W. B. Saunders Co., Philadelphia, 1966, p. 231.

Ujhely, G.: The patient whose symptoms or illness are psychoneurotic or psychosomatic, in The Nurse and Her Problem Patients. Springer Publishing Co., New York, 1963, p. 104.

Wahl, C.: Physical symptoms as a mask of psychiatric disorders in the hospital. Hosp. Med. 1: 28 (Dec.), 1964.

CHAPTER 41

Organic Changes that May Influence Behavior Changes: Nursing Care

Numerous afflictions of the human body may produce toxins, circulatory defects, and other conditions that affect the normal functioning of the brain and result in mental changes that are observable in the patient's behavior. Injury, infection, new growths, glandular disturbances, nutritional deficiencies, poisons, genetic developments, and structural changes in body cells and organs are some of the physical conditions which may, in some individuals, influence behavior reactions. The common basic reaction is known as an acute brain syndrome involving a complex of intellectual impairments that may be reversed when treatment is effective. In these disorders the terms acute and chronic refer to whether the condition is reversible or irreversible. When the syndrome is irreversible, it may develop into a chronic brain syndrome of permanent changes in personality characteristics and functioning. Although the acute syndrome was formerly known as a toxic, delirious reaction, it is not always a sudden flare up of physical and emotional symptoms. It may commence with a change in the physiology of a body system, for example, the glandular system. In many instances, it is a mild or more severe delirium characterized by transient episodes of restlessness, confusion, and incoherent mumbling lasting for a few or more minutes which alternate with rational mental states. When the delirium is severe, disorientation, defects in memory, comprehension, and judgment, delusions, illusions, and hallucinations may be observed. Development of a chronic brain syndrome following the initial physical condition may be a matter of several months, years, or even longer.

Most of the precipitating illnesses that may influence the development of acute and chronic brain syndromes are known by medical and nursing personnel caring for sick people in general hospitals and some other types of health facilities. Alcoholism, drug addiction, convulsive disorders, and senile reactions are also afflictions which may precipitate acute and chronic brain syndromes. Because they are major public health problems, these illnesses are discussed in greater detail in separate chapters (see Chaps. 30 to 33). The content of this chapter will be limited to a discussion of those precipitating disorders which are not as often observed by the average nurse.

EPIDEMIC ENCEPHALITIS

This illness, more commonly known as "sleeping sickness," was caused by a filtrable virus when it occurred in epidemic form in the United States in 1919 and 1925. Encephalitis which is reported from time to time today is caused by other types of bacteria which invade the cephalic area following an upper respiratory infection, mumps, measles, infectious mononucleosis, and other highly infectious diseases. These are known as postencephalitis reactions. During the acute syndrome, the patient's lethargy is manifested in sleep episodes lasting for days or weeks which may be broken at intervals by brief awake periods. The delirium is often overlooked owing to the more obvious stupor. Some individuals also present hyperkinetic symptoms of restlessness, irritability, and excitability in association with the delirious reactions. Jacksonian and grand mal seizures have been known to occur during a hyperkinetic reaction. A postencephalitis parkinsonian syndrome may develop 1 to 20 years after an acute syndrome. Tremors, and muscular and ocular spasms seen in Parkinson's disease characterize the later, chronic reaction. Various mental symptoms may be observed during the chronic syndrome. Depression and feelings of despondency may lead to suicidal attempts by some persons. Intelligence defects do not usually occur except in children having the disorder who may develop serious antisocial behavior problems which do not respond favorably to any treatment approach. It is thought that the behavior of these children constitutes the defenses used by them in reacting to rejection, teasing, taunting, and name calling by members of their peer group who view their physical symptoms of tremors, speech difficulties, and dull facial expressions as peculiar.

BROMIDE INTOXICATION

Bromides contained in several patent medicines and tranquilizing drugs may be taken indiscriminately for the relief of headache, insomnia, and emotional distress. Bromides are excreted slowly from the body and may accumulate sufficiently in the blood to replace its normal sodium chloride content and produce a bromide intoxication. Elderly and arteriosclerotic patients have a poor tolerance for bromides and may demonstrate intoxication symptoms when the blood bromide level is relatively low. The mental reaction observed may be similar to behavior observed in other psychotic disorders. Patients may become overactive, homicidal, and suicidal. Body temperature may be elevated. The differential diagnosis is based upon laboratory reports of blood studies. The bromides are abruptly withdrawn, fluids forced, and the sodium chloride replaced with prescribed drugs. Ammonium chloride, a diuretic, displaces the bromide faster than does sodium chloride. Cathartics are usually necessary to aid in the elimination of bromides from the body. Dialysis, by means of artificial kidney, may be indicated in some instances. As treatment progresses, favorable and often quite striking behavior changes occur, usually within three to ten days.

CEREBRAL ARTERIOSCLEROSIS

Personality changes observed in persons over the age of 50 often indicate the possibility of cerebral arteriosclerosis. It is not so much the sclerotic (hardening) process, as it is a thickening of the artery wall which produces the narrowing of the lumen of the blood vessels. With progressive thickening and diminution in the artery size, the circulation is retarded, and impaired nutrition of the brain results. As a consequence, the ganglion cells of the brain deteriorate and certain areas around the constricted arterioles atrophy. Early symptoms may be fatigue, reduced initiative and attention, emotional instability with periods of weeping or laughing, and sometimes depression. Some patients may be more obviously irritable, quarrelsome, jealous, suspicious, and forgetful. Later progressive symptoms may be manifested in marked confusion, disorientation, apprehension, incoherence, and other psychotic symptoms. Hostile, homicidal, and suicidal behavior may be observed. Convulsions and vascular accidents may complicate the condition.

CENTRAL NERVOUS SYSTEM SYPHILIS

Central nervous system syphilis, caused by the Treponema pallidum organism, usually commences in the frontal lobes, resulting in early impairment of intellectual functions. Early symptoms are said to be an exaggeration of the individual's personality traits. As the disease progresses, it attacks other parts of the brain, manifesting more advanced neurologic signs, disabilities, and behaviors that are psychotic. Irritability, fatigue, difficulty in concentration, confused periods, mild depression, poverty of affect and emotional responses, carelessness in the discharge of one's duties, and a lack of insight into these behavior changes may be observed.

Indulgence in alcoholic beverages and sexual activities may increase. Social and ethical regression takes place. Continued progression of the disorder may be manifested in confabulation, use of poor judgment, grandiose delusions, and expansive schemes. Upon the slightest provocation these persons may become combative, a defense which may be motivated by the need to preserve the integrity which is threatened by disorganization of the personality. Physically and mentally the person shows signs of progressive deterioration, including defects of speech, body system incoordination and pathological reflexes. In the terminal phase, the individual may become critically ill and require careful observation and good bedside nursing care. Treatment may consist of intramuscular injections of penicillin in oil, a regime which may have to be repeated within three to six months after the first series of injections if the infecting organism is discovered to be present following blood-Wassermann and spinal fluid examinations. Some physicians prefer to treat the patient with Aureomycin (chlortetracycline), by intravenous injection or oral capsules, owing to the permeable and diffuse circulatory properties of Aureomycin. Following recovery, spinal fluid examinations should be done every six months for two years, then once a year. Activities requiring complete self-control, such as driving an automobile, should not be undertaken by afflicted persons until the spinal fluid is negative.

HEAD TRAUMA

Transient or complete loss of consciousness may develop following a head injury. There is often an amnesia for the few moments preceding injury and the actual trauma. Some patients pass from an unconscious state into an acute traumatic delirium within a short time following injury. Delirium lasting more than one week is suggestive of considerable brain damage which cannot be completely evaluated for six months. Delirium of more than one month's duration indicates serious tissue destruction which cannot be evaluated for long term expectations of behavior for at least 12 to 18 months. Post-traumatic personality changes which may develop may be a change in the person's disposition and mood, often occurring a considerable time following the injury. The patient suffers from headache frequently, is easily fatigued, irritable, and emotionally unstable. Attention and concentration ability decline and there is marked narrowing of interests. Whenever brain injury involves a severe contusion, or is complicated by hemorrhage, laceration, and tissue destruction, the individual may develop convulsive seizures, aphasia, paralysis, and other neurological conditions, such as deafness or pugilist's encephalopathy (punch-drunk). Chronic personality changes are sometimes detected after complete recovery is pronounced. One may hear family or friends of the patient describe him as different, or queer, since the injury occurred. Symptoms of emotional instability, impaired judgment, irritability, apprehension, fear, depression, fatigue, headache, insomnia, and inability to concentrate may be observed. Occasionally, overindulgence in alcohol, barbiturates and smoking is evident. Treatment consists of absolute bedrest and observation for three days in a quieter environment. Diagnostic tests are done and selective medications prescribed. Neurological and psychological examinations are conducted.

BRAIN TUMORS

New, but abnormal, growths of tissue, such as brain tumors, may produce physical and mental changes which are also observed in psychotic disorders. Establishing an early diagnosis is often difficult and may actually be delayed until more obvious but differential symptoms appear. The early psychologic reactions may simply be an exaggeration of the person's individual personality characteristics, such as irritability, apathy, indifference, euphoria, emotional instability, and mood fluctuations. With the passing of time, other psychic disturbances that are impressive may be observed. Defects in thinking, memory, judgment, reasoning, and calculation may be obvious. As the tumor increases in size, intracranial pressure causes symptoms which vary according to the site, size, and type of growth precipitating the reactions. More serious organic symptoms may develop in the absence of diagnosis and remedial treatment, such as dizziness, headache, and visual disturbances. Nausea, vomiting, increasing stupor, and choked optic disks are grave developments which require emergency treatment approaches. Coma is a most serious terminal phase condition. The nurse's observations and record of the patient's symptoms may be helpful in establishing a correct diagnosis. Following surgical removal of a brain tumor, the patient must be skillfully nursed during the immediate postoperative period and convalescence. There should be careful observation and recording of changes in vital signs and motor abilities.

PARKINSON'S DISEASE

This degenerative disease of the nervous system is often referred to as paralysis agitans or shaking palsy. The onset is usually insidious, but may be observed abruptly, and is characterized by a fine, paroxysmal tremor which begins in the hand or foot. As the disease progresses, muscular weakness, rigidity, and a peculiar gait in which the patient's steps grow faster and the body inclines forward are observed. Tremors gradually expand to a continuous, agitated coarse type involving bundles of muscles. The person's facial expression becomes blank or masklike, the speech retarded and measured. Emotionally, these patients may become irritable, faultfinding, difficult to please, and demanding. They may become fearful and depressed as they become aware of their increasing disabilities and dependence upon others. Suicidal attempts have been made by some of them. Artane (trihexyphenidyl) is the drug most widely prescribed to assist in controlling the tremors, although other drugs may be used for relieving the tremors in some individuals who develop a tolerance for Artane or do not respond favorably to it. More recently it has been reported that the drug L-Dopa has affected significant improvement in some patients. Neurosurgical techniques have also been helpful in controlling the tremors of selective patients. A cold instrument, applied through a surgical opening in the skull, to freeze that portion of the brain considered to be involved in the production of tremors is a favored approach.

HUNTINGTON'S CHOREA

Huntington's chorea is known to be a hereditary, degenerative disease of the central nervous system due to a dominant mutation. More than 1,000 cases of this disorder have been traced back, over a period of 300 years, to a person who emigrated from England to the United States in 1603. Considerable research is presently being conducted in attempts to develop early identification techniques and a cure for the disorder. The gene affected in Huntington's chorea is responsible for controlling the growth of certain cells which regulate the movements of muscles in various parts of the body. In Huntington's chorea these cells die early and cannot be replaced. Symptoms usually appear between the ages of 30 and 45 years but have occasionally been observed earlier. The illness is characterized by involuntary, irregular, jerking movements which commence in the upper extremities, neck, and face. As it progresses, the trunk and lower extremities become involved and a shuffling type of gait develops. Contractions of facial, tongue, lip, and respiratory muscles result in facial grimaces and poorly articulated, often incoherent speech. Involuntary movements subside with sleep but reappear upon the patient's awakening. Personality changes manifested in irritable, obstinate, moody reactions may be observed prior to the development of symptoms or following their onset. A lack of initiative, spontaneity, and concern for the disease develops. There is blunting of the esthetic and ethical senses. More progressive psychologic reactions may be demonstrated in suspicious attitudes, delusions of persecution, hallucinations, combative behavior, and suicidal attempts. Mental and physical deterioration develops; the patient becomes unable to swallow or walk and must be confined to bed. The constant movements eventually exhaust the individual and he usually expires about 16 years after the development of the disorder from upper respiratory or other illnesses. Most patients do not live beyond 50 years of age. Huntington's chorea attacks both men and women and is transmitted directly from parent to child. When it misses a generation, the child having parents free of the disease may not expect to inherit it through the family line.

ALZHEIMER'S DISEASE

This disease is characterized by progressive defects in comprehension, memory, and judgment reminiscent of early, senile deterioration. Some investigators believe that a large number of patients confined to mental institutions under the classification of senile disorders may actually have Alzheimer's disease. These persons may be anxious, active, aggressive, and impulsive. Delusions, hallucinations, and confabulation may be observed. Memory impairment is usually so severe that patients are unable to recall from day to day the various room locations on the ward and have to be led to these areas. Making a positive diagnosis of Alzheimer's disease is said to be impossible except by autopsy. Autopsy reveals the presence of cell changes in both left and right lobes of the brain, usually in the frontal, temporal area. Normal cell structure is replaced by coarse, fibrous, whorled arrangements.

PICK'S DISEASE

Although the evidence is not positive, Pick's disease is thought to be hereditary because several cases of the disorder have been observed in one family. It usually occurs between 45 and 60 years of age but has been observed earlier on occasion and is seen twice as frequently in women as in men. Investigators find it very difficult to distinguish Pick's disease from Alzheimer's disease, but the age of development, the slow progressive course, and the incapacitating effects upon the individual's intellectual abilities are similar in both illnesses. The early symptoms are an emotional blunting, lack of spontaneity, and difficulty in thinking and concentrating. As the illness progresses, the individual becomes increasingly bewildered, unable to perform abstract functions, or manage new situations. Some become suspicious, depressed, and irritable. As the disease advances, speech and memory defects increase, the individual becomes inactive, immobile, and must be confined to bed. Incontinence develops; little nourishment is taken so that malnutrition and a wasting away become obvious. At autopsy, the brain is drastically reduced in size and weight in comparison to the normal brain owing to a severe atrophy of one lobe, usually the frontal or temporal. Structural cell changes are also noted with the disappearance of the chromatin, leaving an empty shell. Some of the cells may be observed to be swollen, but an inflammatory process is absent. The frontal lobe may appear as if a constricting band had been applied to it.

CUSHING'S SYNDROME

This condition, due to hypersecretion of the adrenal cortex, produces such physical changes in the female as obesity, fatigue, inactivity, cessation of menses, a masculine beard, deep tone of voice, and atrophy of the breasts. Patients may become depressed, retarded, irritable, anxious, and uncooperative. Mental symptoms may bear some relationship to adreno-cortical dysfunction and metabolic abnormalities, but the psychological reaction to the development of masculine features would appear to be the most emotionally distressing influence upon the self image.

NURSING CARE

Perhaps the most vital aspect of nursing care involves attitudes. Unfortunately, a legend of chronicity has persisted for many years in a large number of psychiatric hospitals. This hopeless, dismal pessimism has hastened the invalid period of many patients who have, as a result, developed increasing, functional disabilities. A more optimistic attitude toward these patients is necessary. Many of them have the ability to learn, create, and participate in social, therapeutic activities. While some may never recover completely, many can be remotivated and improved in their outlook and capacity to function. Nurses need to intensify their efforts to initiate more social activities on the wards and to visit and work closely with these patients as often as possible. Through individual consideration, attention, and emotional support by the nurse, these patients can often be stimulated and remotivated.

Developmental personality behavior changes should be observed carefully and reported. Chronic, permanent behavior changes may be manifested in problematical behavior which may be approached best when the nurse seeks the physician's guidance.

There should be careful but indirect observation of depressed patients who may harbor suicidal tendencies, as well as those who may be injured during confused, overactive periods.

Delirious patients are often restless, disoriented, and apprehensive. Frequently, they have elevated body temperatures. They require good, bedside nursing care with attention to hygiene, nutrition, fluids, and regular elimination. Care should be taken to provide a quiet environment. Protection of the patient from upper respiratory infection is important. These patients are easily frightened and react fearfully to abrupt approaches and unknown procedures. It is necessary to explain what is to be done and to reassure the patient. Sometimes it is possible to bring the patient into contact for varying periods of time by repeatedly reorienting the individual to the date, time, and circumstances. Reporting the patient's response to medications prescribed is important as some may become further confused and disturbed and require a change in prescription. During the terminal phase of chronic, debilitating disorders, good supportive nursing care is required. Patients need to be assisted with their hygiene, bathing, feeding, and other personal care.

SUGGESTED REFERENCES

Bond, J.: St. Louis encephalitis. Nurs. Outlook 14: 26 (Oct.), 1966.

Butts, C., et al.: The unresponsive patient. Am. J. Nurs. 67: 1886 (Sept.), 1967.

DiPalma, J.: The nurse and carbon monoxide poisoning. R.N. 27: 37 (Oct.), 1964.

Elwood, E.: Nursing the patient with a cerebrovascular accident. Nurs. Clin. N. Am. 5: 47 (March), W. B. Saunders Co., Philadelphia, 1970.

Fangman, A., and O'Malley, W.: L-dopa and the patient with Parkinson's disease. Am. J. Nurs. 69: 1455 (July), 1969.

Frankel, E.: "I spoke with the dead." Am. J. Nurs. 69: 105 (Jan.), 1969.

Freedman, A., and Kaplan, H. (eds.): Comprehensive Textbook of Psychiatry. Williams & Wilkins Co., Baltimore, 1967, p. 460.

Haber, M.: Parkinson's disease—challenge to the health professions. Nurs. Clin. N. Am. 4: 263, (June), W. B. Saunders Co., Philadelphia, 1969.

Hamilton, C., et al.: The nurse's active role in assessment. Nurs. Clin. N. Am. 4: 249 (June), W. B. Saunders Co., Philadelphia, 1969.

Jennings, C.: The stroke patient—his rehabilitation. Am. J. Nurs. 67: 118 (Jan.), 1967.

Kolb, L.: Noyes' Modern Clinical Psychiatry, ed. 7. W. B. Saunders Co., Philadelphia, 1968, pp. 174, 180, 185, 212, and 281.

Leavens, M.: Brain tumors. Am. J. Nurs. 64: 78, (March), 1964.

Matheney, R.: Cerebrovascular accident and personality organization. Nurs. Clin. N. Am. 1: 443 (Sept.), W. B. Saunders Co., Philadelphia, 1966.

Ramsey, I.: The stroke patient is interesting. Nurs. Forum 6: 273 (Summer), 1967.

Seabury, C.: A nurse's observations on post encephalitis patients. Nurs. Outlook 14: 28 (Oct.), 1966.

Ullman, M.: Disorders of body image after stroke. Am. J. Nurs. 64: 89 (Oct.), 1964.

CHAPTER 42

Mental Retardation

Since 1963, impressive progress has been made in understanding human development and the factors which contribute to all types of developmental deviations, including mental retardation. The late President John F. Kennedy and his family had a very deep interest in mental retardation, a major health problem that affects approximately six million people in the United States. Proposals contained in the report to the President by the panel on mental retardation in October, 1962 called for national action to combat mental retardation. Accordingly, financial appropriations were increased and research efforts intensified. Some of these studies involved nursing personnel, resulting in the gain of new knowledge and deeper insights into the behavior, needs, and approaches to the care of the mentally retarded. However, ten years later, some persons who are working with the mentally retarded do not believe that sufficient progress has been made in applying this knowledge and implementing needed change.

Patterson and Rowland say,

During the past decade, many plans that might very well result in improved care and training programs for the retarded have been proposed. Unfortunately, very few of these plans have actually been translated into action. It is no longer true as it was, say 10 years ago, to report that we don't really know what to do; we are actually utilizing no more than 10 per cent of what we already know. New knowledges and skills are simply not filtering down to the people who are in day-to-day contact with retarded individuals.

We seem to be on the edge of remarkable innovation, and yet all across the nation one sees sudden removal of essential financial support. Practically every state department of mental retardation is currently facing austerity measures, budget cuts, and a general lack of substantial support for the implementation of programs. Political figures and many citizens who are yet unable to see the retarded individual as a human being are quite capable of cutting or at least stabilizing the dollar cost of residential services. How long will it take for people to realize that it costs much less to maintain a healthy child than it does to maintain a sick child. This is the dichotomy we face. If programs embodying developmental approaches are not provided in residential facilities for the mentally retarded, we will be faced with an ever-increasing number of individuals who will require increasingly expensive and difficult to staff custodial services—merely to sustain life. Given the economic situation of this society, something must be done within our residential facilities to create a better climate and to reduce the dehumanizing situations which result in such a waste of human potential.[1]

MENTAL RETARDATION DEFINED

Mental retardation refers to subnormal general intellectual functioning which originates during the developmental period and is associated with impairment of either learning and social adjustment or maturation, or both.[2]

CLASSIFICATION CORRELATED WITH INTELLIGENCE QUOTIENTS

Borderline mental retardation	IQ 68–85
Mild mental retardation	IQ 52–67
Moderate mental retardation	IQ 36–51
Severe mental retardation	IQ 20–35
Profound mental retardation	IQ under 20

It is recognized that the intelligence quotient should not be the only criterion used in making a diagnosis of mental retardation or in evaluating its severity. It should serve only to help in making a clinical judgment of the patient's adaptive behavioral capacity. This judgment should also be based on an evaluation of the patient's developmental history and present functioning, including academic and vocational achievement, motor skills, and social and emotional maturity.[2]

Developmental Characteristics of the Mentally Retarded*

Degrees of Mental Retardation	Pre-School Age 0–5 Maturation and Development	School Age 6–20 Training and Education	Adult 21 and Over Social and Vocational Adequacy
Mild	Can develop social and communication skills; minimal retardation in sensorimotor areas; often not distinguished from normal until later age.	Can learn academic skills up to approximately sixth grade level by late teens. Can be guided toward social conformity. "Educable"	Can usually achieve social and vocational skills adequate to minimum self-support but may need guidance and assistance when under unusual social or economic stress.
Moderate	Can talk or learn to communicate; poor social awareness; fair motor development; profits from training in self-help; can be managed with moderate supervision.	Can profit from training in social and occupational skills; unlikely to progress beyond second grade level in academic subjects; may learn to travel alone in familiar places.	May achieve self-maintenance in unskilled or semi-skilled work under sheltered conditions; needs supervision and guidance when under mild social or economic stress.
Severe	Poor motor development; speech is minimal; generally unable to profit from training in self-help; little or no communication skills.	Can talk or learn to communicate; can be trained in elemental health habits; profits from systematic habit training.	May contribute partially to self maintenance under complete supervision; can develop self-protection skills to a minimal useful level in controlled environment.
Profound	Gross retardation; minimal capacity for functioning in sensorimotor areas; needs nursing care.	Some motor development present; may respond to minimal or limited training in self-help.	Some motor and speech development; may achieve very limited self-care; needs nursing care.

* "The Problem of Mental Retardation," Secretary's Committee on Mental Retardation, U. S. Department of Health, Education, and Welfare, Washington, D. C.

INTELLECTUAL DEVELOPMENT

Research indicates that about 50 per cent of a person's intellectual development occurs between conception and four years of age. About 30 per cent takes place between ages four and eight. Developments between the period of gestation and early childhood determine to a large extent the life adjustment potential for all individuals, on all intellectual levels. Some of the factors that play a part in each child's development are heredity, nutrition, living conditions, emotions, physical aspects, interpersonal relationships, and environmental interaction. When something goes wrong, either through human neglect, an error of nature, or an environment which fails to provide opportunities for healthy emotional and mental development, retardation can result.[3]

CAUSES OF MENTAL RETARDATION

Increased research into the etiology of mental retardation and its progression has added to our knowledge of the causes of this condition. Among the most recent and significant discoveries are those associated with genetic defects, inborn errors of metabolism, and environmental stimulation. In some instances, mental retardation may be prevented, reversed, or arrested, dependent upon the identified cause. The following are known to be causes of mental retardation.
1. Congenital numerical deficiency or abnormal arrangement of brain cells.
2. Birth injuries due to pelvic disproportions, premature birth, or forceps delivery.
3. Rh blood-factor incompatibility between mother and child.
4. Infectious diseases, such as German measles, of the mother during the first three months of pregnancy.
5. Infectious diseases during childhood, such as meningitis and encephalitis.
6. Brain injuries occurring during childhood.
7. Endocrine deficiencies, such as thyroid deficiency, known to be the cause of cretinism.
8. Exposure to underprivileged environments with poor housing, poor economic and social conditions.
9. Familial or hereditary causes.
10. Inborn errors of metabolism, such as the inability to metabolize proteins, carbohydrates, and fats.
11. Genetic defects, such as abnormalities in the genes and chromosomes.

NEUROTIC AND PSYCHOTIC BEHAVIOR

When a mentally retarded person becomes neurotic or psychotic it is said to be due to the anxiety and frustrations experienced while attempting to adjust to the conditions of the society and compete with others. Such individuals are unable to manage their social and financial affairs, exercise prudence, and assume ordinary responsibilities.

INCIDENCE

Mental retardation occurs in families of all income levels. It has been observed, however, that the largest number of mentally retarded children are born to parents in poverty. Mothers in these families may receive poor or no prenatal care. Nutrition is often inadequate. Children may receive little affection and intellectual stimulation from overworked mothers who often have large families. Retardation that results from social and cultural deprivation is usually mild or "borderline." It may not be recognized until the child enrolls in school. These children are not able to perform at the level expected of other children in their age group. The standards of achievement used to make such comparative observations are determined largely by the social, educational, and cultural standards of the individual community. For example, a person may be able to make an adequate adjustment to a rural farm and its menial work requirements, but be unable to adjust to and meet the demands of living in a highly competitive urban society. Retarded children who come from deprived social environments can improve their performance when help is given early and followed up with a continuous program of assistance. When such help is not given, a child coming from an environment that stunts mental and social growth tends to drop to even a lower IQ level. Preschool and head start programs aim to provide such children with the kind of stimulation needed to overcome their negative environments. Retardation that is due to biological or organic causes is generally not reversible. Genetic defects, infectious diseases, birth injuries, or brain injury resulting from an accident in later life are among the identified causes of irreversible mental retardation. Most of these individuals have physical as well as mental handicaps. Usually, they are among the most severely retarded.[3]

CLINICAL TYPES

Some groups of mentally retarded individuals are easily recognized because they possess definite and unusual physical characteristics.

DOWN'S SYNDROME (MONGOLISM)

Mongolism was first described by Langdon Down about 100 years ago. During the past ten years, it has been recognized that it is the result of a chromosome abnormality; the presence of an extra chromosome. This may occur in three ways: (1) there may be 47 instead of the normal 46 chromosomes, (2) translocation, the chromosome count is 46 with an extra small chromosome being attached to one of the chromosomes, making the count appear normal, (3) mosaic, when the chromosome count is 46 in some cells and 47 in other cells. The frequency of Mongolism is said to be closely related to the age of the mother. The risk of giving birth to a Mongoloid child rises with the age of the mother.[4]

Physically, Mongoloids resemble Asiatics; this explains the name given to them. Usually, they have small heads, almond shaped, downward slanted eyes, thick lips, short fat hands with usually one palmar line, and a sallow complexion. Their tongues are flabby, with deep grooves and fissures. Personally, they are friendly and love to imitate others. Acute leukemia is more prevalent in them than in the general population.[4] Persons with Mongolism are usually mouth-breathers and are prone to respiratory infections. Prior to the use of antibiotic drugs, most of them died at an early age.

HYDROCEPHALUS (WATER ON THE BRAIN)

There is an increased volume of cerebrospinal fluid within the skull. This accumulation may be within the ventricles or in the subarachnoid space. To accommodate the excess fluid, an infant's head may expand to as much as 36 inches. The normal average adult circumference is 22 inches. Hydrocephalus may be primary or secondary. In primary hydrocephalus developmental abnormalities may result in excessive secretion of the cerebrospinal fluid and a low or absent absorption rate of the secreted fluid. In the secondary condition there may be obstructing lesions within the system of ducts which block the drainage of cerebrospinal fluid. Distention of the brain ventricles by the excess cerebral fluid, causes the surrounding tissue to be replaced with fluid, leading to subsequent pressure upon and destruction of brain tissue. Progressive deterioration producing blindness, deafness, and convulsions may take place. The patient becomes bedridden and paralyzed. Death usually occurs very early in life. The condition is slowly progressive in those who survive, and, if arrested, the patient is left with varying degrees of mental and physical disabilities. Hydrocephalics are usually undersized physically. Muscular weakness and spasticity affecting the legs cause their movements to be awkward and uncoordinated.

MICROCEPHALY

A small cone shaped head is the most outstanding feature of microcephalics. Upon completion of development, the head is less than 17 inches in circumference. In addition, these individuals have a receding forehead, beak nose, and receding chin. The sutures of the skull overlap and thick ridges of bone can be felt. The scalp is sometimes loose and wrinkled longitudinally, having the appearance of being too big for the skull. The majority of these patients are severely mentally retarded. The cause of microcephaly is a single recessive gene which determines the inability of the brain to develop to its normal size.

CRETINISM

Cretinism is due to a lack of thyroid gland secretion resulting from various enzyme disturbances. Usually, the child appears normal at birth, but during the later months, the condition becomes noticeable. Cretins have dwarfed bodies, large heads, and dry, wrinkled skin. As they grow, they develop a thickening of the lips, nostrils, hands, feet, and back of the neck. Prominence of the abdomen with umbilical hernia is often observed. Hair on the scalp and eyebrows is usually scanty. The body temperature is below normal. Behaviorally, they are apathetic, slow, do not smile readily or laugh, and refuse to suck. As time goes on, the child makes no attempt to sit up, stand, or walk. Speech may be delayed until seven or eight years of age. Puberty occurs late and the external genitals remain infantile. Early administration of thyroid extract has helped to improve some of these persons mentally and physically. Untreated cases are usually severely mentally retarded.

PHENYLKETONURIA

Infants with phenylketonuria inherit an inability to metabolize phenylalanine, a constituent of all natural protein foods. The presence of phenylpyruvic acid in the urine as well as a concentration of phenylalanine in the blood is a diagnostic indicator. An early diagnosis is necessary to prevent severe mental retardation. A test of blood drawn from the infant's heel shortly after birth establishes the diagnosis. The onset of mental retardation can be prevented with a diet which is low in phenylalanine, but provides sufficient protein for growth and repair. Patients afflicted with phenylketonuria are nearly always fair haired, have light skin, blue eyes, and widely spaced incisor teeth. They urinate more frequently and in larger amounts than unaffected children. Cyanosis of the hands and feet due to poor circulation is often observed. In appearance, they are dwarfed and may walk with a short stiff gait.

WILSON'S DISEASE

There is a decrease of copper and the copper containing protein caeruloplasmin in the serum. The symptoms of mental subnormality may appear after the age of 10 years. Involuntary choreiform movements with tremors develop and there is progressive deterioration in articulation and swallowing. As the condition progresses, rigidity of the muscles of the limbs, trunk, and face occur, resulting in contractures of the limbs and wasting of muscles. Mental and physical deterioration are progressive. Treatment with penicillamine increases urinary excretion of copper and may be helpful in some cases.

FROLICH'S SYNDROME

Severe mental retardation is caused by insufficient secretion of the pituitary gland. The physical signs include a defective stature, infantile genital organs, and obesity of the abdomen and mammary regions.

AMAUROTIC FAMILY IDIOCY

A single recessive gene is the cause of this rare condition. Deposits of lipid material within the nerve cells leads to their degeneration. Two main types of the disorder are associated with mental retardation, infantile (Tay-Sachs disease) and juvenile (Spielmayer-Vogt disease). In the infantile type the infant is normal at birth, but abnormal signs usually appear about the end of the third month. Progressive muscular weakness leads to an inability of the child to sit up and the head falls backward if not supported. A cherry red spot is observed in the retina of the eye. Death usually occurs before the age of two years. In the juvenile type the onset is between age five and ten years. Mental development is arrested and deteriorates to a state of dementia. Muscular weakness is progressive and impaired vision usually ends in blindness. The course of this type is much slower than the infantile, but it terminates in death.

GALACTOSAEMIA

In this rare and familial disorder, sugar galactose.is not converted into glucose in the normal way due to an enzyme defect caused by a single autosomal recessive gene. An infant thus afflicted appears normal at birth. Loss of appetite and persistent vomiting occur after a few days of milk feedings. Urine examinations show the constant presence of the sugar galactose and an increase in the excretion of amino-acids and protein. Jaundice and enlarged liver and spleen may develop. If diagnosed shortly after birth, milk and milk products are removed from the diet and replaced with soybean or casein hydrolysate substitutes. In severe cases, malnutrition causes death. Infants who survive appear undernourished and smaller than usual at the age of three months. Mental retardation occurs.

GARGOYLISM

This is a rare type of mental subnormality caused by a single recessive gene. Deposits of mucopolysaccharides are found in the tissue cells of the brain, liver, heart, lungs, and spleen. There are two types of gargoylism, one in which both males and females are equally affected and intermarriage with cousins is frequent. Dwarfism and clouding of the cornea occur. In the second type only males are affected, and there is an absence of corneal clouding. Only one third of those afflicted are of small stature, and about half of them are deaf. The strange physical appearance of individuals having gargoylism accounts for the name of this condition. The head is large with a protruding forehead, bushy eyebrows, and saddle-shaped nose. The abdomen protrudes and there is usually an umbilical hernia. There is enlargement of the liver and spleen. No treatment exists at the present time for this disorder.

PREVENTION

Members of the health disciplines recognize that prevention of mental retardation will require extensive research, planning, and education programs that only the government will be able to afford. The following preventive measures can help to reduce the magnitude of this problem

1. Adequate medical care during the prenatal period and birth.
2. Early detection of the various disorders.
3. Immunization against communicable diseases.
4. Educating parents to understand the important concepts of growth and development.
5. Educating family members and society to accept the mentally retarded.
6. Better housing and living conditions.
7. Preschool and head start programs.
8. Improved nutrition through dietary requirement instruction, meal planning, and the provision of breakfast and school lunch programs.
9. Intellectual stimulation through socialization, recreation, play, and learning activities for affected individuals.

DETECTION OF EARLY SYMPTOMS

Detection of early signs of mental retardation may be one of the problems confronting the public-health nurse in the home. A very young baby who appears to be chronically listless, lies quietly, and sleeps for unusually long periods should be carefully observed. Such a child may not notice other persons in the room and may not be aware of light and sound changes in his environment. Most young babies normally reach out and grasp objects within their reach, but the mentally retarded child does not usually do this. Quite often, these children teethe much later than is usual. As the child grows, he appears to be slow and awkward in learning to walk and talk. He may also have great difficulty in learning excretory-function control.

Older children may be given intelligence tests which often prove helpful in establishing the diagnosis. However, it is recognized that test results may be adversely influenced if the child becomes emotionally disturbed during administration of the tests. Emotionally disturbed children may rate unfavorably. Children who belong to the severely underprivileged social and educational groups may also rate unfavorably. It is very important that all of these factors be recognized by the examiner.

NURSING CARE

Parents may feel shock, shame, embarrassment, and have feelings of guilt and personal failure when an abnormal child is born. Guilt feelings about the origin of the abnormality, particularly if they fear it is hereditary, may be expressed. During pregnancy every mother fantasizes about having a perfect child. This expectation is a composite of the images she has of people who are important to her. When the infant is drastically different from the anticipated child, the sudden loss of the idealized child and the demand to accept an abnormal one can be overwhelming. The greater deviation of the child from the normal, the greater is the impact of the experience. Before they can accept the deviant child, the parents need to express the grief they feel for the lost, perfect one. The process of grief involves anger and may be shown toward anyone, including nurses. The nurse has an opportunity to be of assistance to such parents at the time they experience the impact of this event. To utilize this opportunity the nurse must be aware of the concerns such parents are likely to have and their significance to them.

One of the first things a mother wants to know right after the baby's birth is the condition of her child. If people evade her and she is kept waiting for this information she may become anxious and consume energy which will be needed later when the diagnosis is made known. Nurses should make themselves available to parents when the diagnosis of abnormality is communicated. If they can accept anger that may be shown as not being personal and if they are able to support the parents as they express their grief, they will be making a contribution to the parents as well as the infant. Nurses will also be able to pick up cues and make observations about the parent's responses during this time that will be helpful to them in deciding how they can best be of help.[5]

Patterson and Howland believe that the medical model of mental retardation that is so prevalent in our institutions has the effect of reinforcing the dehumanization of the mentally retarded. This model allows the nurse to use a clinical label that emphasizes the deviancy instead of the humanness of the affected person. These are some of the reasons why they do not think the mentally retarded in institutions should be called patients. When the patient does not recover, they say, use of the medical model permits rationalization of the symbolic death of humanness as an act of God. With respect to this viewpoint, there is a trend toward calling these individuals residents.

These same authors state that we should use a vocabulary that reflects the goal of personal and social rehabilitation in contrast to the current "therepeutic" concept. In their view, use of the term "therapy" tends to perpetuate a model of illness which reflects a dependency in the patient.

These specialists have studied job descriptions for nurses in institutions for the mentally retarded and believe they are written in medical instead of nursing terms. Their concept of the nursing job description is that a nurse

evaluates the resident's behavior and assesses his abilities in relation to his physical and developmental needs and checks this evaluation with the assessments made by other members of the multidisciplinary team; participates in the development and implementation of the nursing plan for the training and habilitation of the residents; studies the group structure and its impact upon behavior and physical care and conducts individual and group conferences with nursing and non nursing personnel; observes and evaluates interpersonal relationships among residents and staff and reviews information from other disciplines; interprets and implements physician's orders for physical care.[1]

This description, they point out, shows the nurse to be an educator while not excluding nursing's medical function. Nursing is more clearly differentiated as a science in its own right, with its own objectives and practices. It is not dependent upon or parallel to the practice of medicine.

HELPING PARENTS

One of the most difficult problems for the nurse arises when she is attempting to assist parents to accept a diagnosis of mental retardation in a child. Nurses must be expert in human relations in order to sense the emotional climate and determine the best approach toward parents. There are some mothers and fathers who are extremely sensitive and resent questions about the child's behavior. Other parents are over-anxious and freely seek advice. Guilt feelings and depressive reactions may be obvious in some parents. The whole family life and future seems to revolve around the mentally retarded child; parents have been known to lose sexual interest in each other.

An interesting reaction pattern has been observed in parents, particularly intelligent parents, who find it difficult to accept a diagnosis of mental retardation. Such parents first go through a period of frantic searching for proof that the child is not abnormal. To secure this proof they write letters to authorities in the field of abnormal psychology and visit psychiatrists and specialists all over the land until their financial resources are exhausted. Still not convinced, the mother next devotes her every waking hour in attempts to train the child. Family and social relationships are excluded during her efforts. The third stage comes only when both parents accept their child as being abnormal and plan constructively for their own and the child's future.

Nurses have the opportunity to work very closely with parents, doctors, the clergy, and social workers when helping parents accept a diagnosis of mental retardation and recommendations for institutionalization of a child. Team harmony must prevail if assistance to these parents is to be successful. All members of the team must be in agreement so that the parents will not become confused and indecisive.

CRITERIA FOR INSTITUTIONALIZATION

Four guiding suggestions for deciding whether or not the mentally retarded child should be institutionalized are suggested by the National Mental Health Foundation. Institutionalization is recommended:

1. *When the child is without a home or is not well taken care of in his home.*
2. *When he overburdens his mother and the rest of the family.*
3. *If the community or school lacks a training program for the mentally retarded.*
4. *If the child cannot be managed at home or in the community and tends to be a danger to himself or others.*[6]

COMMUNITY ASSISTANCE

Day nurseries for mentally retarded children are suggested as one way to provide some change and relief for mothers who care for such children in their homes. Mothers may form a group and take daily turns in caring for the children in each one's home so that it is possible for the group members to socialize and carry on normal lives in the community. There is a national association of parents and friends of the mentally retarded with local chapters in every state. Foster-home parents have had success in supervising and training a mentally retarded child who could not be helped by his own parents. Permanent or traveling clinics in state sections have been suggested. Schools and social agencies may coordinate their efforts to discover the mentally retarded, provide training programs to develop their limited abilities, give guidance to parents, seek institutional placements, educate the general public toward an understanding and sympathetic attitude, and prevent antisocial behavior. The philosophy of interested persons is that we must stop talking about what the mentally retarded are not, and help them become what they can be. It is said that the mentally retarded constitute a group of solid citizens whose value to the community lies in their faithful performance of the routine and monotonous jobs that must be done by someone.

TEACHING PARENTS TO PROTECT AND ASSIST THE CHILD

The following helpful suggestions concerning the guidance and supervision of mentally retarded children may be useful to the public-health nurse and to nursing personnel engaged in the institutional care of such children:

1. Protect the child from danger. Keep pins, matches, medicine bottles and other hazardous articles out of his reach.

2. Attempt to make the child as independent as his condition will permit. When possible, teach him to care for his personal needs.

3. Teach him small social graces and manners which are a tremendous factor in helping the child to be accepted by others. They can be taught to greet persons cordially, bid them good-by, say "thank you," "please," "good morning," "good night," etc.

4. Many of these children have a tendency to hold their mouths open which gives them a dull appearance. They can be taught to refrain from this practice.

5. Personal appearance is another important factor which helps to increase the child's acceptance by others. Attention to selection of attractive, well-fitted clothing, hair styling, and good hygienic practices are positive approaches toward gaining acceptance for the child.

6. Undesirable social traits, such as touching their noses and ears, scratching, and so on, may be eliminated through proper guidance and teaching.

7. Teach the child only one thing at a time.

8. Whenever possible, demonstrate what you are teaching.

9. Pictures are valuable visual aids in teaching the mentally retarded.

10. Start teaching the child simple accomplishments. Gradually progress to more complex learning experiences.

11. Patience and repetition are necessary virtues for those who teach the mentally retarded.

12. Teaching should be timed. Prolonged teaching sessions do not produce learning, as retarded individuals easily become fatigued.

13. Scolding is a negative approach which blocks learning and instills fear.

14. Compliments, when deserved, are a motivating force.

15. Never exhibit fear yourself (for example, fear of mice, thunder), as this emotion will be transferred to the child.

16. Recognize a temper tantrum as, quite often, a child's attempt to meet some underlying emotional need such as attention, affection, and security, or as the expression of the child's dislike for an activity. Perhaps a suggestion for the child to do something different will be helpful during such outbursts. If this approach is not successful, the child may be left alone until he has released the emotion experienced.

17. These children have a tendency to express jealousy. Recognize these reactions as an indication that the child needs to have some demonstration of affection.

18. Protect the child from teasing and taunting. Other children may sometimes be appealed to to show more consideration for the mentally retarded child.

19. Play activities are enjoyed and may be a teaching experience. Many of these children can be taught to trace designs, write their own names, recite simple rhymes, and so on.

EMPLOYMENT

When assisting the mentally retarded in securing employment, proper guidance and selection are important. Usually these individuals are able to perform only one kind of work and find it very difficult to change jobs. Since they are unable to exercise quick or fine judgments, they should not be placed in hazardous situations. For instance, the operation of certain intricate machinery might prove to be a very dangerous occupation for a mentally retarded person. The mentally retarded need to be under the guidance and supervision of a patient, understanding person who will not overwork or exploit them and who will protect their welfare so that they do not become social failures.

SUGGESTED REFERENCES

Barnard, K. (ed.): Symposium on mental retardation. Nurs. Clin. N. Am., Vol. 1, #4 (Dec.), W. B. Saunders Co., Philadelphia, 1966.

Employing the mentally handicapped (Editorial). Ment. Hosp. 6: 7 (June), 1965.

Forbes, N.: The nurse and genetic counseling. Nurs. Clin. N. Am. 1: 679 (Dec.), W. B. Saunders Co., Philadelphia, 1966.

Forbes, N., and Shaw, K.: Maternal phenylketonuria. Nurs. Outlook 14: 40 (Jan.), 1966.

Hallas, C.: The Care and Training of the Mentally Subnormal. John Wright & Sons, Bristol, England, 1967.

McCarty, K., and Chisholm, M.: Group education with mothers of retarded children. Nurs. Clin. N. Am. 1: 703 (Dec.), W. B. Saunders Co., Philadelphia, 1966.

Murray, B., and Barnard, K.: The nursing specialist in mental retardation. Nurs. Clin. N. Am. 1: 631 (Dec.), W. B. Saunders Co., Philadelphia, 1966.

Noble, M.: Nursing's concern for the mentally retarded is overdue. Nurs. Forum 9: 192 (Spring), 1970.

Patterson, E., and Rowland, G.: Toward a theory of mental retardation nursing: an educational model. Am. J. Nurs., 70: 531 (March), 1970.

Paulus, A.: A tool for the assessment of the retarded child at home. Nurs. Clin. N. Am. 1: 659 (Dec.), W. B. Saunders Co., Philadelphia, 1966.

Powell, M.: An interpretation of effective management and discipline of the mentally retarded child. Nurs. Clin. N. Am. 1: 689 (Dec.), W. B. Saunders Co., Philadelphia, 1966.

Ragsdale, N., and Koch, R.: Phenylketonuria detection and therapy. Am. J. Nurs. 64: 90 (Jan.), 1964.

Teague, B.: Implementing changes in the traditional institutional environment of the mentally retarded. Nurs. Clin. N. Am. 1: 651 (Dec.), W. B. Saunders Co., Philadelphia, 1966.

The president's message on mental illness and mental retardation (Editorial). J. Psychiat. Nurs. 1: 310 (Jul.), 1963.

Tizard, J.: Community Services for the Mentally Handicapped. Oxford University Press, New York, 1964.

U.S. Department of Health, Education, and Welfare: The Problem of Mental Retardation.

Waechter, E.: The birth of an exceptional child. Nurs. Forum 9: 202 (Spring), 1970.

Whitney, L.: Behavioral approaches to the nursing of the mentally retarded. Nurs. Clin. N. Am. 1: 641 (Dec.), W. B. Saunders Co., Philadelphia, 1966.

Wright, M.: Nursing services in a mental retardation clinical research unit. Nurs. Clin. N. Am. 1: 669 (Dec.), W. B. Saunders Co., Philadelphia, 1966.

FOOTNOTES

1. Patterson, E., and Rowland, G.: Toward a theory of mental retardation nursing—an educational model. Am. J. Nurs. 70: 533 (March), 1970.
2. Committee on Nomenclature and Statistics: Diagnostic and Statistical Manual of Mental Disorders. American Psychiatric Association, Washington, D.C., 1968, p. 14.
3. Secretary's Committee on Mental Retardation: The Problem of Mental Retardation. U. S. Department of Health, Education and Welfare, Washington, D.C.
4. Hallas, C.: The Care and Training of the Mentally Subnormal. John Wright & Sons, Bristol, Eng., 1967, p. 27.
5. Waechter, E.: The birth of an exceptional child. Nurs. Forum 9: 202 (Spring), 1970.
6. National Mental Health Foundation: Forgotten Children (pamphlet), pp. 18-19.

CHAPTER 43

Nursing in Children's and Adolescents' Psychiatric Services

ESTABLISHMENT AND MAINTENANCE OF SERVICES

A children's psychiatric hospital or hospital unit is a medical facility established for the diagnosis and treatment of children suffering from psychiatric disorders, in which the psychiatrist carries medical and corresponding legal responsibility for the diagnosis and treatment of the patient. It may be an independent institution or an identifiable medical unit in a medical or nonmedical agency.[1]

Adolescent units may also be established for the same purposes in these locations under the supervision of a responsible psychiatrist. Unit locations are based upon the premise that they should be an integral part of community mental health facilities.

SOURCES OF REFERRAL

Community general hospitals, clinics, welfare institutions, foster homes, children's courts, guidance counsellors, physicians, and psychiatrists refer children and adolescents to these services for diagnosis, treatment, and recommendations for after-care following their discharge from the medical facility.

GROWTH AND DESIGN OF SERVICES

During the past decade the number of children's and adolescents' services has increased steadily with a corresponding growth in the number of professional nurses and members of allied disciplines participating as team members in the study and treatment of emotionally disturbed and mentally ill patients referred to these agencies.

Some experiments have been conducted to test the efficacy of having children and adolescents reside in the same wards as those occupied by adult patients. However, the majority of these special services are designed to house together in a unit the members of peer groups. A ward may be maintained to care for 3 to 8-year-old children, 8 to 12-year-old patients, or adolescents in the 12 to 16 year age group. Some well-organized children's services have also established day-care treatment plans whereby a few children may come daily to the service from their homes in the community. Qualified teachers may plan and conduct an educational program in the hospital setting or some of the patients may attend classes in community schools.

ADMISSION PROCEDURE

The admission procedure in children's and adolescents' psychiatric services usually reflects the administrative medical staff's philosophy as well as the objectives associated with the type of services provided. Hospitals may maintain the privilege of refusing to admit patients merely upon the examination of an application. Confinement of patients may be limited and vary in time from a stated number of weeks to more than one year. Research centers may house patients for longer periods than is ordinarily approved in other locations.

Applications for admission often exceed the available patient capacity. To prevent overcrowding as well as to make decisions regarding which children need and can benefit most through the services provided by the particular facility, the chief psychiatrist and social worker may visit the home of a patient referred for admission by a community agency. Considerable data may be gathered during the visit and discussed later in a ward team conference. If and when the patient is admitted to the service, the staff is already acquainted with many details concerning the individual's disorder.

CLASSIFICATION AND DYNAMICS OF DISORDERS

Agreement has not been reached concerning the standardization of diagnostic terminology in child psychiatry. Different schools of thought, educational centers, and individual psychiatrists tend to use diagnostic terms which reflect their respective theoretical approaches. For example, a diagnosis of "pregenital behavior disorder" reflects a particular theoretical frame of reference. A diagnosis of "parent-child relationship disturbance" reflects only the diagnostician's concept of faulty interpersonal relationships. There is disagreement concerning whether the diagnostic nomenclature used in child psychiatry should be based on the presenting symptoms, on etiology, on prognosis, or on more than one of these factors.[2]

Children, adolescents, and adults may be afflicted with the same classification of emotional and mental disorders. Although members of the various age groups suffer the same afflictions, the symptomatic expressions observed differ according to the stage of physical and intellectual growth attained by the individual patient as well as the unique life experiences to which the person has been exposed and reacted. More important than diagnostic classification is the careful study conducted by competent team members of the patient's growth, development, and life situations which have influenced the emergence and persistence of abnormal behavior reactions. This information provides knowledge of the physical as well as the social psychological aspects of the patient's illness which are reflected in the psychodynamic interpretations made concerning the patient's ability to organize his experiences and achieve personality integration within the environment. Dynamic treatment approaches evolve from an identification and understanding of the relative forces, including the mental mechanisms of defense, underlying the patient's symptomatic behavior.

The following general frame of reference may be helpful in clarifying the types of illnesses which may afflict children, adolescents, and adults. Differences in the expressions of symptoms should be viewed in relation to the individual patient's physical, intellectual, and social growth.

Organic Defects or Changes

A primary organic defect or change is considered to be the frank cause of impairments manifested in convulsive seizures, speech, aphasias, learning and hearing incapabilities, etc. There may or may not be a superimposed psychotic or personality disorder, such as schizophrenia or sociopathic behavior, presenting additional, observable symptoms.

Psychosomatic Disorders

A body organ expresses its reaction to a distressing life situation through symptoms associated with the organ's malfunctioning. Body elimination disturbances, allergic reactions, emesis, etc., may represent an organ's reaction to some situation.

Psychoneurotic Disorders

Anxious, phobic, hysterical, or compulsive patterns of behavior may be symbolic of an unconscious, conflictual life situation which threatens the individual's self-security and need to control the environment.

Personality Disorders

Sociopathic and delinquent behavior may be expressed through anti-social or dysocial behavior actions which, it is thought, cannot be held in check owing to the patient's lack of an internal impulse-controlling appara-tus.

Transient Situational Personality Disorders

Reactions to environmental situational stress and strain may be ex-pressed through temporary episodes of excitability, apathy, feeding and sleeping difficulties, nail-biting, thumb-sucking, enuresis, masturbation, tantrums, restlessness, stammering, stuttering, and difficulties in learning, adjusting to new experiences and other persons, etc. Organic defects are absent in these situations.

Psychotic Disorders

Remote as well as immediate circumstances and events may influence the emergence of abnormal behavior symptoms of withdrawal, phantasy, autism, delusions, hallucinations, overactivity, homicidal and suicidal ac-tions, etc.

Mental Retardations

An intellectual defect which may be mild, moderate, or severe in degree. There may or may not be a superimposed psychotic or personality disorder present.

NURSING SKILLS

Nursing of children and adolescents has its rewards and its challenges. Its rewards lie in the successful treatment and rehabilitation of patients. Reaching this goal is actually the prevention of more severe, disintegrating disorders. Its achievement is as dependent upon the development of skill in detecting evidences of healthy personality development potentials in patients as well as that of being able to identify and cope well with problematical situations which develop in the clinical settings maintained for these patients. Anticipating and focusing upon normal as well as abnormal manifestations of behavior are prerequisites for successful treatment and rehabilitation.

Erik Erikson's concepts of personality development strivings may be a useful frame of reference for making interpretations of behavior leading to decisions which influence nursing approaches. According to Erikson, all individuals strive through eight successive stages of growth to develop basic senses of (1) trust, (2) autonomy, (3) initiative, (4) industry, (5) identity, (6) intimacy, (7) generativity, and (8) integrity.

When attempting to identify an inherent striving in behavior observed, the nurse may make self-directed queries such as the following: Is the patient testing my trustworthiness? Attempting to strengthen his personal or sexual identification? Aiming to establish friendly social relations? Expressing creativity or vocational potentials? Is this persistence of behavior the development of personal integrity? When behavior is interpreted in relation to Erikson's frame of reference, nursing personnel may be helped to recognize healthy as well as abnormal aspects of personality functioning.

STAFF FEELING COMMUNICATIONS

Staff members who fail to explore the motivation and meaning of behavior may unwittingly communicate to other personnel their personal feeling reactions towards a patient's persistent behavior manifestation. Infectious communications should be recognized and avoided because they can seriously deter the making of dynamic interpretations leading to therapeutic nursing approaches.

PERSONAL FEELING REACTIONS

It is helpful for nurses to be as aware of their personal feeling reactions as they should be of the approaches to behavior which may be predetermined by the staff. The nurse's personal feelings may interfere with the implementation of recommended staff approaches and consistency. Undesirable behavior responses of patients may become intensified instead of being modified or changed. For this reason, the selection of nursing staff members in well-organized children's and adolescents' psychiatric services is aimed to eliminate the employment of persons who are experiencing problematical behavior with their own children.

INTERPRETATIONS OF SOME BEHAVIORS

The following discussion will focus upon the dynamics underlying some behavior situations which appear to be universal developments in children's and adolescents' wards. In addition to those selected for discussion, behaviors do occur which require interpretations of the dynamic forces underlying unique situations.

CHILDREN

INITIAL CONTACTS WITH CHILDREN

Children may respond to initial nursing approaches by being inattentive, being unresponsive to verbal communications, making unfriendly gestures or critical remarks, or physically repulsing the nurse. If the nurse recognizes and respects the child's striving to establish a sense of trust, contact may be and often is established subsequently through the child's friendly overtures. Unexpectedly, the nurse entering the ward one day may discover that the child rushes a greeting, brushes affectionately against her, asks where she came from or what she is going to do or makes other advances. When one considers the traumatic social environment, with its deprivations, that many of these children come from, the observation made by Anna Freud is significant when making initial contacts. According to Anna Freud, the more tenderly a little child is attached to its mother, the fewer friendlier impulses it has towards strangers. This reaction may be observed in the baby who shows anxious rejection towards everyone other than its mother or nurse. Conversely, children who are accustomed to receiving and showing little love and affection in the home often establish most quickly a positive relationship with the analyst. They obtain from the analyst what they have expected in vain from the original love object.[3]

PEER GROUP IDENTIFICATION

A therapeautic nurse-patient activity may suddenly be rejected and abandoned by the child if members of the peer group appear on the scene. Some nurses having strong mothering needs may become distressed as the child changes to the peer group activity in his striving for personal identification. Children may feel affection for adults, including nurses, but the degree of the emotion felt as well as the therapeutic affectiveness of the nurse-patient relationship cannot be judged by the time spent in nurse-patient activities or the preferences for individuals shown by the child.

AGGRESSIVE BEHAVIOR

Quarreling and fighting are commonly observed among children and may develop rapidly. Competitive aspects of autonomy, initiative, and industry strivings may be inherent in aggressive behavior, dependent upon the particular form of its expression. Some situations may not be threatening physically to the individuals involved. Children matched in physical prowess can protect themselves as they fight it out and learn through the experience. But the child who is not the physical equal of another or who is too ill to meet aggression successfully needs to be protected through the nurse's intervention. The nurse must have the ability to judge whether or not rational appeals or explanations to the aggressor and others involved will be meaningful and effective in helping these patients to develop internal impulse controls. On some occasions, the mere act of separating the children involved will convey the meaning underlying the nurse's approach even though its limitations are recognized. On other occasions, verbal communications are necessary to help children learn socially acceptable behavior, knowledge of which helps to build inner-impulse controls.

Children sometimes persist in maintaining the exclusive right to a particular toy or play equipment, or in having first turn or the leader role in certain activities. Some of these developments may be reduced in number or intensity when a nurse is assigned to remain with the group. The nurse's presence may be sufficient to set limitations and curb excessive manifestations of these behaviors. On occasions, the nurse observing the group may have to intervene to set the limitations which help children to learn how to share and to refrain from carrying out threats towards other persons.

PROFANE COMMUNICATIONS

Profane language spoken by children is usually the language to which they have been exposed in their cultural environments. They lack understanding of this language's real meaning and social inacceptance. Hostility is expressed and others are made to feel uncomfortable in the child's presence through his or her use of profane communications. This form of aggressive behavior is sometimes motivated by strivings to achieve recognition of the individual child's presence or identity in relation to the group. On occasion it may be an autonomous response toward actions instituted by other patients or staff members which limit or curb the patient's expressions of initiative or industry strivings. Basically, such actions may ignore the child's potentialities and needs, upset the prevailing status quo, or place unwelcome demands upon the patient. Sometimes the nurse may discover the motivational aspects of profane communications by remarking, "Those are strong words," and then observing carefully what the child says and does. There may be times when the nurse will determine that it is appropriate to say to the child, "We do not allow those words to be said in this place. We like you, but we do not like those words." If a child persists in using profane language, the nurse may consider it appropriate to exclude the child from a group play activity which he values. The child should be told why the privilege has been withdrawn. If these approaches are ineffective, the nurse may show the child to a room and tell him that if he feels he must speak as he does, he may do so freely in the room apart from the group. She may tell him that when he has finished speaking the words that are not allowed, he may return to the group activity.

EATING HABITS

Awkward eating mannerisms of children are related to the physical capacity achieved from the growth stage attained. Corrective approaches are useless and produce only negative responses from the child.

A child who is overly stimulated during meal periods to a degree which interferes with his partaking of the meal may be allowed to eat by himself in another room. From time to time the child may be brought to the regular dining room to determine whether or not he may remain with the peer group or requires the quiet environment.

Some children manifest selective eating patterns which are not unusual for members of their peer group. They may eat the same food for successive days but in sufficient quantity to meet their nutritive requirements. Children eat what gratifies their hunger instinct. When hunger has been satisfied, children usually change their food preferences.

NURSERY-SCHOOL ACTIVITIES

Nursery-school activities cannot be structured in the children's psychiatric service according to planned learning experiences having educational objectives. Each child's ability to evoke or retain interest and to intellectualize an experience varies and may be related also to the illness process. Psychotic children and those having organic brain damage are often limited in these capacities. Nursery-school experiences are helpful when they are liberalized so that individual children may select their interests and move about freely as desired. Children in the classroom at the same time may all engage in different experiences. One teacher is kept busy helping two or three children who may change their interest at frequent intervals or roam about the room. The degree to which limitation settings may be instituted and be therapeutic in the nursery-school environment reduces the number of children that can be given assistance or tolerated within the peer group during one session.

Nursery-school experience is ineffective when children are fatigued. Because only two or three children may be assisted at one time in the classroom, it may be necessary to plan afternoon periods for some of the group. A rest period following morning activities and lunch is essential to avoid fatigue and to effect a therapeutic nursery-school experience for the afternoon group.

RESPONSIBILITY ASSIGNMENTS

Some, but not all, children respond well to the assignment of small tasks which help them to learn to assume responsibility while strengthening their basic senses of personal identification, initiative, industry, and generativity (creativity). Children may be asked to assemble the materials for an activity, collect and store items of play equipment, help a less capable child with some aspect of dressing or toileting, rearrange a room that has been used for activities, and perform similar tasks. When the tasks are completed, it is therapeutic for the children to be complimented by the nurse for their accomplishments or the assistance given to another child. Children who do not respond to such assignments may be observed turning away without comment from task suggestions, sometimes verbalizing refusal, or on occasions releasing hostile feelings by pushing equipment around or out of place and disrupting a situation. Dependent upon the dynamic interpretation of the individual behavior expressed in reaction to the request, the nurse may make one of the following possible approaches or any other approach based upon the underlying dynamics. She may quietly and without further comment carry out the task by herself, recognizing the child's striving for autonomy. Or, perhaps the child is unable to intellectualize and enact the suggestion. If the nurse believes that it will not be emotionally distressing for the child who has not responded favorably, she may seek the assistance of another child who may respond well. When assigning tasks to children, the nurse may find it helpful to include an incentive, such as stating that a specific play activity will be commenced as soon as the task is completed. With children who are capable of competing, the nurse may introduce a happy element of competition by converting the task into a playful race in which she may participate.

ENURESIS

Enuresis may be related to feelings of insecurity due to unmet needs for attention and affection. Various writers have discussed enuresis and demonstrated how the meeting of the individual's needs has reduced or eliminated the symptom. When bed-wetting occurs the nurse may transfer a feeling of understanding and trust by refraining from comments as she helps the child to remove soiled clothing and put on dry apparel and provides fresh bedding. If the child whimpers and appears to be distressed, the nurse may soothe the situation with a tender stroking of the child's head as she comments to the effect that she knows the child could not help himself and that with a change of clothing he will feel better. She may humor the occasion with a playful challenge such as, "Let's see how fast you can jump into bed! Jumpity, jump, jump, there you go! My, what a fine jumper you turned out to be." It is such little pleasantries in the nurse's approach which replace fear and insecurity with trust and which children love and respond to well.

OVERT INTIMATE RELATIONSHIPS

Some children have experienced severe emotional deprivation due to a lack of sufficient early physical contact with parental, especially mothering, figures. In other instances, children have been seduced sexually at an early age. Both types of relationship increase bodily tensions, heightening the need for tension release. Strivings for intimacy by children having such early traumatic experiences may be manifested overtly in masturbation or bodily contact with another child. An approach toward another child of either sex in the peer group for physical contact may be resisted sufficiently to thwart a mutual relationship. If the child who is approached is physically incapable of resisting or if a mutual relationship is apparent, the nurse should intervene to separate the children. The nurse's brief comment, "We do not allow that here," is sufficient to indicate the social undesirability of such actions. The same comment may be made to a child who masturbates openly. Further discussion is unnecessary unless the nurse is pressed into further explanations. Group activities which introduce some competition as well as a challenge to exercise initiative and industry are substitute nursing approaches which help to release pent-up bodily tensions. The nurse's participation in activities, combined with a show of acceptance and genuine liking for the children, is also helpful in gratifying their need for relationships with others.

DISCIPLINE

When a child is singled out to lose a privilege owing to some unacceptable mode of behavior, it is important that the nurse identify the right child. Some children are as expert in provoking situations as they are in being able to move out of them in time to cause another child to be identified as the offender from whom the nurse may withdraw a privilege. This may cause the child from whom the privilege is taken to lose face, feel rejected, and believe that punishment is unfair. Such reactions often lead to increased aggressive behavior with hostile-feeling expressions by the child disciplined as well as to a loss of confidence in the nurse.

ADOLESCENTS

Adolescent patients often act out their underlying feelings of insecurity, rejection, deprivation, and low self-esteem and identification with significant surrogate figures through situations which are often provoking and challenging to other persons, especially those who have no understanding of the motivation, meaning, and purpose of the behavior. For this reason, nurses caring for adolescents need to develop skill in making interpretations of patients' conversations and other aspects of their behavior. Lack of understanding and skill may cause the nurse to be manipulated by these patients to the extent of sometimes making responses to behavior which are not therapeutic. Some of the situations which the nurse may meet in caring for this group will be discussed so that an understanding may be gained of some typical behavior incidents which occur.

REACTIONS FOLLOWING ADMISSION

It is not unusual for adolescents admitted to the psychiatric service to test early the reactions of nursing personnel as they seek evidences of acceptance by others as well as a trusting relationship. While organizing their personal defenses in the new environment, these patients may refuse to associate with others or to partake of food. Food may be refused at meal time for the first two or three days. When the staff is aware of the meaning of the behavior, an accepting response towards it leads to the development of a trusting relationship. The patient may begin to relinquish his defenses, commence to seek out companions, and establish his identity in the peer group.

Early elopements or escape from the hospital ward are part of the testing pattern. These occasions are often indications that the patient wants to be sought after and returned to the ward. When located, it is not unusual for a patient to remark, "I just wanted to see if you would come after me, if anyone really cared."

ROLE CONCEPTS

As adolescent patients and youthful-appearing members of a nursing staff interact, their concepts of each other's role may influence the course of the patients' behavior as well as the responses made to their behavior situations by individual nurses. The natural tendency to be attracted to persons of one's age group and experiences may cause young nursing personnel members to over-identify with adolescent patients. Conversely, the youthful-appearing nurse may be viewed by adolescent patients as a member of their peer group instead of a member of the professional staff. There are occasions when the behavior of adolescents on the hospital ward requires that the nurse set limitations. If the nurse fails to make a strong identification with her professional role in an adolescent unit, she may be unable to set the limitations which adolescents often need and want. External controls often help these patients to feel secure because so many of them have not developed an internal control-regulating apparatus which would make them capable of setting their own limits. It is helpful for nurses to attend professional ward team conferences where they can identify with the professional group and its therapeutic aims. During conferences, nurses have opportunity to become acquainted with the dynamics of behavior observed. They may also develop an awareness of the personal feeling reactions which they have developed in response to the behavior discussed. From the professional staff the nurse may learn of approaches which she may make towards behavior situations which will transfer to the patient a realistic concept of the nurse's professional role.

COMMUNICATION SITUATION

Adolescents often complain that nobody listens to them. As their strivings for intimate associations develop, one of their greatest needs is to have other persons listen. Some nurses have a natural affinity for establishing the kind of relationships which provide opportunities for the patient to verbalize freely. While listening to conversations which may be those having connotations of complaints, boasting, opinions, and the like, the nurse is very much attuned to the underlying dynamics of the conversation as well as to its meaning and is guided in her responses according to the interpretations made.

When a patient has gained feelings of trust in a nurse he may commence to reveal confidences to her. On occasions, what the patient has to tell may be for him anxiety-producing. The nurse may be the communication channel through which the patient is attempting to convey information to the doctor. It is not unusual to have a patient terminate a confidential communication session with the comment, "But don't tell my doctor." Nurses having the ability to interpret communications well can identify the motivation and need associated with such a comment. They can recognize when the patient's purpose in revealing confidences is actually to have the information relayed to the doctor.

Sarcastic remarks, through which hostile feelings are released, may be motivated by former environmental relationships which have left their imprint upon the personality structure of the patient. Owing to former observations of untruthfulness and disloyalty an adolescent may develop the belief that these character traits may be expected to emerge automatically from other persons with whom they relate. While struggling to resolve inner strivings for intimate associations with individuals, which are often fraught with fearful feelings of rejection and mistrust, the patient may test the nurse's truthfulness as well as her loyalty through the voicing of complaints about some aspect of the institution. For instance, if the patient remarks, "This is a lousy meal!" and there is some justification for the truthfulness of the statement, the nurse's response is important. She may comment in return, "Well, I agree with you. It's not so good this time, but we do have some good meals in this hospital." Such a response may be helpful in causing the patient to change his character concepts of other persons and his capacity to trust and expect truth as well as loyalty from others.

ARGUMENTS

Arguments between members of the patient group may reflect strivings for trust, autonomy, identification, and the like. These patients may quarrel and threaten each other over situations which some persons would consider trivial enough to avoid or ignore. They may become embroiled in reactions to differences of opinions concerning the selection of a television program, someone discovered cheating in a game, a remark, teasing of an individual, and so on. These situations are sometimes resolved by permitting the group to argue it out. However, if the nurse observing the situation concludes that someone may get hurt physically, she will have to terminate the activity, be firm in her directions for ending the controversy, and may possibly have to withdraw privileges from one or more group members.

If a patient threatens or challenges the nurse to fight, the nurse must recognize the need to establish her identification and reorient the patient to her professional role. Argument should be avoided. In a serious, calm voice the nurse may impress the patient by remarking, "I'm not here to fight. I will not allow fighting. I must see to it that you and no one else gets hurt."

PROFANITY, SMOKING

Some adolescents have been reared in cultures in which profane language and smoking are acceptable at an early age. When profanity and smoking are observed among teenage patients, little can be accomplished by a nurse through attempts at direct corrective approaches. Instead, attempts to control behavior, which for some adolescents is normal culturally, usually causes the patient to become increasingly hostile. If the staff concludes that corrective approaches should be made, they are more likely to succeed when the patient's doctor makes them during a personal interview. Smoking may be limited according to a schedule arranged by the physician and profanity may be discouraged. The degree to which these limitation approaches are successful will depend upon the manner in which the reasons for the undesirability of the actions in the hospital culture is presented by the doctor to the patient as well as the rapport and identification which exists between doctor and patient. While many adolescents appear to be accustomed to profane language, sometimes a particular patient is so excessively profane that even the members of the peer group cannot tolerate its expression. The group may then set the limitations upon the patient's behavior by avoiding his or her association.

FLIRTATIOUSNESS AND SEDUCTIVENESS

Complex communications may be inherent in the flirtatious, seductive behavior manifested by adolescents towards adult team members. Adolescent girls, especially, have been known to make subtle, sophisticated "vamping" approaches toward members of the treatment team who are of the opposite sex. This behavior may be due to conflictual frightening feelings that arise from heightened sexual impulses and are interwoven with the adolescent's strivings for intimacy. Such comments, as "He's just like all men" [or "women"], may be generalizations related to identifications with parental figures. Flirtatious, seductive approaches may also be unconsciously practiced to ward off relationships with adult members of the treatment team. The therapeutic relationship response to be made in each situation is determined by the therapist, dependent upon the dynamics of the behavior. For example, is the patient attempting to ward off the team member, strengthen his or her sexual identification in relation to the opposite sex, or to feel at ease and comfortable in a heterosexual relationship?

INSTIGATING BEHAVIOR OF PEERS

An adolescent may incite a disorganized peer into acting out or into engaging in unacceptable behavior. The instigator achieves vicarious gratification as he attempts to divert the attention of the professional staff toward the acting-out patient. Interpretations of the underlying motivation of the instigator's behavior may be made by the doctor to the patient. These may be helpful in convincing the instigator that the physician is acquainted with the reality of the situation. This approach orients the patient to the reasons for his behavior as well as acquaints him with the fact that it is understood by the treatment team. It may help to change the patients behavior when the patient realizes the requirements necessary to be accepted and trusted in a group.

COMPETITION FOR ATTENTION

Adolescents sometimes compete with each other for their doctor's attention. A patient may provoke or create a situation which necessitates a personal visit with the doctor. The nurse may overhear competitive members discussing the number of interviews held with their physicians. When such situations are recognized by the nurse, she should be alert to behavior which appears to be competition motivated and designed to achieve a special visit from the doctor.

EVENING RETIREMENT: MORNING ARISING

When a patient or group of patients refuses to retire at night or to arise in the morning according to the hour set for these occasions, it is well for the nurse to convey the impression that cooperation is anticipated. At the appointed evening hour the nurse may commence to perform functions associated with retiring, such as turning off the television set and the living-room lights and asking patients to assist with rearranging the furniture and storing away games that have been used. In the morning the nurse may enter the patient's room to raise the window shades as she pronounces the initial greeting of the day. These actions by the nurse may be based upon an interpretation that often the refusal to cooperate during the hours of retirement and arising are an expression of the patients' identifications and reactions towards authority figures, as well as strivings for autonomy.

ENURESIS

When a patient manifests a problem of enuresis, it is helpful to appreciate the importance of preserving the individual's self-esteem. Awaken the patient earlier than the rest of the group, commence preparation of a bath, then place fresh linen on the bed. Comments concerning the incident should be avoided unless the patient initiates discussion of it. The nurse's actions will convey to the patient an understanding of the individual's inability to control elimination. Eventually the patient may feel secure enough to establish personal control of this function.

NURSING PERSONNEL

Skillful management of adolescent behavior can be achieved best through careful selection of nursing staff members. Nursing personnel should be free of similar problematical behavior with their own children, because they may identify, during their nursing practice, with their personal problems and be unable to carry out therapeutic approaches. It is helpful to have the staff meet and talk out their feelings about certain types of behavior, such as personal attitudes felt toward teenagers, smoking, and use of profane language. Discussions may lead to the development of self-awareness of how and why individual staff members are reacting to certain aspects of adolescent behavior. Meetings may be helpful in getting nursing personnel to recognize the need to change when change is indicated.

SUGGESTED REFERENCES

Bindman, A.: Programs for disturbed children: Problems in planning, implementing and evaluating special education and community mental health. J. Psychiat. Nurs. 2: 540 (Nov.-Dec.), 1964.

Chapman, A.: Management of Emotional Problems of Children and Adolescents. J. B. Lippincott Co., Philadelphia, 1965.

Christ, A., Critchley, D., et al.: The role of the nurse in child psychiatry. Nurs. Outlook 13: 30 (Jan.), 1965.

Coffman, J.: Anger: it's significance for nurses who work with emotionally disturbed children. Perspect. Psychiat. Care 7: 104 (May-June), 1969.

Finch, S.: Fundamentals of Child Psychiatry. W. W. Norton & Co., New York, 1960.

Goodman, J.: Short term treatment in child psychiatry. Ment. Health Dig. 3: 37 (June), 1971.

Harley, A.: Group psychotherapy for parents of disturbed children. Ment. Hosp. 14: 14 (Jan.), 1963.

Jones, C.: A day-care program for adolescents in a private hospital. Ment. Hosp. 12: 4 (Oct.), 1961.

Kolb, L.: Noyes' Modern Clinical Psychiatry, ed. 7. W. B. Saunders Co., Philadelphia, 1968, p. 526.

Planning Psychiatric Services for Children in the Community Mental Health Program. American Psychiatric Association, Washington, D.C.

Psychiatric Treatment Center Staff: A design for adolescent therapy. Ment. Hosp. 12: 20 (Sept.), 1961.

Public Health Service: Mental Health of Children. U.S. Department of Health, Education, and Welfare, Bethesda, Maryland, Dec., 1965.

Randell, B.: Short term group therapy with the adolescent drug offender. Perspect. Psychiat. Care 9: 23 (May-June), 1971.

Rouslin, S.: The adolescent in psychotherapy. Perspect. Psychiat. Care 7: 263 (Nov.-Dec.), 1969.

Strutzel, E.: A disturbed adolescent. Nurs. Clin. N. Am. 6, No. 4, p. 727. W. B. Saunders Co.,
Philadelphia, Dec. 1971.
Turner, R.: A method of working with disturbed children. Am. J. Nurs. 70: 2146 (Oct.), 1970.
Weinberg, S., Schonberg, C., and Grier, D.: Seminars in nursing care of the adolescent. Nurs.
Outlook 16: 18 (Dec.), 1968.

FOOTNOTES

1. Robinson, J. Franklin (ed.): Psychiatric Inpatient Treatment of Children. American Psychiatric Association, Washington, D. C., 1957, p. 4.
2. Chess, S.: An Introduction to Child Psychiatry. Grune & Stratton, New York, 1959, p. 85.
3. Freud, Anna: The Psycho-analytical Treatment of Children. Image Publishing Co., London, 1946, p. 34.

For reviewing this chapter, grateful acknowledgment is made to Mrs. Esther Mackenzie,
R.N., Miss Elizabeth Maloney, R.N., Doctor Rochus Stiller, and Miss Rita Tempia, R.N.

Appendix

The Diagnostic Nomenclature
List of Mental Disorders*

I. MENTAL RETARDATION

Borderline
Mild
Moderate
Severe
Profound
Unspecified

With each: Following or associated with
Infection or intoxication
Trauma or physical agent
Gross brain disease (postnatal)
Disorders of metabolism, growth, or nutrition
Unknown prenatal influence
Chromosomal abnormality
Prematurity
Major psychiatric disorder
Psychosocial (environmental) deprivation
Other condition

II. ORGANIC BRAIN SYNDROMES (OBS)

A. Psychoses
Senile and Presenile Dementia
Senile dementia
Presenile dementia

*DSM-11 Diagnostic and Statistical Manual of Mental Disorders, ed. 2. Prepared by the Committee on Nomenclature and Statistics of the American Psychiatric Association, Washington, D.C., 1968, pp. 5-13.

Alcoholic Psychosis
  Delirium tremens
  Korsakoff's psychosis
  Other alcoholic hallucinosis
  Alcohol paranoid state
  Acute alcohol intoxication
  Alcoholic deterioration
  Pathologic intoxication
  Other alcoholic psychosis

Psychosis Associated With Intracranial Infection
  General paralysis
  Syphilis of central nervous system
  Epidemic encephalitis
  Other and unspecified encephalitis
  Other intracranial infection

Psychosis Associated With Other Cerebral Condition
  Cerebral arteriosclerosis
  Other cerebrovascular disturbance
  Epilepsy
  Intracranial neoplasm
  Degenerative disease of the CNS
  Brain trauma
  Other cerebral condition

Psychosis Associated With Other Physical Condition
  Endocrine disorder
  Metabolic and nutritional disorder
  Systemic infection
  Drug or poison intoxication (other than alcohol)
  Childbirth
  Other and unspecified physical condition

B. Nonpsychotic OBS
  Intracranial infection
  Alcohol (simple drunkenness)
  Other drug, poison, or systemic intoxication
  Brain trauma
  Circulatory disturbance
  Epilepsy
  Disturbance of metabolism, growth, or nutrition
  Senile or presenile brain disease
  Intracranial neoplasm
  Degenerative disease of the CNS
  Other physical condition

III. PSYCHOSES NOT ATTRIBUTED TO PHYSICAL CONDITIONS LISTED PREVI-
OUSLY

Schizophrenia
  Simple
  Hebephrenic
  Catatonic
        Catatonic type, excited
        Catatonic type, withdrawn
  Paranoid
  Acute schizophrenic episode
  Latent
  Residual
  Schizo-affective
        Schizo-affective, excited
        Schizo-affective, depressed
  Childhood
  Chronic undifferentiated
  Other schizophrenia

Major Affective Disorders
  Involutional melancholia
  Manic-depressive illness, manic
  Manic-depressive illness, depressed
  Manic-depressive illness, circular
        Manic-depressive, circular, manic
        Manic-depressive, circular, depressed
  Other major affective disorders

Paranoid States
  Paranoia
  Involutional paranoid state
  Other paranoid state

Other Psychoses
  Psychotic depressive reaction

IV. NEUROSES

  Anxiety
  Hysterical
  Hysterical, conversion type
  Hysterical, dissociative type
  Phobic
  Obsessive-compulsive
  Depressive
  Neurasthenic
  Depersonalization
  Hypochondriacal
  Other neuroses

V. PERSONALITY DISORDERS AND CERTAIN OTHER NONPSYCHOTIC MENTAL DISORDERS

Personality Disorders
  Paranoid
  Cyclothymic
  Schizoid
  Explosive
  Obsessive-compulsive
  Hysterical
  Asthenic
  Antisocial
  Passive-agressive
  Inadequate
  Other specified types

Sexual Deviation
  Homosexuality
  Fetishism
  Pedophilia
  Transvestitism
  Exhibitionism
  Voyeurism
  Sadism
  Masochism
  Other sexual deviation

Alcoholism
  Episodic excessive drinking
  Habitual excessive drinking
  Alcohol addiction
  Other alcoholism

Drug Dependence
  Opium, opium alkaloids and their derivatives
  Synthetic analgesics with morphine-like effects
  Barbiturates
  Other hypnotics and sedatives or "tranquilizers"
  Cocaine
  Cannabis sativa (hashish, marihuana)
  Other psycho-stimulants
  Hallucinogens
  Other drug dependence

VI. PSYCHOPHYSIOLOGIC DISORDERS

  Skin
  Musculoskeletal
  Respiratory
  Cardiovascular
  Hemic and lymphatic
  Gastrointestinal
  Genitourinary
  Endocrine

Organ of special sense
Other type

VII. SPECIAL SYMPTOMS

Speech disturbance
Specific learning disturbance
Tic
Other psychomotor disorder
Disorders of sleep
Feeding disturbance
Enuresis
Encopresis
Cephalalgia
Other special symptom

VIII. TRANSIENT SITUATIONAL DISTURBANCES

Adjustment reaction of infancy
Adjustment reaction of childhood
Adjustment reaction of adolescence
Adjustment reaction of adult life
Adjustment reaction of late life

IX. BEHAVIOR DISORDERS OF CHILDHOOD AND ADOLESCENCE

Hyperkinetic reaction
Withdrawing reaction
Overanxious reaction
Runaway reaction
Unsocialized aggressive reaction
Group delinquent reaction
Other reaction

X. CONDITIONS WITHOUT MANIFEST PSYCHIATRIC DISORDERS AND NON-SPECIFIC CONDITIONS

Social Maladjustment Without Manifest Psychiatric Disorder
Marital maladjustment
Social maladjustment
Occupational maladjustment
Dyssocial behavior
Other social maladjustments

Nonspecific Conditions
Nonspecific conditions
No Mental Disorder
No mental disorder

XI. NONDIAGNOSTIC TERMS FOR ADMINISTRATIVE USE

Diagnosis deferred
Boarder
Experiment only
Other

Index